FETAL AND NEONATAL HAEMATOLOGY

Dedicated to the memory of
Barney and Winifrid
and to the future of
Eleanore and Alistair

FETAL AND NEONATAL HAEMATOLOGY

Edited by

I.M. HANN

Consultant Haematologist, The Hospitals for Sick Children, London

B.E.S. GIBSON

Consultant Haematologist, Royal Hospital for Sick Children, Glasgow

E.A. LETSKY

Consultant Haematologist, Queen Charlotte's Maternity Hospital, London

Baillière Tindall

London Philadelphia Sydney Tokyo Toronto

This book is printed on acid free paper.

Baillière Tindall 24–28 Oval Road
W.B. Saunders London NW1 7DX, UK

The Curtis Center, Independence Square West
Philadelphia, PA 19106–3399, USA

55 Horner Avenue
Toronto, Ontario M8Z 4X6, Canada

Harcourt Brace Jovanovich Group (Australia) Pty Ltd
30–52 Smidmore St, Marrickville NSW 2204, Australia

Harcourt Brace Jovanovich Japan, Inc.
Ichibancho Central Building, 22–1 Ichibancho
Chiyoda-ku, Tokyo 102, Japan

First published 1991

British Library Cataloguing in Publication Data is available

ISBN 0–7020–1406–0

Typeset by Columns of Reading
and printed in Great Britain at the
University Press, Cambridge

Contents

Contributors

B.E.S. GIBSON
Consultant Haematologist, Royal Hospital for Sick Children, Yorkhill, Glasgow, Scotland, G3 8SJ.

I.M. HANN
Consultant Haematologist, The Hospitals for Sick Children, Great Ormond Street, London, WC1N 3JH.

E.A. LETSKY
Consultant Haematologist, Queen Charlotte's Maternity Hospital, Goldhawk Road, London, W6 0XG.

D.J. WEATHERALL
Institute of Molecular Medicine, John Radcliffe Hospital, Headington, Oxford, OX3 9DD.

Preface

At no other time is there such a dramatic change in the blood picture as occurs during the first few weeks of life. Haematologists dealing with babies often find this to be a perplexing problem, which is understandable when one considers the dynamic nature of the situation and the major differences that occur with varying degrees of immaturity and stress, for example the respiratory distress syndrome. That this is not a new problem is evident from George Frederic Still writing in 1927:

> The blood in infancy and early childhood is not the same as in older children or in adults. I mention this point *in primis* for it is sometimes forgotten, and what is perfectly normal in a young child is mistaken for some abnormal condition of the blood. At birth the blood shows certain peculiarities which are quite transitory, lasting only a few days or weeks; the most noticeable are the large number of white cells and the high proportion of haemoglobin.

Our aim has been to provide for haematologists, paediatricians and other hospital staff caring for babies, a guide through the complexities of normality and abnormality. Current lack of knowledge about development of blood in the fetus makes this an area of medicine upon which light is being shed painfully slowly. An understanding of the variations between normality and abnormality is facilitated by this type of study. In addition, the recent explosion in the science of immunology and in antenatal diagnosis depend at least in part upon this basic work. We have concentrated upon the rapid developments in antenatal diagnosis, neonatal clotting and blood transfusion, in a way which we hope will help the reader with patient management. The thorny topics of AIDS and other potentially transfusion-related infections have been addressed. Developments in the technology of neonatal clotting tests have provided us with the ability to study this difficult area in the routine laboratory; the application of new micro-methods is fully discussed.

Much of our knowledge of the normal neonatal blood picture stems from a fertile period after the First World War. A paediatric textbook of this period stated that

> the adaptation to the postnatal period begins during the last month or two of fetal life. During this period the red count and the haemoglobin diminish; iron from the destruction of red cells begins to accumulate in the liver; nucleated red cells diminish in the peripheral circulation. After birth, these changes occur more rapidly.

We owe a great debt to the authors of this and subsequent eras — Williamson, Lucas, Lippman, Forkner, Blackfan, Diamond, Gairdner, Oski, Naiman, Stockman and many others.

We would personally like to thank the doctors, nurses and hospital staff at the Royal Hospital for Sick Children and the Queen Mother's Hospital, Glasgow, and the Hospitals for Sick Children and Queen Charlotte's Maternity Hospital, London, without whose help and inspiration this work would be impossible. We are greatly indebted to Dr Jon Pritchard and Dr P. Morris Jones for the pictures of children with neonatal tumours, and to Dr V. Broadbent for advice on the neonatal tumour chapter.

E.A. Letsky
I.M. Hann
B.E.S. Gibson

1

Development of blood in the fetus

I.M. Hann
The Hospitals for Sick Children, London

THE ONTOGENY OF BLOOD FORMATION

The beginnings

Within a few days of implantation, angioblastic tissue separates from the wall of the blastocyst and spreads into the developing body stalk and yolk sac wall. Solid masses of cells called blood islands form within the yolk sac, and by the 14th day of gestation these have hollowed out, with peripheral cells forming the vascular endothelium and central cells the first blood cells. Clefts appear between the blood cells to form the vascular lumen. Growth and union of the blood islands result in a plexus of channels. By the 25th day, these differentiation processes within the mesenchyme make up the vascular system of the embryo (Keleman *et al.*, 1979).

Erythropoiesis in the yolk sac produces macrocytic, nucleated red cells that have a polychromatic cytoplasm and a fine nuclear chromatin pattern and which are not under the control of erythropoietin. These distinct differences between yolk sac ('primitive') nucleated red cells and mature ('definitive') normoblastic cells, gave rise to the hypothesis that the primitive cells have an ephemeral lifespan and have no role in 'seeding' the sites of production that appear later in ontogeny. However, studies in mice have demonstrated that the development of haemopoietic organs (liver, spleen and bone marrow, Figure 1.1) is probably dependent on colonization by circulating cells derived from the yolk sac (Moore and Metcalfe, 1970). Fresh human samples obtained at fetoscopy have shown very high levels of committed erythroid and granulocytic/macrophage progenitors (Linch *et al.*, 1982); this gives some support to the hypothesis, though these studies have been carried out at a later stage of fetal development. Blood obtained from aborted mid-trimester fetuses confirms the very high levels of committed and pluripotent (colony forming unit, granulocyte, erythroid, megakaryocyte, monocyte; CFU-GEMM) progenitors (Hann *et al.*, 1983) (Figure 1.2).

The next stage of haemopoietic development is also outside the bone marrow (extramedullary) being of hepatic derivation (Figure 1.1). Extramedullary haemopoiesis may persist until shortly after birth, if there is excessive blood destruction and haemopoietic drive, as in Rhesus disease. It can recur in later life when the marrow is unable to cope with increased

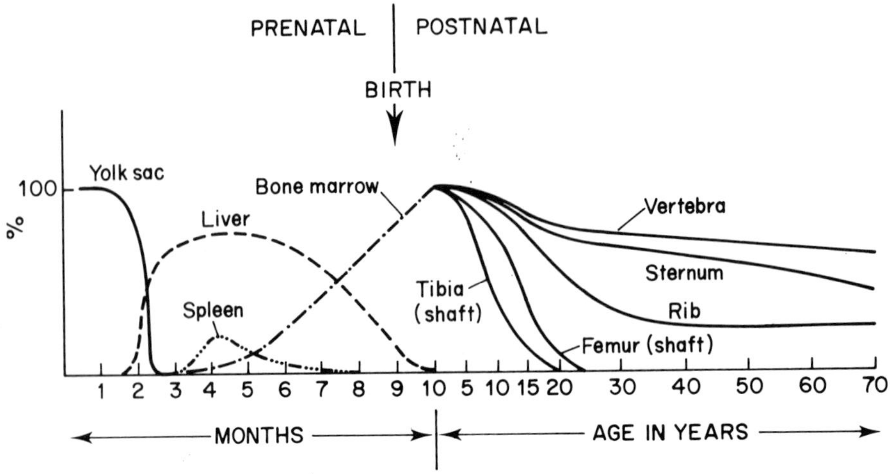

Figure 1.1 The sites of haemopoietic tissue in the fetus and adult life. The other flat bone (e.g. skull and pelvis) are also haemopoietic, similar to the vertabrae and sternum. The ordinate refers, in the fetus, to the contribution to total haemopoiesis and, in postnatal life, to the proportion of the bone marrow at the various haemopoietic sites (the remainder being fat). (From A.V. Hoffbrand and S.M. Lewis, eds, 1981, *Postgraduate Haematology* 2nd edn, with permission of Heinemann Medical Books.)

demand, for example in severe haemolysis, bleeding or megaloblastic anaemia.

It is likely that all haemopoietic cells are derived from pluripotent stem cells (Figure 1.2). Until recently, these cells could only be studied *in vitro* in lethally irradiated mice spleen colonies (CFU-S), but it is now possible to study them in human tissues, using long-term marrow cultures on top of stromal cells in tissue culture flasks. The stem cells are able to self-replicate as well as give rise to daughter cells that are committed to differentiation along one or more haemopoietic lines. Additionally, a pluripotent progenitor cell that is at a slightly later stage in differentiation (CFU-GEMM) can be grown in semi-solid culture, as can the committed erythroid (BFU-E, CFU-E) and granulocytic/macrophage (CFU-GM) colonies. These early haemopoietic precursors are morphologically undistinguished, resembling small or intermediate sized lymphocytes.

The liver and haemopoiesis

The fetal liver becomes haemopoietic between the 6th and 10th weeks of gestation. This phase of blood production overlaps with yolk sac activity, but the liver is the major site of production by the 10th week. Its importance diminishes after the mid-trimester and ceases at term. Large numbers of pluripotent and committed progenitor cells can be demonstrated in cultures

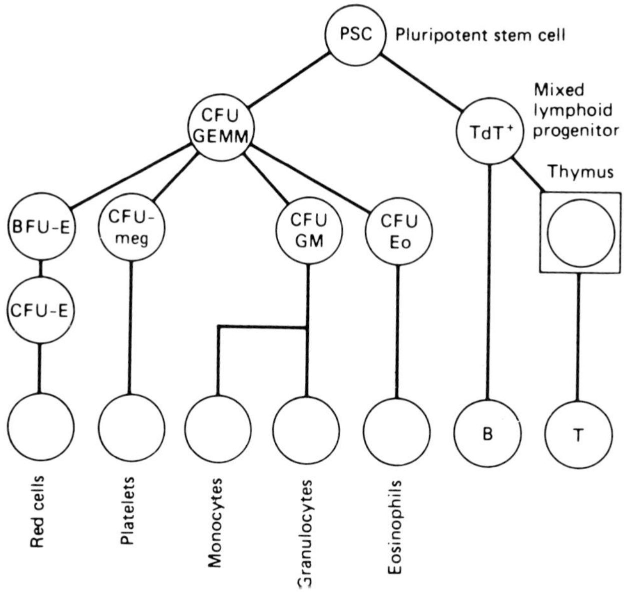

Figure 1.2 A scheme of haemopoiesis. The pluripotent stem cell (PSC) gives rise to a series of committed progenitors defined by cultural characteristics in semisolid medium. CFU-GEMM = colony-forming unit, granulocyte, erythroid, megakaryocyte, monocyte; BFU-E = burst-forming unit, erythroid; GM = granulocyte/monocyte; meg = megakaryocyte; Eo = eosinophil; tdt = terminal deoxynucleotidyl transferase.

from fetal liver throughout the mid-trimester (Hann *et al.*, 1983; Porcellini *et al.*, 1983).

The number of haemopoietic cells in fetal liver has been determined relative to the number of parenchymal cells, usually by counting 1000 cells in histological sections. Haemopoietic cells account for 10% of the total at 5 weeks, rising rapidly to a plateau of 60% at 7–15 weeks and then slowly declining. 'Primitive' erythroblasts form about half the haemopoietic cells up to the 7th week, falling to 10% by the 10th week and being rare thereafter.

Granulocytes are found in small numbers during the first 15 weeks and then increase, particularly after the 21st week. They are located in the connective tissue of the portal spaces; neutrophils and eosinophils at various stages of maturation are seen. Lethally irradiated animals are not protected by transfusions of fetal liver, suggesting that the haemopoietic stem cells of the fetal liver are not capable of forming adequate numbers of mature leukocytes to protect against infection. This contrasts with the finding many precursor colonies committed to granulopoiesis in tissue-culture systems. A large proportion of macrophages is present from the start, rising to 69% of non-hepatic tissue cells and diminishing rapidly after the 6th week.

Megakaryocytes are seen among the hepatocytes and occasionally in the venous sinuses. They account for about 2% of haemopoietic cells at about 5 weeks, falling to about 0.5% by 6 weeks and stabilizing at that point. They exhibit a morphological 'shift to the right'.

Some lymphocytes appear by 7 weeks, but they do not rise above 1% until 13 weeks. Unclassified blasts are seen at high levels (5–8%) in 4 to 6-week-old fetuses and later fall below 1%. Stem cells and committed progenitors probably make up part of these 'lymphoid' and blast cell populations.

Throughout the early part of the hepatic phase of haemopoiesis, high levels of CFU-GEMM, BFU-E and CFU-GM circulate in fetal blood, and it is now assumed that these cells 'seed' the bone marrow and spleen. It is known that to repopulate the lethally irradiated adult, 100-fold fewer nucleated blood cells are needed from fetal than from adult mice (Peschle *et al.*, 1981).

The bone marrow and haemopoiesis

The initiation of bone-marrow formation varies from the 7th or 8th (clavicle) to the 18th or 19th (sternum) week of gestation. The blood cell-forming marrow consists of a vascularized stromal matrix derived from perichondrial cells and haemopoietic parenchyma.

The marrow becomes populated with progenitor cells at about the 15th or 16th week of gestation. A fascinating recent finding is that before any haemopoietic progenitors are found in tissue culture of marrow, the cultures show a profuse growth of stromal cells. These cells may either be the 'seed-bed' upon which circulating stem cells are 'sown'; alternatively, stem cells may produce these marrow elements, as well as reproducing themselves as daughter cells committed to differentation.

The percentage of red cell precursors is about 35% up to the 12th week, and about 20–30% thereafter. In earlier fetuses, most of these cells are 'primitive' erythroblasts, being replaced rapidly by 'definitive' erythroblasts during the 11th week. Neutrophils and granulocytes constitute 30–40% of marrow cells between the 10th and 13th weeks. The percentage of promyelocytes and myelocytes then increases from below 10% to 15–20% after the 14th week.

Eosinophils constitute 1–2% of cells up to 16 weeks, rising to 5% subsequently. Basophils are scarce and remain so. Histiocytes and macrophages are more abundant during the 10th to 16th weeks (4–6%) than later on (about 1%), while monocyte counts rise to 2% at 12 weeks and remain at about this number. Megakaryocytes are present in all fetuses studied (between 0.3% and 1.3% of cells). Lymphocytes make up 12% of cells until the 12th week, increasing to 20–30% subsequently. Large numbers of unclassified blasts (about 15%) are present between weeks 10 and 14, but by the 16th the level begins to fall and reaches a value of 2% at 21 weeks. These cells may include 'stem cells'. Throughout infancy and much of childhood, the entire bone marrow is haemopoietic, comprising 50% haemopoietic tissue and 50% fat. Thereafter, fat progressively takes over the marrow of the small bones of the hands and feet and the shafts of the long bones. This process is complete by the mid-teens.

The spleen as a haemopoietic organ

At 8 weeks of fetal development, this organ consists of a densely packed population of mesenchymal cells without evidence of blood cell formation. By the 12th to 14th weeks, the mesenchymal cells form a syncytial network with erythroblastic islands, megakaryocytes and scattered lymphocytes. By the 15th week, lymphocytes are seen in the surroundings of arteries, and red pulp contains vessels with nucleated red cells. Lymphocyte cell counts increase from about 17% at 11 weeks to 57% at 17 weeks and 70% at 22 weeks. Undifferentiated blast cells are found in most sections of spleen and account for 1% of nucleated cells.

Splenic haemopoiesis has proved difficult to investigate because of the poor viability of aborted tissues. However, it appears from culture studies that haemopoisis begins at about the 19th to 20th weeks, slightly later than the bone marrow, and continues throughout the second trimester. These results are slightly at variance with studies of haemoglobin synthesis, which suggest a simultaneous bone marrow and spleen commencement at about 15–16 weeks.

The thymus

From the 8th week onwards, the thymus epithelium transforms into a meshwork of stellate cells attached by desmosomes. Within this 'mesh' lymphocytes proliferate. By the end of the 3rd month, the thymic tissue forms a dense cortex rich in small lymphocytes and a looser medulla containing thymic corpuscles, lymphocytes at different stages of maturation and some large mononuclear cells. Thymic development is completed with the formation of a capsule, trabeculae and lobules. Groups of erythroblasts and granulocytes are seen in the loose connective tissue of the trabeculae. The thymus and lymph nodes are thought to act as 'supplementary' sites of haemopoiesis during the third trimester. There have been no functional studies of haemopoietic precursors in lymph nodes, but one study was unable to demonstrate any erythroid or myeloid activity in the mid-trimester human fetal thymus (Hann *et al.*, 1983). The lymphopoietic role of this latter organ is discussed below.

Lymph nodes

During the third month, lymph glands develop along the course of peripheral lymphatics. Their development is characterized by a lymphatic plexus associated with mesenchymal tissue and populated by lymphocytes. At 12–14 weeks, small and large lymphocytes and some blast cells can be distinguished. They very rarely contain cells other than lymphocytes; the occasional finding of other haemopoietic cells is a result of migration from the blood or adjacent loose connective tissue. Lymphopoiesis is further discussed below.

The blood

Primitive erythropoetic cells constitute nearly all of the nucleated blood cells from the 4th to the 8th week of gestation (Thomas and Yoffey, 1962). By the 9th to 10th weeks this falls to 88%, and thereafter the proportion of primitive erythroblasts falls very rapidly and they are not found in blood after 12 weeks. Non-nucleated red cells begin to appear in small numbers from the 7th week, increasing rapidly thereafter (Figure 1.3). Megaloblasts and occasional giant erythrocytes are seen from the 4th to 10th weeks. Numerous polychromatic erythrocytes and occasional Howell–Jolly bodies are observed in 11 to 21-week blood smears.

The concentration of red cells in fetal blood increases throughout intrauterine life, being 1×10^{12} per litre at 10 weeks and a mean of 5.1×10^{12} per litre at 40 weeks. The increase in red cell numbers shows a rapid rise in the first trimester, stabilizing in the second trimester and increasing rapidly again to term. These changes are paralleled by haemoglobin content (mean 6.0 g dl^{-1} at 10 weeks and 18.4 g dl^{-1} at term). The packed cell volume (PCV) rises from a mean of 20% to a mean of 60% over this period. Large numbers of nucleated red cells circulate at the 12th week (up to 5×10^{10} per litre), decreasing rapidly to 1×10^{9} per litre at mid-gestation and staying at this level to term. The red cell size in the fetus is larger than in adults and in full-term neonates; the mean cell volume (MCV) is 108 fl which falls to a mean of 78 fl at one year. Normal values were until recently largely dependant upon small series of abortuses and cord bloods of premature babies (Table 1.1). In consequence, there was a dearth of reliable values below 30 weeks of gestation. This situation has now been rectified, following the development of fetoscopic blood sampling (Forestier *et al.*, 1986). Table 1.2 shows the evolution of haematological values in 163 normal

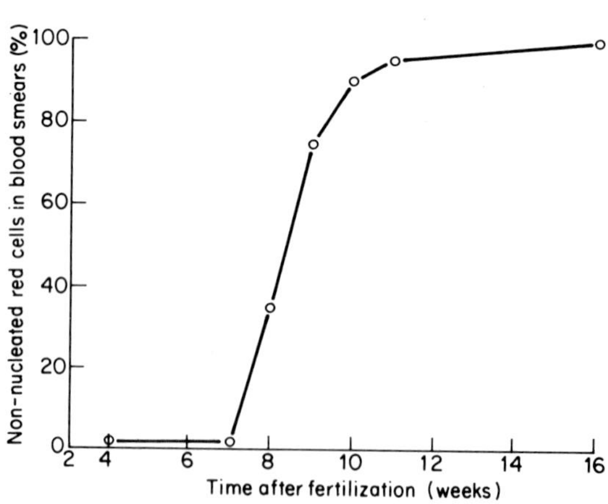

Figure 1.3 The percentage of non-nucleated red cells in blood films at different stages of human embryonic and fetal development. (From E. Keleman *et al.*, 1979, *Human Haemopoietic Development*, with permission of Springer Verlag.)

Table 1.1 Mean red cell and values during gestation (abortuses and hysterotomy).*†

Age (weeks)	Hb (g dl^{-1})	PCV%	RBc ($\times 10^{12}$ per litre)	MCV (fl)	MCH (pg)	Reticulocytes (%)
12	8–10	33	1.5	180	60	40
16	10	35	2.0	140	45	10–25
20	11	37	2.5	135	44	10–20
24	14	40	3.5	123	38	5–10
28	14.5	45	4.0	120	40	5–10
34	15.0	47	4.0	118	38	3–10

* Adapted from F.A. Oski and J.L. Naiman, 1982, *Haematological Problems in the Newborn*, vol. IV, W.B. Saunders.
† Hb = Haemoglobin, MCV = mean cell volume, MCH = mean corpuscular haemoglobin, PCV = packed cell volume (haematocrit).

fetuses between 18 and 30 weeks of gestation. Table 1.3 shows the results of the other large group at King's College Hospital. Although there is some duplication, this latter table contains the results of 116 fetuses in the earlier period of 15–21 weeks' gestation (excluding abnormal fetuses and those with chromosomal abnormalities). The rise in red cell count (RBC) and reciprocal fall in MCV with a consequent fall in mean cell haemoglobin (MCH) is well illustrated. The haemoglobin level remains constant whilst reticulocyte and normoblast levels fall. There is no statistically significant change in platelet numbers.

Granulocytes are circulating in very small numbers in early fetuses ($< 1 \times 10^9$ per litre). Neutrophils, promyelocytes and myelocytes make up 0.2% of all nucleated cells at 7 weeks and 3% at 21 weeks. Band forms and mature neutrophils only begin to appear at 9–10 weeks and form 4% of nucleated cells by 12 weeks, rising to 16% at 21 weeks. At term they rise to a mean of 6.0×10^9 per litre Eosinophils form 0.5% of nucleated cells from 16 weeks on and basophils appear at 14 weeks (0.3% of nucleated cells). Occasional monocytes are seen at 4–5 weeks and they form 1–4% of nucleated cells by 11 weeks. Histiocytes and macrophages are present in the earliest blood samples up to 14 weeks but are not found later.

Large lymphocytes make up 3–5% of nucleated blood cells from the 11th week. Small lymphocytes are found in much larger numbers, from 0.2% at 9 weeks to 30% at 14 weeks. The lymphocyte count at 20 weeks is at a mean of 1.5×10^9 per litre rising to 2.5×10^9 per litre at term.

Megakaryocytes are present in the yolk sac at 5 weeks and in the blood at 8 weeks. Platelets are seen in the blood at 5 weeks and large platelets occur in 16 to 21-week-old fetuses. Undifferentiated blast cells can be seen in 4 to 5-week-old embryo blood in small quantities (0.2–2.0% of nucleated cells).

Table 1.4 gives differential white cell counts taken at fetoscopy during weeks 18–30 (Forestier *et al.*, 1986). Neutrophils were low throughout the period although there was a slight increase from 0.2×10^9 to 0.4×10^9 per litre, with about half of these being present as band forms. Eosinophil and monocyte counts remained constant, as did lymphocyte counts, although

Table 1.2 Haematological values in mid-trimester fetoscopic samples.*†

Gestation (weeks)	n‡	WBC ($\times 10^9$ per litre)	Platelets ($\times 10^9$ per litre)	RBC ($\times 10^{12}$ per litre)	Hb (g dl^{-1})	PCV (%)	MCV (fl)	MCH (pg)
18–20	25	4.20 ± 0.83	242 ± 35	2.66 ± 0.29	11.5 ± 0.8	36 ± 3.3	134 ± 8.8	43 ± 2.7
21–22	55	4.19 ± 0.84	258 ± 54	2.96 ± 0.26	12.3 ± 0.9	39 ± 3.2	130 ± 6.2	41 ± 3.3
23–25	61	3.95 ± 0.69	260 ± 43	3.06 ± 0.26	12.4 ± 0.8	39 ± 2.4	126 ± 6.2	40 ± 2.9
26–30	22	4.44 ± 0.85	254 ± 37	3.52 ± 0.32	13.4 ± 1.2	42 ± 3.3	118 ± 5.8	38 ± 3.7

* Adapted from: F. Forestier *et al.*, 1986, *Paediatric Research* **20**: 342.
† Values quoted are mean ± SD from studies performed with a Coulter S Plus 2.
‡ n = Number of fetuses studied.

Table 1.3 Mid-trimester red cell and platelet values (SD in parentheses) at fetoscopy.*

	Gestational age (weeks)						
	15	16	17	18	19	20	21
Haemoglobin (g dl^{-1})	10.9 (0.7)	12.5 (0.8)	12.4 (0.9)	12.4 (1.2)	12.3 (1.2)	13.0 (1.1)	12.3 (0.8)
Total red cells ($\times 10^{22}$ per litre)	2.43 (0.26)	2.68 (0.21)	2.74 (0.23)	2.77 (0.33)	2.92 (0.27)	3.12 (0.36)	3.07 (0.42)
Haematocrit (%)	35 (3.6)	38 (2.1)	37 (2.1)	37 (4.1)	38 (3.1)	39 (4.1)	37 (3.5)
Mean cell volume (fl)	143 (8)	143 (12)	137 (8)	135 (9)	129 (6)	126 (6)	123 (8)
Mean cell haemoglobin (pg)	45.4 (3.9)	46.6 (3.5)	45.4 (2.5)	44.7 (2.7)	42.5 (2.6)	41.8 (2.4)	40.6 (3.7)
Nucleated red cells ($\times 10^9$ per litre)	2.1 (0.8)	3.6 (1.8)	2.5 (0.9)	2.7 (2.2)	2.6 (1.7)	2.4 (1.2)	3.7 (0.8)
Reticulocytes ($\times 10^9$ per litre)	0.63 (0.15)	0.43 (0.07)	0.43 (0.08)	0.36 (0.09)	0.36 (0.01)	0.32 (0.17)	0.23 (0.08)
Platelets ($\times 10^9$ per litre)	190 (31)	208 (57)	202 (25)	192 (45)	211 (48)	170 (60)	223 (61)
Number of fetuses	6	5	16	18	29	12	13

* Adapted from Miller *et al.*, eds, 1985, *Blood Diseases of Infancy and Children*, 5th edn, with permission of C.V. Mosby Company.

Table 1.4 Differential white cell counts from 18 to 30 weeks' of gestation.*

Gestation (weeks)	*n*‡	Lymphocytes (%)	Neutrophils (%)	Eosinophils (%)	Monocytes (%)	NRBC† (%)
18–20	25	80.0 ± 9.0	5.0 ± 2.0	1.5 ± 2.5	1.5 ± 2.0	12.0 ± 8.0
21–22	55	81.0 ± 7.0	5.5 ± 3.5	1.0 ± 1.0	1.5 ± 1.5	11.0 ± 7.0
23–25	61	82.0 ± 6.0	7.5 ± 4.5	2.0 ± 2.0	1.5 ± 1.5	7.0 ± 4.0
18–20	22	84.0 ± 6.0	8.5 ± 2.5	2.0 ± 1.0	1.5 ± 1.0	4.0 ± 3.5

* From F. Forestier *et al.*, 1986, *Paediatric Research* **20**: 342. Results are the mean of 163 normal fetuses ± SD.
† NRBC = Nucleated red blood cells.
‡ *n* = Number of fetuses studied.

some of the lymphocytes appeared to be large and have basophilic cytoplasm.

Another study of fetoscopic samples, made by Millar *et al.* (1985), in the earlier period of 15–21 weeks, was more detailed. At 15 weeks, very low total white blood cell (WBC) counts were seen, the lowest being 0.8×10^9 per litre (Table 1.5). The counts rose during the period studied and all fetuses had a WBC of more than 1.0×10^9 per litre at 21 weeks. This study confirmed the low neutrophil counts demonstrated by Forestier *et al.* (1985) and showed a trend of rising counts for neutrophils, lymphocytes, monocytes and eosinophils. Millar *et al.* (1985) also found a very small proportion of more immature cells, which apparently decreased with increasing gestational age.

Regulation of fetal haemopoiesis

Erythroid progenitors (BFU-E and CFU-E) present in the fetal liver during the 7th to 15th weeks of gestation have been studied in semi-solid tissue culture. Regulation of all these red cell precursors was shown to be under the control of erythropoietin (Epo) and burst-promoting factor (BPF), as in postnatal life, though fetal BFU-E and CFU-E may be more sensitive to the control of erythropoietin and BFF. However, there are big differences between red cell precursors in other regulatory aspects. Differentiation of 'adult' precursors entails a gradual increase in proliferative rate, whilst all fetal progenitors are characterized by maximal cycling activity. In addition, ontogenetic maturation of the erythron is associated with a progressive decline in proliferative activity of early and intermediate erythroid progenitors and cell doubling time in erythropoietic differentiation. Finally, the main source of erythropoietin is probably hepatic in the fetus (Zanjani *et al.*, 1977), whereas 'adult' regulators are derived from the kidneys and probably from T-lymphocyte-macrophage complexes. Recent evidence from Flake *et al.* (1987) suggests that the liver and kidney 'switch' during ontogeny is a genetically predetermined event rather than a result of postnatal environmental factors.

Table 1.5 Mid-trimester red cell and platelet values (SD in parentheses) at fetoscopy.*

	Gestational age (weeks)						
	15	16	17	18	19	20	21
Total WBC	1.6 (0.7)	2.4 (1.7)	2.0 (0.8)	2.4 (0.9)	2.5 (0.8)	2.6 (1.2)	2.7 (0.7)
Neutrophils	0.11 (0.07)	0.2 (0.2)	0.13 (0.06)	0.16 (0.06)	0.13 (0.08)	0.13 (0.08)	0.19 (0.01)
Lymphocytes	1.36 (0.62)	2.17 (1.63)	1.7 (0.7)	2.12 (0.85)	2.16 (0.7)	2.33 (1.16)	2.33 (0.52)
Monocytes	0.06 (0.03)	0.02 (0.02)	0.07 (0.5)	0.07 (0.05)	0.11 (0.07)	0.11 (0.09)	0.11 (0.09)
Eosinophils	0.009 (0.01)	0.02 (0.02)	0.02 (0.02)	0.02 (0.02)	0.03 (0.03)	0.05 (0.04)	0.1 (0.1)
Basophils	0.002 (0.004)	—	0.02 (0.02)	0.01 (0.2)	0.02 (0.02)	0.01 (0.02)	0.02 (0.02)
Metamyelocytes	0.004 (0.01)	0.003 (0.006)	0.001 (0.004)	0.009 (0.02)	0.002 (0.005)	0.003 (0.008)	—
Myelocytes	0.005 (0.008)	—	0.002 (0.008)	0.006 (0.01)	—	0.003 (0.008)	—
Blasts	0.02 (0.01)	0.01 (0.02)	0.02 (0.03)	0.02 (0.02)	0.02 (0.02)	0.01 (0.02)	0.01 (0.02)
Number of fetuses	6	5	16	18	29	12	13

* Adapted from: Miller *et al.*, eds, 1985, *Blood Diseases of Infancy and Children*, 5th edn, with permission of C.V. Mosby Company.

Table 1.6 The stromal cells, extracellular matrix, growth factors and monokines and lymphokines on which haemopoiesis depends.*

Stromal cells	Extracellular matrix	Growth factors	Monokines and lymphokines
Macrophages	Fibronectin	Multipotent	Interleukin-1
Fibroblasts	Laminin	Multi-CSF	Interleukin-2
Reticulum ('blanket') cells	Collagen	(interleukin-3; BPA)	Interferons α and γ
Fat cells	Proteoglycans (acid mucopolysaccharides)	GM-CSF	Tumour necrosis factor
Endothelial cells		Committed	B cell stimulating factor 1 (IL-4)
		G-CSF	B cell growth factor (IL-5)
		M-CSF (CSF-1)	B cell differentiation factor (IL-6)
		Eo-CSF	Migration inhibition factor
		Erythropoietin	
		? Thrombopoietin	

* From A.V. Hoffbrand and J.E. Pettit, 1987, *Clinical Haematology Illustrated*, Churchill Livingstone.

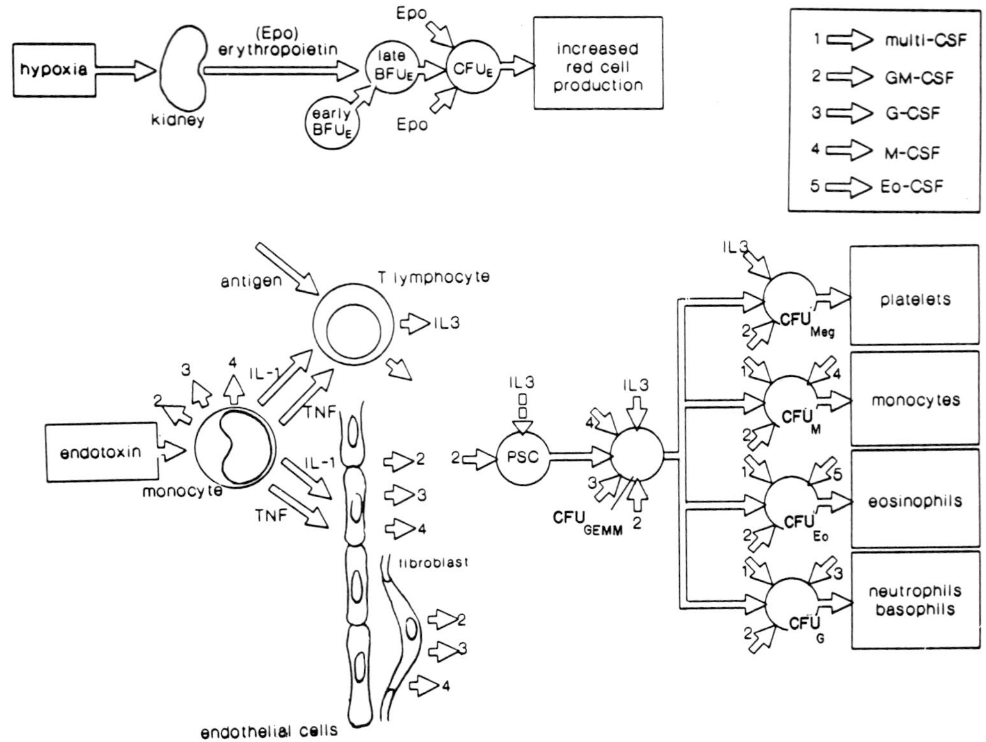

Figure 1.4 Regulation of haemopoiesis: pathways of stimulation of leucopoiesis by endotoxin, for example from infection, and of erythropoiesis by hypoxia. It is likely that endothelial and fibroblast cells release basal quantities of GM-CSF and G-CSF in the normal resting state and that this is enhanced substantially by the monolines TNF and IL-1 released in response to infection. IL-1 and TNF also stimulate T cells, and antigen may stimulate T cells directly. The action of multi-CSF on human pluripotent stem cells has not been proven. (From A.V. Hoffbrand and J.E. Pettit, 1988 *Sandoz Atlas of Clinical Hematology*, Sandoz Ltd/Gower Medical Publishing.)

Regulation of postnatal haemopoiesis

Haemopoiesis is regulated by a series of glycoproteins which are listed in Table 1.6. Their cellular origin and target cells are shown in Figure 1.4. It is likely that their action in causing cellular proliferation and differentiation depends upon a close cell-to-cell interaction and also interaction with the extracellular matrix (marrow stroma). The growth factors also affect the functions of the more mature cells, for example phagocytosis, motility, killing and chemotaxis.

Human urinary erythropoietin was first purified in 1977, and the complete primary sequence of the protein and the gene sequence have now been reported. The gene is organized into five exons and four intervening sequences (introns) and exists as a single copy in the human genome, located on the long arm of chromosome 7. The erythropoietin gene encodes a 193 amino acid polypeptide, the first 27 amino acids of which represent the secretory leader sequence that is cleared upon secretion of the hormone. This yields a mature protein of 165 amino acids with two internal disulphide bonds and four carbohydrate chains. The circulating glycosylated hormone has a molecular weight of 36 000 Da. The recombinantly produced hormone is indistinguishable from the native human urinary hormone both biologically and immunologically and is structurally very similar (Eschbach and Adamson, 1988).

THE ONTOGENY OF HUMAN FETAL LYMPHOPOIESIS

The appearance of identifiable B and T cells in the haemopoietic organs is summarized in Table 1.7. There have been only a few studies of the ontogeny of lymphoid precursor cells and lymphocytes in human fetal tissue, most studies being confined to rodents and chickens. The enzyme terminal deoxynucleotidyl transferase (tdt) has been a useful marker of lymphoid precursor cells and immature T lymphocytes (Bollum, 1979). Cells containing tdt in adults are confined to: (1) bone marrow, where they express HLA-DR (Ia) antigen and the common acute lymphoblastic leukaemia antigen (cALLA) and include pre-B cells, that also show cytoplasmic immunoglobulin (Ig), as well as common lymphoid progenitors, and (2) the cortical areas of the thymus. Tdt-positive cells are not observed in normal peripheral lymphoid organs such as lymph nodes, blood, spleen and tonsils. The function of tdt is to generate diversity in the lymphoid system by inserting new DNA bases into immunoglobulin T cell receptor genes during the phase of lymphoid development at which rearrangement of these genes take place (Alt and Baltimore, 1982). The gene for tdt has now been shown to be localized to the region q23–q25 of chromosome 10 (Isobe *et al.*, 1985).

The liver and bone marrow from second trimester fetuses are highly enriched for tdt^+ cells and, like pluripotent and myeloid progenitor cells, tdt^+ cells circulate in the peripheral blood (Bodger *et al.*, 1983; Bonati *et al.*, 1983; Brashem *et al.*, 1983). The majority of tdt^+ cells in the bone marrow express the p24 antigen, a marker for B lymphoid precursor cells that is

Table 1.7 Early events in the development of lymphocytic cell systems.*

Site and event	week(s) of gestation
Yolk sac and other extraembryonic sites	
Lymphopoiesis was not found	
Liver	
Appearance of:	
E-Rosette forming T cells	7
MLC responsive cells	8
Ig-Bearing B cells	8
The number of T and B cells is less than 1% up to the 12th week and 1–4% (of all nucleated haemopoietic cells) after the 12th week	
Thymus	
Appearance of:	
Lymphopoiesis	7–10
E-Rosette forming T cells	9
Ig-Bearing B cells	11.5
Well-developed population of T cells	12
More than 90% of lymphoid cells have T or B characteristics	16
Blood	
Appearance of:	
T-Lymphocytes	7–8
B-Lymphocytes	12
Small lymphocytes:	
1 × 10 μ/l	12
10 × 10 μ/l	20–25
More than 90% of lymphoid cells have T or B characteristics	16
64Gut-associated lymphoid tissue	
Lamina propria	7–10
Peyer's patches	11–15
Palatine tonsils	10–14
Appendix	11–15
Bronchial Lymphocytes	
Lamina propria	7–10
Lymph plexuses — lymph nodes	
Primordia, jugular region	7–8
Retroperitoneal region	11
Lymphoid development	8–12
Bone marrow	
B and T lymphocytes	12
'Negative' (null) lymphocytes (= B + T)	12
Spleen	
Appearance of T and B lymphocytes	10–12
Lymphocyte aggregates	12–14
More than 90% of lymphoid cells have T or B determinants	16

* From Keleman *et al.*, 1979. *Atlas of Human Hemopoietic Development*, with permission of Springer Verlag.

detected by monoclonal antibody CD9 (Brashem *et al.*, 1983).

The lymphoid progenitor cells generate pre-B cells (which express intracytoplasmic, but not surface, Ig) and B cells in the liver (Kamps and Cooper, 1982) which then probably seed to the bone marrow. The first B cells, at 9 weeks, show surface IgM but, subsequently, cells with surface IgG, IgA and IgD appear, some fetal cells showing more than one class of surface Ig. The characteristic feature of the precursor B cell is that it rearranges its genes for immunoglobulin synthesis. In all other body cells, these genes remain in the germline configuration. Rearrangement of the heavy-chain gene occurs first, then of the κ light-chain gene and lastly of the λ light-chain gene (Figure 1.5). The rearrangement takes place by the joining together of the different segments of each gene, with splicing out of the intervening sequences. For the heavy chain, the coding sequences include V regions, diversity (D), joining (J), and constant (C) regions (Figure 1.6). The final gene produced codes for the particular immunoglobulin that the individual B cell will produce. Diversity between different B cells is introduced by variation of which of the V, D, J and C regions are used to join each other, and also by tdt, which inserts new bases (N regions) into the V–D or D–J junctions at the time of rearrangement. When the genes are functionally rearranged, a mRNA is produced that still contains RNA transcribed from an intron between the J and C region. This RNA is spliced

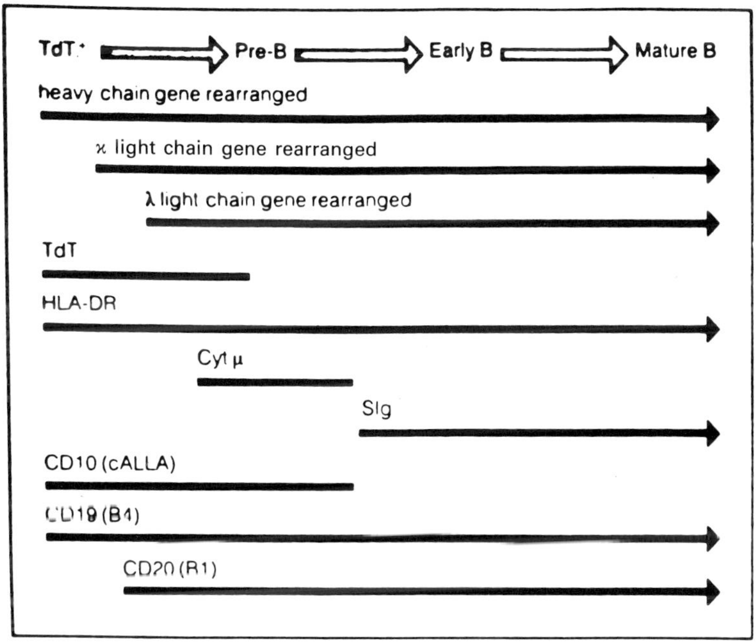

Figure 1.5 The sequence of immunoglobulin gene rearrangement, antigen and immunoglobulin expression during early B cell development. S = surface. Cyt = cytoplasmic. Intracytoplasmic CD22 is also a feature of very early B cells. (From A.V. Hoffbrand and J.E. Pettit, 1988, *Sandoz Atlas of Clinical Hematology*, with permission of Sandoz Ltd/Gower Medical Publishing.)

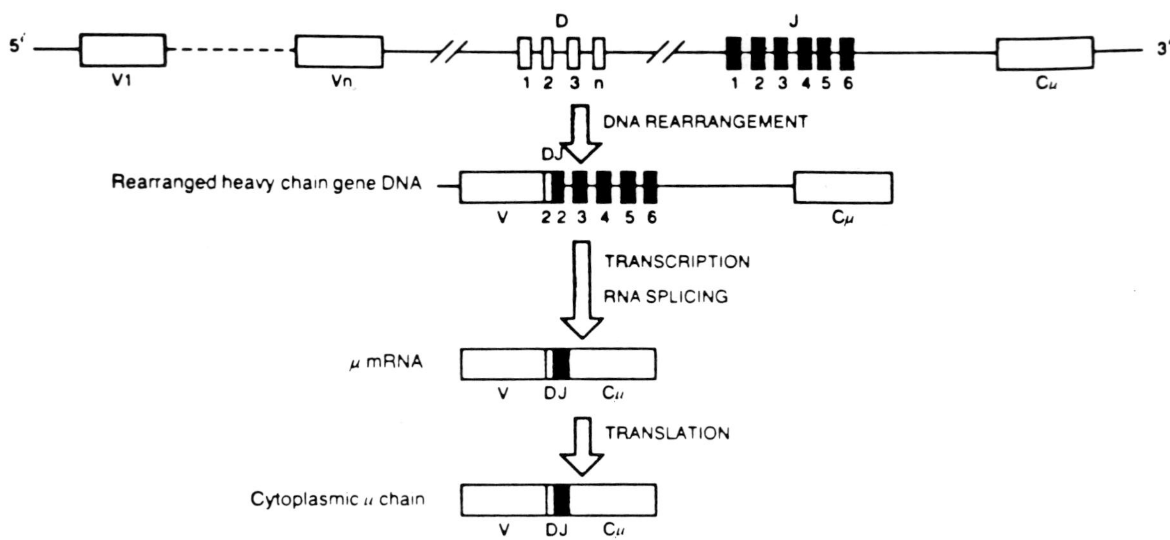

Figure 1.6 Rearrangement of a heavy chain immunoglobulin gene. One of the V segments is brought into contact with a D, a J, a C (in this case Cμ) segment, forming an active transcriptional gene from which the corresponding mRNA is produced. The DJ rearrangement precedes VDJ joining. (From A.V. Hoffbrand and J.E. Pettit, 1988, *Sandoz Atlas of Clinical Hematology*, with permission of Sandoz Ltd/Gower Medical Publishing.)

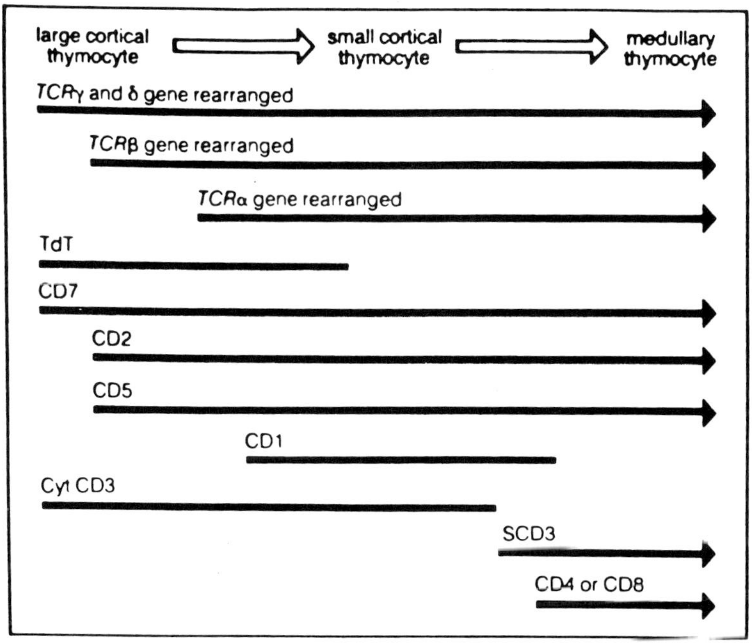

Figure 1.7 The sequence of T cell gene rearrangments and antigen expression during early T cell development. (From A.V. Hoffbrand and J.E. Pettit, 1988, *Sandoz Atlas of Clinical Hematology*, with permission of Sandoz Ltd/Gower Medical Publishing.)

so that a continuous peptide heavy chain is synthesized. The cells first express cytoplasmic heavy chain (pre-B cells) and, subsequently, surface immunoglobulin. The switch from IgM synthesis utilizing the $C\mu$ locus to synthesis of other heavy chains (e.g. IgD, IgA, IgE or IgG) requires usage of the different C region loci, e.g. δ, α, ε, τ, respectively. This requires deletion of constant chain loci other than the one to be used. At an early stage, the CD19 antigen is expressed on the surface of the pre-B cells, surface CD22 in the cytoplasm and, subsequently, surface CD10 and other B cell antigens (Figure 1.6).

The site where these cells are formed in fetal life is initially the liver and then the marrow. Immunoglobulin gene rearrangement occurs at both these sites, since surface IgM appears as early as 9 weeks of gestation in the human, with subsequent cells showing IgG, IgA, IgD or combinations. Plasma cells are not seen in the fetus, however, in the absence of intrauterine infection.

T cells are rare in liver from 7 to 14 weeks, but appear in low numbers (0.5–1.0%) in the bone marrow at around 16–22 weeks. T cells and their precursors are characterized by rearrangement of one or other of two sets of genes. These codes for the two heterodimer T cell receptors (TCR) either the α and β or γ and δ receptor (Figure 1.7). In all other body cells, these genes remain in the germline configuration. The TCR α/β cells are the major population of T cells in late fetal and post-natal life.

The TCR (α/β or γ/δ) is associated on the T cell surface with the CD3 complex. This is made up of five polypeptide CD3 units; γ, δ, ε, ζ and η. The CD3 complex is thought to be involved in transmitting the antigenic signal from the TCR to the cell interior. The intracytoplasmic expression of CD3ε, when it is assembled in the endoplasmic reticulum before its insertion into the membrane, is one of the earliest and most reliable features of T cell commitment.

Rearrangment of the TCR genes occurs in the same way as that of the immunoglobulin genes, with splicing out of those segments not required in the finished gene and reassembly of the remaining segments. The same enzymatic machinery is thought to be involved, recombinases recognizing certain heptamer and nonamer sequences at the 5′ and 3′ ends of the V, D and J sequences. TDT is also expressed in the cells rearranging their TCR genes and, as in B cells, contributes to the diversity of gene structure. The δ gene is situated within the α gene cluster on chromosome 14, so deletion or rearrangement of the α gene necessarily deletes the δ gene.

The site at which T cells develop from stem cells appears to be first in the liver, which is populated in the 7th week with $CD7^+$ lymphoid cells. By the 9th week, $CD7^+$ cytoplasmic $CD3^+$, TDT^- cells appear. $TCR\beta^+$ membrane $CD3^+$ cells appear from the 11th to the 20th week. TDT appears first at the 20th week. Surface CD7 may act as a homing device for liver or marrow prothymocytes to the thymus. $CD7^+$ cytoplasmic $CD3^+$ or $CD7^+$ $CD3^-$ cells colonize the thymus at 8–9 weeks; they then express CD2 (the sheep red cell receptor). A wave of TCR γ/δ, TDT^- cells is followed by waves of TCR α/β cells, initially TDT^- and their TCR, then TDT^+. Rearrangement of the TCR α/β or γ/δ chains may occur outside the thymus, especially in the bone marrow.

The earliest thymic cells are localized in the subscapular region of the thymic cortex and move through the cortex to the medulla, encountering cortical thymic nurse cells, dendritic cells and medullary epithelial cells, and they are then exported to the blood. Within the thymus, selection of T cells occurs, 99% being eliminated, including all those that would recognize self. T cell associated antigens (e.g. CD7, CD2, CD5, CD1) are expressed and the mature T cells divide into helper ($CD4^+$) or supressor ($CD8^+$) cells.

The thymus ultimately contains three population of cells: large subcortical blasts, typical cortical thymocytes (both TDT^+) and TDT^- medullary thymus lymphocytes divided into $CD4^+$ $CD8^-$ helper cells and $CD4^-$ $CD8^+$ supressor cells.

In the mouse, TCR γ/δ cells are found in the skin and intestinal epithelium especially, but whether they form the receptor in the thymus and then home to these sites, or whether prothymocytes home there and then arrange the TCR^- γ/δ genes is not clear.

There is an orderly acquisition of major histocompatibility complex antigens and myeloid and B cell antigens expressed on myeloid and lymphoid cells in liver, bone marrow and spleen during fetal maturation (Rosenthal *et al.*, 1983). This is not observed in the T cell population, which remains consistently low during maturation. The surface phenotype of mid-trimester thymocytes is very similar to that of neonatal thymocytes and includes a substantial number of cells that have acquired mature T cell antigens.

The phenotypic analysis of peripheral blood mononuclear cells sampled *in utero* from normal fetuses aged 20–26 weeks has recently been reported (Rainaut *et al.*, 1990). T cells accounted for 40–45% of the mononuclear cells and were significantly decreased in comparison with the percentage of T cells in neonatal (71%) and adult (75–80%) peripheral blood. The combined percentage of CD4 and CD8 cells was higher than either the percentage of CD3 or CD2 (pan T cell antibodies) T cells, which suggest that some fetal T cells co-express the CD4 and CD8 antigens. However, the ratio of CD4:CD8 cells in fetal blood (5.7) was significantly higher than in adult peripheral blood (3.1), but not significantly different from that in neonatal peripheral blood (5.0). B cells accounted for 4–5% of the circulating mononuclear cells. Whereas CD16 (natural killer, NK, cells), CD14 (myeloid cells), CD5 and CD20 (B cells) accounted for almost 100% of the cells in adult peripheral blood, the same combination of monoclonal antibodies accounted for only 80% of fetal peripheral blood cells. The high percentage of HLA-DR$^+$ cells (29%) in fetal blood suggests that many of the CD16, CD14, CD2, CD20 cells could be immature myeloid cells and haemopoietic progenitor cells. High numbers of haemopoietic progenitor cells are found in the peripheral blood during the second trimester (Linch *et al.*, 1982; Hann *et al.*, 1983).

Lymph nodes

In early fetal lymph nodes (16th week), 70% of lymphoid cells found are T cells, the remainder being IgM$^+$ B cells diffusely distributed and mixed. The lymph node B cells react with monoclonal antibodies that characterize peripheral, but not bone marrow, lymphocytes in the infant and adult, and also express IgD as well as IgM.

A population of almost pure B cells with surface IgM develop from about 17 weeks gestation, in fetal lymph nodes around developing follicular dendritic reticulum cells inside small primary nodules. These 'virgin' B cells are not found in fetal liver or bone marrow, and they show antigenic determinants detected by monoclonal antibodies not present on marrow lymphoid cells, and have the same phenotype as the cells found in adults with chronic lymphatic leukaemia.

Severe combined immune deficiency (SCID)

Some infants are born without T or B cells and with sparsely populated thymus or lymph nodes. There are probably a number of inborn errors of metabolism causing this. One of the most frequent is deficiency of adenosine deaminase (ADA), an ezyme that is essential in purine degradation. Deficiency of the related enzyme, purine nucleoside phosphorylase (PNP) causes a more selective T cell deficiency.

METABOLIC CHANGES IN FETAL RED CELLS AND CHANGES IN RED CELL METABOLISM

The pathways of glucose metabolism in mature red cells are shown in Figure 1.8. Pure fetal blood obtained at fetoscopy in mid-trimester is available for the study of glycolytic enzymes (Lestas *et al.*, 1982; Table 1.8). the availability of these normal ranges should allow prenatal detection of severe enzyme deficiencies of, for example, triose-phosphate isomerase, pyruvate kinase or hexokinase. The activities of all glycolytic enzymes in fetal erythrocytes (except phosphofructokinase, PFK, and 6-phosphogluconate dehydrogenase, 6PGD) are higher than those of adults or term or premature infants. The mean age of fetal red cells is much less than neonatal or adult erythrocytes, partly explaining some of the higher enzyme activities, especially for those enzymes that are highly age-dependent (e.g. hexokinase, pyruvate kinase, PK, aldolase and glucose-6-phosphate dehydrogenase, G6PD).

Fetal levels of PFK and 6PGD are similar to adult values and thus are less than in adult cells of comparable mean age. This is consistent with the finding of a low level of PFK in neonatal red cells and a 6PGD activity in neonatal cells comparable to that of adult cells of similar mean age. The low

Table 1.8 Enzyme activities (EU g^{-1} Hb) in the erythrocytes of fetal and adult subjects.*

	Fetal (EU g^{-1} Hb)		Adult (EU g^{-1} Hb)		
Enzyme	Mean ± SD	*n*‡	Mean ± SD	*n*‡	$M_F - M_A$†
Hexokinase	2.91 ± 0.55	14	0.85 ± 0.10	20	+20.6
Glucosephosphate isomerase	59 ± 5	13	34 ± 3	16	+5.3
Phosphofructokinase	8.3 ± 1.3	21	8.4 ± 0.8	13	−0.1
Aldolase	3.0 ± 0.25	14	1.9 ± 0.26	20	+4.2
Triosephosphate isomerase	1722 ± 114	14	1347 ± 83	12	+4.5
glyceraldehyde-3-phosphate dehydrogenase	195 ± 18	13	136 ± 20	20	+3.0
Phosphoglycerate kinase	353 ± 17	13	231 ± 14	16	+8.7
Diphosphoglyceromutase	5.5 ± 0.4	14	3.2 ± 0.35	20	+6.6
Monophosphoglyceromutase	25.5 ± 3.4	14	16.8 ± 2.3	12	+3.8
Enolase	10.6 ± 1.25	14	3.6 ± 0.3	16	+23.3
Pyruvate kinase	19.4 ± 3.2	19	9.2 ± 1.8	24	+5.7
Lactate dehydrogenase	149 ± 10	14	113 ± 7	22	+5.1
Glucose-6-phosphate dehydrogenase	15.8 ± 1.1	14	6.2 ± 0.7	20	+13.7
6-Phosphogluconate dehydrogenase	5.9 ± 0.4	14	6.0 ± 0.4	20	−0.2

* From Lestas *et al.*, 1982, *British Journal of Haematology 50*: 439, with permission of Blackwell Scientific Publications.
† Number of standard deviations characterizing the difference between fetal and adult mean activities for each enzyme; denoted as '+' if the fetal is higher than the adult, and '−' if it is lower.
‡ Number of blood samples investigated for each enzyme.

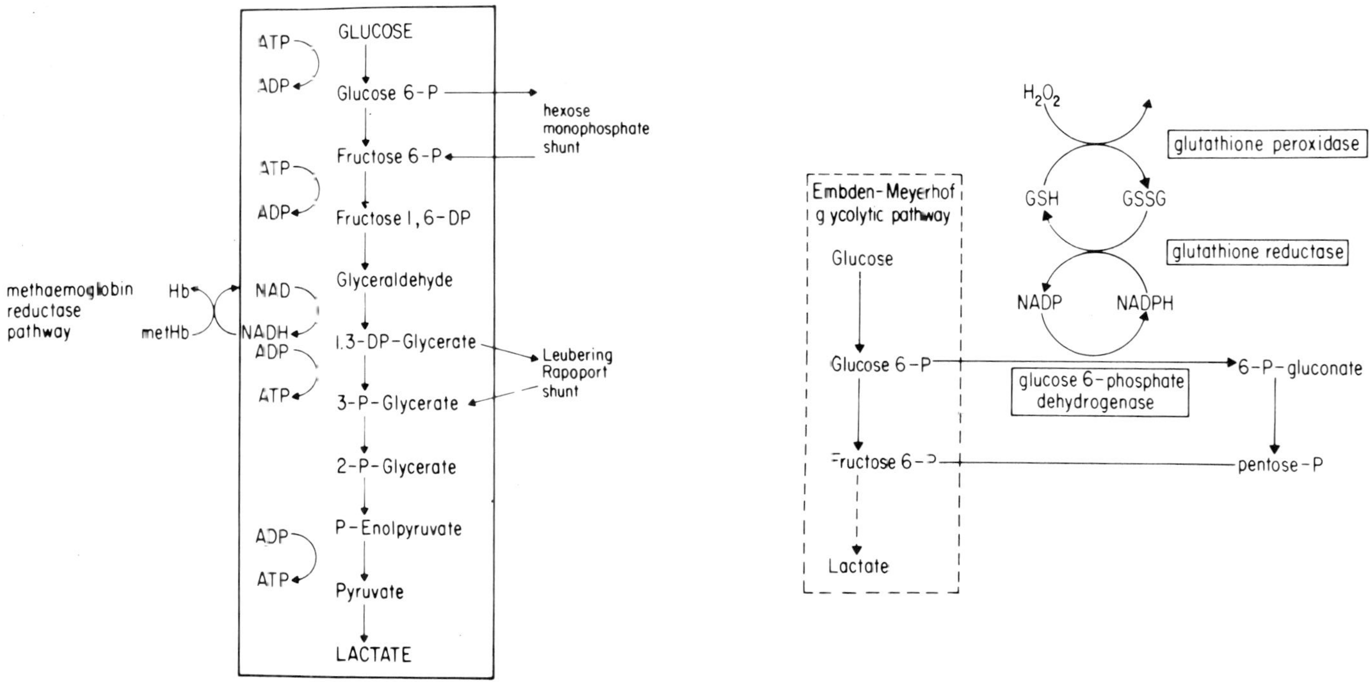

Figure 1.8 Pathways of glucose metabolism in the red cell. Left: Embden–Meyerhof pathway, methaemoglobin reductase pathway and Leubering Rapoport (2,3-DPG shunt). Right: Hexose monophosphate shunt. For enzyme abbreviations see Table 2. (Adapted from A.V. Hoffbrand and J.E. Pettit, 1984, *Essential Haematology*, 2nd edn, with permission of Blackwell Scientific Publications.)

level of PFK in neonatal samples is probably responsible for the decreased glycolysis of red cells in newborns.

The age range studied by fetoscopic sampling is restricted to a short period (weeks 17–24), and over this range no significant changes in enzyme levels with age have been detected. Clearly it would be of interest to look at levels at other fetal ages.

The activities of glucose-phosphate isomerase, glyceraldehyde-3-phosphate-dehydrogenase, phosphoglycerate kinase and enolase are increased in cord blood samples. The levels of 2,3 diphosphoglycerate (2,3-DPG) are similar in cord and adult blood, despite the lowered affinity of haemoglobin F for this compound and the fact that 2,3-DPG is a potent inhibitor of its own formation. This finding has not been explained. Galactose metabolism, unlike glucose metabolism, is enhanced in neonatal blood, with an increased galactokinase activity.

The susceptibility of neonatal red cells to oxidant injury leads to glutathione instability, methaemoglobinaemia and Heinz body formation. The reason for this is uncertain, though it is probably the result of a number of factors: inappropriately low levels of glutathione peroxide for the metabolic age of the red cells; reduced levels of methaemoglobin reductase and catalase; reduced levels of methaemoglobin reductase and catalase; reduced levels of membrane-SH groups, associated with low levels of membrane antioxidants such as vitamin E.

ATP levels are elevated in cord blood, but to a level consistent with mean cell age. Other cord red cell enzyme changes which have been documented are low levels of acetyl cholinesterase and adenylate kinase, and a very marked reduction of the two red cell carbonic anhydrases (but all four enzymes are adequate to maintain normal function).

HAEMOGLOBIN SYNTHESIS IN THE FETUS

Globin

Interest in fetal haemoglobin has been aroused because of the availablity of blood samples obtained at fetoscopy and from placental stabs, both of which can be used in antenatal diagnosis (see Chapter 10). Moreover, the possibility of switching on haemoglobin F (HbF) synthesis as a means of treating severe inherited disorders of haemoglobin synthesis continues to excite research throughout the world. However, the mechanism for the switch from fetal to adult haemoglobin production is still unknown.

A variety of globins, each molecule comprising four polypeptide chains, are synthesized throughout fetal and postnatal life. In the earliest fetuses examined (approximately 5 weeks into gestation), Hb Gower 1 ($\zeta_2\varepsilon_2$) comprises 42% and Hb Gower 2 ($\alpha_2\varepsilon_2$) 24% of the total haemoglobin, the remainder being mainly HbF ($\alpha_2\gamma_2$) (Figure 1.9). Gower 1 and 2 haemoglobins decline to zero by the time that the crown rump length reaches 6 cm. Haemoglobin Portland ($\zeta_2\gamma_2$) comprises 5–20% of haemoglobin at 8 weeks and virtually disappears after 10 weeks, although very small amounts (up to 0.2%) occur in normal cord blood. Subsequent work has shown that

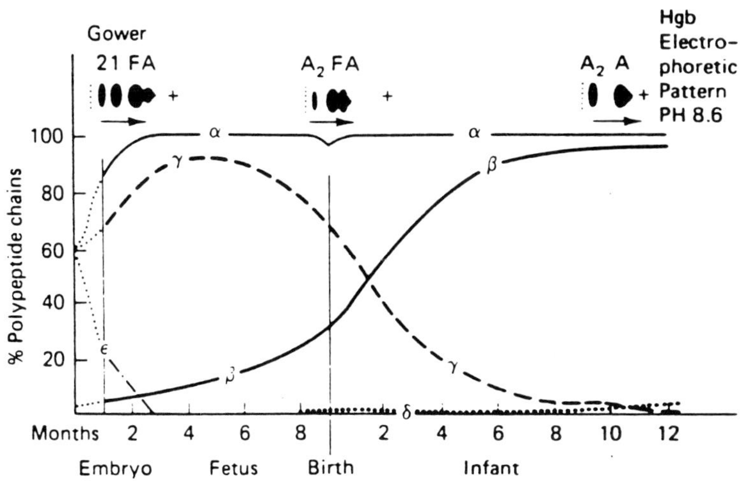

Figure 1.9 Proportion of the main haemoglobin polypeptide chains found in blood throughout embryonic and fetal life and the first year of life. In embryonic life Gower 1 ($\zeta_2\varepsilon_2$) and Gower 2 ($\alpha_2\varepsilon_2$) or Portland ($\zeta_2\gamma_2$) are found. The haemoglobin electrophoretic patterns typical for each period are shown. (From H.A. Pearson, 1966, *Recent Advances in Haematology*, 473, with permission of C.V. Mosby Company.)

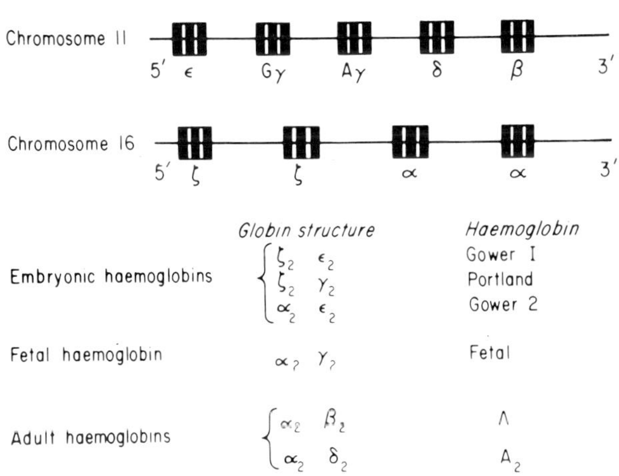

Figure 1.10 Diagram of the globin gene clusters on chromosomes 11 and 16; 5′ and 3′ refer to the position of the sugar-phosphate bonding in the backbone. There is duplication of the α gene. The genes are switched on during fetal life in the 5′ (upstream) to 3′ (downstream) direction. (From A.V. Hoffbrand and J.E. Pettit, 1984, *Essential Haematology*, 2nd edn, with permission of Blackwell Scientific Publications.)

the ξ chain resembles the globin α chain and both genes are on chromosome 11, while the chain resembles β globin, which like the δ and γ genes is on chromosome 16 (Figure 1.10).

Haemoglobin F comprises about 30% of the total haemoglobin in the earliest fetuses studied (5 weeks) and by 8 weeks comprises 90%. For the remainder of intrauterine life, it is the major haemoglobin type. There are two types of HbF, differing only in the presence of glycine or alanine at position 136 of the peptide chain — Gγ and γA, respectively. The ratio of these two types is 3:1 throughout gestation.

'Adult' HbA ($\alpha_2\beta_2$) is found throughout fetal development, although it is difficult to visualize in early fetuses on electrophoresis because of the presence of Hb Portland $\zeta_2\gamma_2$. This necessitates the use of citrate agar gels or preferably globin-chain synthesis, which detects HbA in 6–8 week fetuses. The amount produced remains stable at 5–10% throughout gestation, but its presence is essential for antenatal detection of haemoglobinopathies affecting α and β globin chains using globin chain synthesis studies.

Haemoglobin synthesis is not site-restricted in the switch from fetal to adult haemoglobin production. The proportion of HbF and HbA does not differ in the various haemopoietic organs during gestation. However, there is some evidence that yolk sac megaloblasts produce only Gower haemoglobins, with little or no HbF being produced.

Abnormal haemoglobin patterns occur in two chromosomal abnormalities, affecting somatic cells. In D1 trisomy, small amounts of Hb Gower 2, Hb Portland 1 and Hb Barts (γ_4) are found in cord blood along with high HbF levels. In C/D translocation, one infant with a HbA of 70% in cord blood has been described. These findings suggest that a D-group chromosome may be involved in the regulation of haemoglobin production. In addition to these two disorders, a large number of structural variants of the γ chain have been described.

The thalassaemias are disorders with abnormal globin synthesis rates (Weatherall and Clegg, 1981). Because the α and γ chains form the dominant fetal globin, only thalassaemias affecting these globin chains will produce problems during gestational life. Homozygous α-thalassaemia results from a deletion of all four α-chain genes and is responsible for the Hb Barts hydrops fetalis syndrome. Babies with this disorder do not survive after delivery. Their haemoglobin consists of Hb Barts (γ_4), HbH (β_4) and Hb Portland (10–15% of the total). Haemoglobin H disease results from deletion of three α-chain genes and is less severe clinically. Large amounts of γ and β tetramers are formed along with smaller amounts of HbF and HbA. Children with this disease survive and suffer a life-long anaemia. The heterozygous α-thalassaemia 1 (two deletions) and α-thalassaemia 2 (one deletion) conditions present with 5–6% and 1–2% Hb Barts, respectively, in cord blood. A microcytic hypochromic blood picture, usually with anaemia, occurs throughout life. α-Thalassaemia is commonest in South-east Asian people, and Bart's hydrops remains one of the commonest causes of stillbirth in that part of the world.

The relative increase in HbA in relation to HbF (the 'switch') takes place at about 32–36 weeks, concomitant with a decrease in HbF. By 4 months after delivery, the amount of HbF is less than 10% and declines gradually to the adult level of 1%, often remaining above this level well into childhood.

This fall in the HbF level is accompanied by a reversal of the G:A ratio from 3:1 to 2:3. When there is a reversion to a fetal type of erythropoiesis in postnatal life, for example in juvenile chronic myeloid leukaemia, there is a rise in HbF level accompanied by a reversal to the fetal type of γ chain ratio (and to other characteristics of fetal erythropoiesis, e.g. fetal carbonic anhydrase, I red cell antigen, etc.).

The 'switch' involves stem cells which probably have the ability to produce HbA and F at all stages of fetal maturation. There is increasing evidence that adult F cells come from the same stem cell pool as HbA-containing cells. Studies on cord blood samples from 26 to 43-week gestation infants suggest that the switch is related to the relative maturity of the fetus and not to the actual birth process. Finally, it has not been possible to demonstrate the presence of the minor adult HbA_2 ($\alpha_2\delta_2$) in fetuses. The cord-blood HbA_2 level is 0.2%, or a ratio of HbA:HbA_2 of 100:1 compared with 40:1 in adults. Thus, the production of β and δ chains is asynchronous and the control mechanisms for each are probably separate. Following birth, the normal adult HbA_2 level of 2.5% is reach at about 3–4 months of age.

Understanding the mechanism for the switch from HbF to HbA remains an elusive goal, mainly because of the lack of a suitable animal model. At the molecular level, various theories exist, such as the presence of controller genes between the globin structural genes during the first trimester of pregnancy. There is now evidence available that granulocyte–macrophage colony-stimulating factor (GM-CSF) reactivates HbF synthesis in erythroid progenitors in normal adults (Gabbianelli *et al.*, 1989). The implication derived from this is that the 'switch' to HbF synthesis may not only be time-related in the stem cell but may be mediated partly by a perinatal fall in placental GM-CSF (and possibly other cytokines as well). In addition, it has been shown that trans-activation contributes to the tissue and developmental specificity of regulation of human haemoglobin genes. Various agents such as the simian virus SV40 T antigen, the adenovirus E1a protein and tax1 from HTLV-1 (human T cell leukaemia virus) have been studied and are found to be involved in normal regulation of globin genes (Fox *et al.*, 1989). A critical question is whether a switch can be induced in an individual stem cell. If, as seems likely, it cannot, efforts to control the haemoglobinopathies may be directed towards augmentation of the contribution of HbF clones in adults by arresting the switch from HbF to HbA in neonates.

Haematinics

Iron

Serum iron and ferritin levels in cord blood are always higher than the corresponding maternal levels and are not depleted unless there is extreme maternal deficiency. Thus, the fetus enjoys a favoured status, usually protecting it from maternal deficiencies.

Neonatal iron content of about 80 mg kg^{-1} is correlated with fetal weight because most of the stores are in the circulating red cell mass, which is related to blood volume. At delivery, about 67% of total placental–fetal blood is in the fetus, but within three minutes, uterine contractions force placental blood via umbilical veins into the fetus, so the infant's blood volume increases from about 70 to 93 ml kg^{-1}. Clamping the cord immediately after delivery may, therefore, lead to a substantial fetal blood (and therefore iron) deficit.

The serum iron levels in cord blood range from 27 to 45 μmol l^{-1} (150–250 μg dl^{-1}). The cord-blood ferritin level in full-term infants is approximately three times maternal levels. One study showed a mean of 183 ± 43 μg l^{-1} in maternal serum at the end of pregnancy. The mothers had all received prophylactic iron. There is no correlation between individual mothers and babies. Some workers, but not all, have found lower serum ferritin levels in babies than in normal adults. These fall rapidly in the first few weeks so that levels are halved by 3 months. In premature babies, decreases in serum ferritin levels are steeper. Postnatal deficiency disorders are discussed in Chapter 4.

Vitamin B_{12}

Vitamin B_{12} is involved in conversion of methyl THF (from plasma) with active folate coenzymes. It is also involved in the isomerization of methylmalonyl coenzyme (Co) A to succinyl CoA. Vitamin B_{12} deficiency is rare in early postnatal life because of the ample body stores gained from the mother. The adult daily need for B_{12} is 1–2 μg, and the average Western diet contains much more than this. Stores are 2–3 mg, and it takes several years to develop B_{12} deficiency because of malabsorption or a totally inadequate diet. In pregnancy, increased demands often cause a slow fall in serum B_{12} levels which, in about a third of subjects, are subnormal by normal adult standards. This does not reflect tissue deficiency, but instead a more rapid turnover with consequently lower circulating levels. Serum B_{12} rises to normal within a week of delivery. Vitamin B_{12} accumulates in the placenta and fetus and at term the fetus contains about 50 μg B_{12}. Cord blood levels of B_{12} are higher than levels in normal adults due to active transfer across the placenta. In normal blood, B_{12} is largely attached to a transport glycoprotein, transcobalamin I (TCI) derived from leucocytes and probably other tissues. A similar binder is present in milk, saliva and other body fluids. A similar protein, transcobalamin III (TCIII), also occurs in serum, but is largely unsaturated. A third protein, TCII (synthesized by macrophages), largely unsaturated with B_{12} is nevertheless responsible for B_{12} entry to blood cells and for transfer of B_{12} across the placenta (see Chapter 4 for details of deficiency disorder). In pregnancy, all the serum binders increase, and in the fetus TCIII seems to be particularly raised.

REFERENCES

Alt FW and Baltimore D (1982) Joining of immunoglobulin heavy chain gene fragments: implications from a chromosome with evidence of 3D-J_H fusions. *Proceedings of the National Academy of Sciences, USA* **79**: 4118.

Bodger MP, Janossy, G, Bollum FJ *et al.* (1983) The ontogeny of terminal deoxynucleotidyl transferase positive cells in the human fetus. *Blood* **61**: 1125.

Bollum FJ (1979) Terminal deoxynucleotidyl transferase as a hematopoietic cell marker. *Blood* **54**: 1203.

Bonati, C, Casoli C, Starich B and Buscaglia M (1983) Terminal deoxynucleotidyl transferase (tdt) in human fetuses. *Scandinavian Journal of Immunology* **31**: 447.

Brashem C, Kersey JH, Bollum FJ and Lebien TW (1983). Ontogenetic studies of lymphoid progenitor cells in human bone marrow. *Experimental Haematology* **10**: 886.

Eschback JW and Adamson JW (1988) Recombinant human eyrthropoietin: implications for nephrology. *American Journal of Kidney Diseases* **11**: 203.

Flake AW, Harrison MR, Adzick MS and Zanjani ED (1987) Erythropoietin production by the fetal liver in an adult environment. *Blood* **70**: 542.

Forestier F, Daffos F, Galacteros F *et al.* (1986) Haematological values of 163 normal fetuses between 18 and 30 weeks of gestation. *Paediatric Research* **20**: 342.

Fox HB, Gutman PB, Dave HP *et al.* (1989) Trans-activation of human globin genes by HTLV-1 Tax1. *Blood* **74**: 2749–2754.

Gabbianelli M, Pelosi E, Bassono C *et al.* (1989) GM-CSF reactivates fetal haemoglobin synthesis in erythroblast clones from normal adults. *Blood* **74**: 2657–2667.

Hann IM, Bodger MP and Hoffbrand AV (1983) Development of pluripotent hemopoietic progenitor cells (CFU-GEMM) in the human fetus. *Blood* **62**: 118.

Hokland P, Rosenthal P. Griffin JD *et al.* (1983) Purification and characterization of fetal hematopoietic cells that express the common acute lymphoblastic leukaemia antigen (CALLA). *Journal of Experimental Medicine* **157**: 114.

Isobe M, Huebner K, Erikson J *et al.* (1985) Chromosome localization of the gene for human terminal deoxynucleotidyl transferase to region 10q23-q25. *Proceedings of the National Academy of Sciences, USA* **82**: 5836.

Janossy G, Tidman, Papageorgiou ES, Kung PC and Goldstein G (1981) Distribution of T lymphocyte subsets in human bone marrow and thymus: an analysis with monoclonal antibodies. *Journal of Immunology* **126**: 1608.

Kamps WA, Cooper MD (1982) Microenvironmental studies of pre-B and B cell development in the human and mouse fetuses. *Journal of Immunology* **129**: 526.

Keleman E, Calvo W and Fleidner TM (1979) *Atlas of Human Hemopoietic Development*. Berlin: Springer Verlag.

Kimura, N, Yamano Y, Niko Y and Yanase T (1983) Multipotent haemopoietic progenitors (CFUmix) in human fetal liver. *Experimental Haematology* **11**: 849.

Lestas AN, Rodeck CH and White JM (1982) Normal activity of glycolytic enzymes in fetal erythrocytes. *Blood* **50**: 439.

Linch DC, Knott LJ, Rodeck CH and Huehns ER (1982). Studies of circulating hemopoietic progenitor cells in human fetal blood. *Blood* **59**: 976.

Mibashan R and Modell B (1982). Antenatal diagnosis of haemoglobinopathies. In *Haematology and Oncology* (Willoughby MLN and Siegel SE, eds), pp 167–195. London: Butterworth Scientific.

Millar DS, Davis LR, Rodeck CH *et al.* (1985) Normal blood cell values in the early mid-trimester fetus. *Prenatal Diagnosis* **5**: 367.

Moore MAS and Metcalfe D (1970) Ontogeny of the haemopoietic system: yolk sac origin of in vivo and in vitro colony forming cells in the developing mouse and embryo. *British Journal of Haematology* **18**: 279.

Peschle C, Migliaccio AR, Migliaccio G *et al.* (1981) Identification and characterisation of three classes of erythroid progenitors in human fetal liver. *Blood* **58**: 565.

Porcellinia A, Manna A, Manna M *et al.* (1983) Ontogeny of granulocyte–macrophage progenitor cells in the human fetus. *International Journal of Cell Cloning* **1**: 192.

Rainaut M, Forestier F, Daffos F *et al.* (1990, in press) Characterisation of mononuclear cell subpopulations in normal human fetal peripheral blood. *Prenatal Diagnosis*.

Rosenthal P, Rimm IJ, Umiel T, Griffen JD, Osanthanondh R and Schlossmann SF (1983) Ontogeny of human haemopoietic cells: analysis utilizing monoclonal antibodies. *Journal of Immunology* **31**: 232.

Thomas BD and Yoffey JM (1962) Human foetal haemopoiesis: the cellular composition of foetal blood. *British Journal of Haematology* **8**: 290.

Weatherall DJ and Clegg JB (1981) *The Thalassaemias* (3rd edn). Oxford: Blackwell Scientific.

Wood WG (1976) Haemoglobin synthesis during human fetal development. *British Medical Bulletin* **32**: 282.

Yoffey JM (1971) The stem cell problem in the fetus. *Israel Journal of Medical Sciences* **7**: 825.

Zanjani ED, Poster J, Burlington K *et al.* (1977) Liver as the primary site of erythropoietin formation in the fetus. *Journal of Laboratory and Clinical Medicine* **89**: 640.

2

The normal blood picture in neonates

I.M. Hann

The Hospitals for Sick Children, London

The bone marrow of the newborn is very active and involves most of the body's marrow spaces. The consequence of this is that marrow stress, as can occur for instance in haemolytic disease, leads to expansion of the marrow cavity and extramedullary haemopoiesis in liver, spleen and lymph nodes. Study of marrow in the neonatal period has been restricted by difficulties in procuring adequate marrow aspirate samples. It can be difficult to obtain non-diluted smears, but the posterior superior iliac spine usually yields good samples and it is rarely necessary to use the tibia or other sites.

In 1952 Gairdner *et al.* (1952a, 1952b) showed that bone marrow cellularity falls in the first week of life, followed by a slow rise to approximately adult cellularity between the first and third month. Premature babies usually have more cellular marrows, but their relative cell proportions do not differ from full-term babies; approximate percentages of the marrow elements are given in Table 2.1. The myeloid:erythroid ratio changes from 1.5:1.0 at birth to 6:1 at the end of the first week and to 3:1 by the end of the second month,

Table 2.1 Range of bone marrow differential counts in the neonatal period.*

	Age			
Cell type	0–24 hours	7 days	1 month	Adult
Myeloblasts	0–2	0–3	0.4–1.9	0.7–1.1
Promyelocytes	0.5–6.0	0.5–7.0	1.0–2.5	1.8–2.0
Myelocytes	1–9	0.6–11	2.5–7.2	2.4–19.0
Metamyelocytes	4–19	2–30	3.1–9.1	3–24
Bands	10–30	13–43	17–32	7–20
Neutrophils	10–40	10–39	9–30	10–15
Eosinophils	1–3	1–3	2–5	5–7
Basophils	0.0–0.2	0.0–0.2	0.0–0.2	0.2–1.8
Red cell precursors	19–51	0–16	12–26	20–32
Lymphocytes	4–8	3.7–8.0	10–19	14–28
Monocytes	2–6	2.0–7.3	3–10	2–12
Plasma cells	—	—	0.0–0.2	0.6–0.9
Myeloid:erythroid ratio	1.5.1.0	6.5:1.0	2.0:1.0	2.7:1.0

* Values are all percentages apart from the M:E ratio.

which approximates to the normal adult ratio. In addition, lymphocytes increase in number to reach about 50% of marrow nucleated cells by the third month. This number may be even higher in the face of infection, often with a small percentage of lymphoblasts. This has undoubtedly led to the erroneous diagnosis of leukaemia in the past, and marrow reporting must be circumspect and associated with modern immunological techniques in this age-group. Plasma cells are only infrequently seen in the newborn marrow (less than 0.02%). Megakaryocyte numbers appear normal at birth.

NORMAL HAEMOGLOBIN AND RED CELL VALUES

Haemoglobin

The blood picture at birth is primarily dependent upon the maturity of the baby. In this chapter the differences that occur during the neonatal period, and how they are affected, are discussed. Several technical and obstetric factors can also considerably alter the picture. One technical problem that arises is differences in haemoglobin depending on the method of sampling. Capillary samples have a consistently higher haemoglobin concentration than venous samples, usually a difference in the order of 5–10%. Moe (1967) showed a similar problem when considering cord-blood samples, with levels as much as 8 g dl^{-1} lower than simultaneous capillary samples. In his study of 41 neonates, only 14 would have been considered to be anaemic by capillary samples whereas 25 were actually so by cord blood samples. The largest differences occur in babies born before 30 weeks of gestation. Recently, Thurbeck and McIntosh (1987) showed that in pre-term (24–32 week) babies both haemoglobin and total neutrophil counts were higher in capillary than in arterial samples (mean 16.4 ± 2.9 versus 14.1 ± 2.1 for haemoglobin and 5.5 ± 3.0 versus 3.7 ± 1.5 for neutrophils). Arterial and venous samples were comparable for neutrophil counts, but the venous haemoglobin was higher (13.8 ± 3.0 versus 13.3 ± 3.0).

An increase in haemoglobin coincentration is a uniform phenomenon in the first few hours after birth, even in infants where the cord has been clamped as rapidly as possible. In 1958 Gairdner showed that there was a mean rise of 2.5 g dl^{-1} in this group. In other infants the rise can be as great as 6 g dl^{-1}, partly as a result of the perinatal placental transfusion and partly because of a rapid decrease in plasma volume in the face of a stable red cell volume. Thus, there is an associated rise in packed cell volume and red cell count. Yao *et al.* (1969) reviewed the effect of umbilical clamping on haematological values (Figure 2.1). They demonstrated that there could be an increase of blood volume as great as 61% on delayed clamping. The figure demonstrates that progressive emptying of the placental vessels is associated with progressively larger increases in blood volume. The actual amount of blood in the placental vessels has been estimated to be 75–125 ml, which approximates to between a quarter and a third of the fetal blood volume. The rate of transfer of this blood varies and is enhanced by ergotamine treatment of the mother. However, approximately a quarter is transfused within 15 s and a half by 1 min. In addition, because the umbilical arteries clamp down soon after birth, there is no reverse flow.

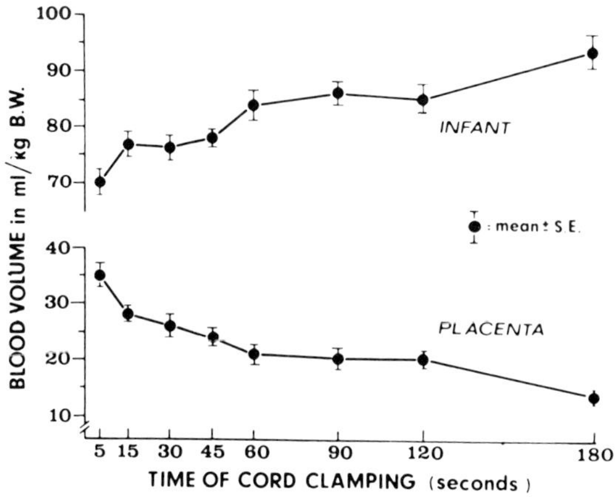

Figure 2.1 Changes in blood volume related to the time of cord clamping. (From Yao *et al.*, 1969, *Lancet*, *2*: 891.)

Also, the umbilical veins remain dilated allowing flow by gravity. Thus, it is advisable to hold the infant below the level of the placenta even during caesarean section delivery.

The consequence of all this is that infants with delayed cord clamping have an average blood volume of 93 ml kg^{-1} compared with an immediate clamping level of 82 ml kg^{-1}. There is a wider discrepancy in haemoglobin values because the volumes tend to even out by a more rapid fall in plasma volume in the delayed clamping group. In various studies on full-term babies, the haemoglobin level showed mean values of 15.6 g dl^{-1} in early clamping versus 19.3 g dl^{-1} for the delayed group, measured at 1 day of age. On the third day the level is 17.4 versus 20.8 g dl^{-1} and by 6 weeks of age there was no longer a difference.

Blood volume

As stated previously, the blood volume may vary greatly in the newborn in relation to the method of cord clamping, the presence of intra-uterine asphyxia and maternofetal blood loss. At birth the mean is 85 ml kg^{-1}, with a range of 50–100 ml kg^{-1}. The mean with early cord clamping is 78 and 99 mk kg^{-1} where delayed clamping was practised. Infants with delayed clamping had much larger red cell volumes. In premature babies during the first few days of life, volumes vary between 89 and 105 ml kg^{-1}. In this case, the higher of the two quoted values is mainly due to increased plasma volume. The increase in plasma volume falls with increasing gestational age, but babies with intra-uterine growth retardation have greater plasma volumes. By 1 month of life the mean blood volume is between 73 and 77 ml kg^{-1} (normal adult mean = 77 ml kg^{-1}) Measurements of red cell mass at different gestational ages are given in Figure 2.2. A rise of 1.5% per day is shown from the 28th gestational week onwards. It can be calculated from the mean cell life that red cell mass production at term is 3.6–4.2% per day. This shows that the rate of red cell production during the last 2 gestational months is three to five times that of the adult.

Differences in blood volume occur in certain circumstances. Blood volume is reduced in asphyxiated children, and respiratory distress syndrome (RDS) is also associated with low volume.

Early studies in the 1950s produced a range of normal values for cord haemoglobin in term infants, varying from 15.7 to 17.9 g dl^{-1}. More recent studies have produced a tighter range of 16.6–17.1 g dl^{-1} with an overall mean of 16.8 g dl^{-1}, 95% of values falling between 13.7 and 20.1 g dl^{-1}. However, some proportion, at least, of these lower values are probably due to transplacental haemorrhage as evidenced by a compensatory rise in numbers of reticulocytes and nucleated red blood cells. Similarly there is some evidence that high values may be related to maternal cigarette smoking.

There has in the past been some controversy as to whether the haemoglobin of pre-term babies is lower at birth than for full-term babies. In fact studies show that there is little difference (Table 2.2). However, the rapidity of the postnatal decline is greater for pre-term babies, with increasing degrees of immaturity, related to the shorter red cell survival of the extremely premature baby. A study by Stockman *et al.* (1984), looking at babies of less than 1500 g, showed that during the anaemia of prematurity erythropoietin is produced in response to altered oxygen availability, i.e.

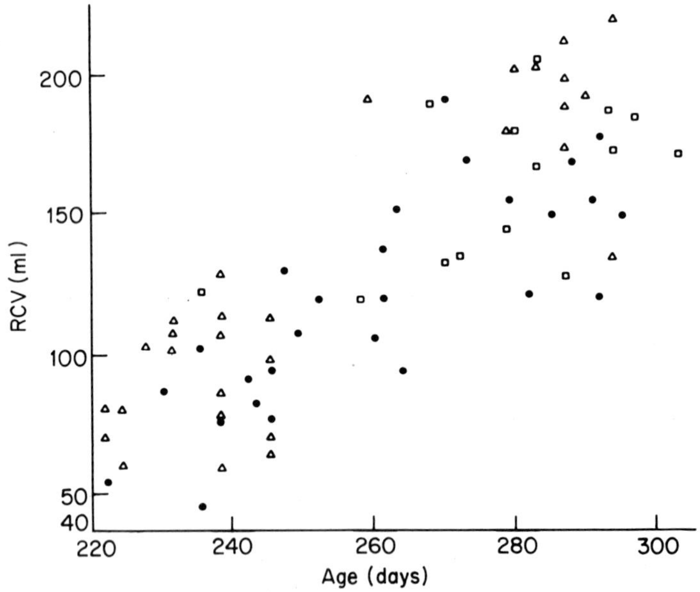

Figure 2.2 The circulating red cell mass in newborn babies related to their gestational age. ●, ^{51}Cr-dilution method; △, □, from plasma volume measurements. (From Bratteby, 1968, *Acta Paediatr*, *57*: 132.)

Table 2.2 Normal pre-term haemoglobin levels (g dl^{-1}).*

Birth weight (g)	Postnatal age (weeks)				
	2	4	6	8	10
800–1000	16.0 (14.8–17.2)	10.0 (6.8–13.2)	8.7 (7.0–10.2)	8.0 (7.1–9.8)	8.0 (6.9–10.2)
1001–1200	16.4 (14.1–18.7)	12.8 (7.8–15.3)	10.5 (7.2–12.3)	9.1 (7.8–10.4)	8.5 (7.0–10.0)
1201–1400	16.2 (13.6–18.8)	13.4 (8.8–16.2)	10.9 (8.5–13.3)	9.9 (8.0–11.8)	9.8 (8.4–11.3)
1401–1500	15.6 (13.4–17.8)	11.7 (9.7–13.7)	10.5 (9.1–11.9)	9.8 (8.4–12.0)	9.9 (8.4–11.4)
1501–2000	15.6 (13.5–17.7)	11.0 (9.6–14.0)	9.6 (8.8–11.5)	9.8 (8.4–12.0)	10.1 (8.6–11.8)

* Mean values quoted, with ranges in parentheses. From Williams *et al.* (1975).

Table 2.3 Normal haematological values during the first 12 weeks in full-term infants.*

Age	HB (g dl^{-1})	RBC ($\times 10^{12}$ per litre)	PCV (%)	MCV (fl)	MCHC (g dl^{-1})	Reticulocytes (%)	NRBC (per millilitre)
Days							
1	19.0 ± 2.2	5.14 ± 0.7	61 ± 7	119 ± 9.4	31.6 ± 1.9	3.2 ± 1.4	500
2	19.0 ± 1.9	5.15 ± 0.8	60 ± 6	115 ± 7.0	31.6 ± 1.4	3.2 ± 1.3	
3	18.7 ± 3.4	5.11 ± 0.7	62 ± 9	116 ± 5.3	31.1 ± 2.8	2.8 ± 1.7	0–5
4	18.6 ± 2.1	5.00 ± 0.6	57 ± 8	114 ± 7.5	32.6 ± 1.5	1.8 ± 1.1	
5	17.6 ± 1.1	4.97 ± 0.4	57 ± 7	114 ± 8.9	30.9 ± 2.2	1.2 ± 0.2	
6	17.4 ± 2.2	5.00 ± 0.7	54 ± 7	113 ± 10.0	32.2 ± 1.6	0.6 ± 0.2	
7	17.9 ± 2.5	4.86 ± 0.6	56 ± 9	118 ± 11.2	32.0 ± 1.6	0.5 ± 0.4	0
Weeks							
1–2	17.3 ± 2.3	4.80 ± 0.8	54 ± 8	112 ± 19.0	32.1 ± 2.9	0.5 ± 0.3	
2–3	15.6 ± 2.6	4.20 ± 0.6	46 ± 7	111 ± 8.2	33.9 ± 1.9	0.8 ± 0.6	
3–4	14.2 ± 2.1	4.00 ± 0.6	43 ± 6	105 ± 7.5	33.5 ± 1.6	0.6 ± 0.3	
4–5	12.7 ± 1.6	3.60 ± 0.4	36 ± 5	101 ± 8.1	34.9 ± 1.6	0.9 ± 0.8	
5–6	11.9 ± 1.5	3.55 ± 0.2	36 ± 6	102 ± 10.2	34.1 ± 2.9	1.0 ± 0.7	
6–7	12.0 ± 1.5	3.40 ± 0.4	36 ± 5	105 ± 12.0	33.8 ± 2.3	1.2 ± 0.7	
7–8	11.1 ± 1.1	3.40 ± 0.4	33 ± 4	100 ± 13.0	33.7 ± 2.6	1.5 ± 0.7	
8–9	10.7 ± 0.9	3.40 ± 0.5	31 ± 3	93 ± 12.0	34.1 ± 2.2	1.8 ± 1.0	
9–10	11.2 ± 0.9	3.60 ± 0.3	32 ± 3	91 ± 9.3	34.3 ± 2.9	1.2 ± 0.6	
10–11	11.4 ± 0.9	3.70 ± 0.4	34 ± 2	91 ± 7.7	33.2 ± 2.4	1.2 ± 0.7	
11–12	11.3 ± 0.9	3.70 ± 0.3	33 ± 3	88 ± 7.9	34.8 ± 2.2	0.7 ± 0.3	

* Values given are means ± SD. Adapted from Mathoth *et al.* (1971).

Table 2.4 Red cell values in 40 premature babies with birth weights of less than 1500 g.*

Day of postnatal life	Hb ($g\ dl^{-1}$)	MCV (fl)	MCH (pg)	MCHC (%)	RBC ($\times 10^{12}$ per litre)
1	18.2 ± 2.7	115 ± 5	38.9 ± 1.7	33.5 ± 1.2	4.71 ± 0.75
3	16.2 ± 2.9	112 ± 4	39.0 ± 3.4	33.8 ± 1.0	4.40 ± 0.83
7	16.3 ± 2.9	110 ± 5	37.3 ± 1.8	33.9 ± 1.3	4.45 ± 0.83
14	14.5 ± 2.4	106 ± 5	36.3 ± 1.9	33.9 ± 1.0	4.10 ± 0.69
21	12.9 ± 2.0	102 ± 5	35.3 ± 2.2	34.2 ± 1.1	3.71 ± 0.59
28	10.9 ± 1.9	100 ± 5	35.1 ± 1.9	33.4 ± 1.0	3.17 ± 0.60
35	10.0 ± 1.4	98 ± 5	34.4 ± 1.5	34.5 ± 0.7	2.97 ± 0.45
42	9.5 ± 1.5	97 ± 5	32.2 ± 1.7	33.7 ± 0.9	2.92 ± 0.49
49	10.1 ± 1.7	95 ± 5	32.1 ± 1.6	33.5 ± 1.0	3.21 ± 0.59

* Data are means ± 1 SD. Taken from Stockman and Oski (1980).

lowered central venous oxygenation produces a response increasing erythropoietin production. Although absolute amounts are lower than in other types of anaemia, for example Blackfan–Diamond anaemia, the regulatory mechanisms responding to venous oxygen tension are operative. However, it is doubtful that these mechanisms are sufficient to prevent clinical problems as there is some evidence for symptomatic changes when haemoglobin and available oxygen reach their lowest values.

The changes in haemoglobin, red cell indices, reticulocytes and nucleated red cells during the first 12 weeks of the term neonate and immature babies are shown in Tables 2.3 and 2.4, respectively.

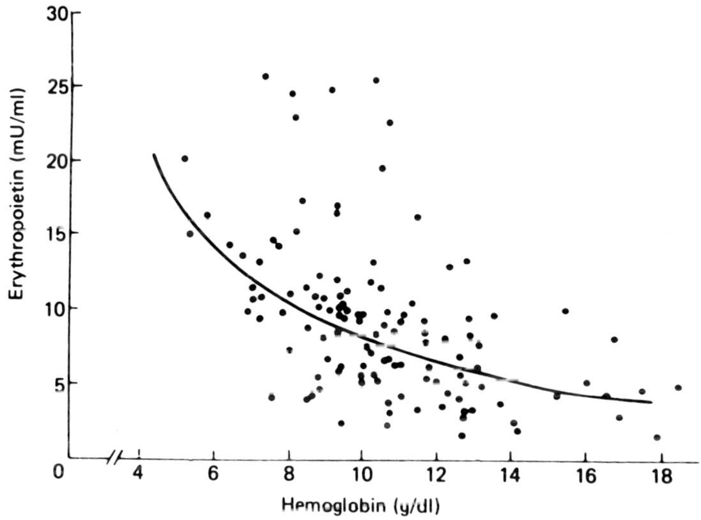

Figure 2.3 The changes in plasma erythropoietin related to haemoglobin levels in pre-term babies of birthweight < 1500 g. (From Stockman *et al.* 1977, *New Engl. J. Med.*, *296*: 647.)

A progressive fall in haemoglobin begins by the second or third day, in relation to a marked decrease in erythopoietic activity. Although cord blood contains increased amounts of erythropoietin, no bioavailable activity is detected in urine or blood from the second day. This and the improved oxygenation account for the decreased red cell production, possibly with some suppression by erythropoietin inhibitors. Biological erythropoietin activity returns by 2–3 months, when the haemoglobin is at its nadir but, using newer radioimmunoassays, small amounts can now be detected throughout infancy. The level is inversely correlated to the haemoglobin level (Figure 2.3).

The packed cell volume

Normal values for packed cell volume (PCV) in cord blood have varied in different series from a mean of 51.3% to 56%. The sharp rise during the first few hours after birth parallels that of the haemoglobin; it is followed by a decline such that by the end of the first week it approximates again to cord levels. Thereafter the level declines to a mean of 31% by the second month at its nadir, increasing to 35% at 1 year and 38% by 3 years, and not reaching adult levels until adolescence.

Red cell count and indices

The red cell count in cord blood has also varied between different series, the mean level being as low as 4.6×10^{12} and as high as 5.2×10^{12} per litre. As with haemoglobin and PCV there is also a rapid rise of the order of 0.5×10^{12} per litre during the first few hours of life and, at the end of the first week, the mean level is at 4.86×10^{12} per litre. As can be seen in Table 2.4, newborn babies have large red cells (mean corpuscular volume 119 fl and average diameter 8.3 μm, adult mean 7.5 μm). There is also a remarkable variability in size (anisocytosis), with a maximum difference between largest and smallest that is of the order of 8 μm. Special stains and microdensitometery have shown that the macrocytic cells contain significantly less fetal haemoglobin (HbF) than the small red cells.

The mean corpuscular volume (MCV) and mean diameter fall rapidly over the first weeks of life, reaching an MCV of 93 fl by 9 weeks (normal adult values = 82–92 fl). Using electronic methods, values of 94 fl or less in term infants at birth have been shown to be strongly suggestive of the α thalassaemia trait or of iron deficiency. In a group of premature babies with an average birth weight of 1300 g the mean MCV was 115 ± 5.0 fl on the first day, falling to 95 ± 4.0 by the seventh week (Stockman and Oski, 1980).

The mean corpuscular haemoglobin (MCH) is also increased at birth, with ranges of 33.5–41.4 pg (adult range = 27–32 pg). The mean corpuscular haemoglobin concentration is, however, similar to or slightly lower than adult values, with a mean value of 31.6 ± 1.9 g dl^{-1} (adult mean = 33 g dl^{-1}). This reflects the similar concentration of haemoglobin in individual red cells (MCHC = Hb/PCV). The high MCH represents the average increased quantity of haemoglobin in individual red cells (MCH = Hb/RBC) and the decline parallels the decline in MCV fairly closely.

Reticulocytes and nucleated red blood cells

As with most normal values in the neonatal period there is a wide range in the quoted values for reticulocytes. The average values have varied between 1.6 and 6.2%. The three most recent studies quote 3.2 ± 1.4, 5.1 ± 1.1, and 4.7 ± 1.9% at term. Premature infants show higher values reflecting the rapid fall in numbers occurring during fetal life (see Chapter 1) being in the order of 6–10% at 30- to 36-week babies; there are slight but significant increases in reticulocytes where early cord clamping is practised. Thereafter, in all babies not subjected to erythropoietic stress, the percentage falls abruptly after the third day of life to reach values of about 0.5% by the end of the first week.

Nucleated red blood cells (NRBCs), or normoblasts, are usually seen on the first day of life in all babies. At birth the number is around 200–500 NRBC mm^{-3} of blood; in other words, one in a 1000 red cells are nucleated. It is not helpful to quote this figure in relation to the number of white blood cells (WBCs) because of the wide variability in the number of the latter. However, on an individual basis, it is important to work out this relationship so that the white cell count from electronic counters can be adjusted (average 7.3 NRBCs per 100 WBCs). These counters produce a total nucleated count, which is assumed to equal the white cell count. By 12 hours after birth the number falls by half, and at 2 days of age the level is usually about 20–30 NRBC mm^{-3}. By the fourth day of life it is unusual for any NRBCs to be present.

Premature babies again show greater numbers, NRBC counts in the order of 1000–1500 per millitre being common, decreasing with increasing maturity. On the blood film there are an average 20 NRBCs per 100 WBCs. Although there is a rapid decline during the first week, many very premature babies will still have the occasional normoblasts in their red cell film at 1 week of age. Clearly, increased numbers of reticulocytes and NRBCs are seen in babies who have haemolytic disease, haemorrhage, hypoxia and other stress.

RED CELLS

Surface morphology and inclusions

Conventional light microscopy, interference phase microscopy, electron microscopy and other techniques have all shown that red cells of normal newborns have some unusual characteristics, which are a consequence of differences in the red cell membrane.

Zipursky (1977) studied red cell shape in wet preparations of red cells suspended in 0.2% glutaraldehyde. In adults, 70% of cells appeared as biconcave discs and 27% as 'bowl' forms, with 3% assorted spherocytes and poikilocytes. However, full-term infants displayed only 41% biconcave discs and as many as 14% spherocytes and poikilocytes. Premature babies (mean birth weight 1400 g) had 43% discs, 30% bowls and 27% unusual red cell forms, of which the echinocyte (spiky form) was the most common.

Holroyde (1969) used interference phase microscopy to show that red cells from neonates have a 'pocked' appearance. Normal adults show 2.6% pits or craters 0.2–0.5 μm in diameter, whereas premature babies have a mean 47.2% and term babies 24.3%. The full-term neonate will revert to adult levels by 2 months of age, and the premature baby will do so several weeks later. These appearances, which are caused by the presence of vacuoles and internal structures just below the membrane, are similar to those seen where there is splenic hypofunction, for example in coeliac syndrome or sickle cell disease, or following splenectomy. Thus the theory is that they represent impaired splenic function in the neonate. This is also reflected in the increased number of siderocytes in the normal newborn, averaging 3.16% compared with a mean of 0.09% in adult males. All of the above features help to explain why many haematologists find the neonatal red cell film so bizarre. Fortunately, the instances in which study of the film are of diagnostic importance are severely limited; they are discussed in subsequent chapters.

Red cell osmotic fragility in newborns is abnormal in that they are generally slightly more resistant to lysis (mean 50% lysis in 0.422% saline) and there is a small population of cells with increased fragility. The latter disappear from the circulation within the first few days of life, and the osmotic fragility curve is similar to adults by 4–6 weeks of age.

Examination of neonatal red cell membrane proteins by polyacrylamide gel electrophoresis shows no differences from the normal adults. However, there does appear to be increased membrane fluidity. Full-term neonates have increased quantities of red cell total lipid, lipid-phosphorus and cholesterol, although the overall percentages are similar to adult red cells. In addition, there is a greater percentage of sphingomyelin and less lecithin, as proportions of total phospholipid. Fatty acid patterns show increased percentages of palmitic, stearic, arachidonic and combined 22C and 24C fatty acids, and less oleic and linoleic acid. The cells are consequently much more prone to lipid peroxidation upon oxidant challenges. They are also more prone to acid lysis, and show increased rates of potassium influx and altered kinetics of glucose, glycerol and thiourea transfer.

There are major differences in blood group antigens of the neonatal red cell membrane. The A and B antigens are weakly expressed, as is the I antigen with relative excess of *i*. Red cell antigens of the MN, Kell, Duffy and Vel systems are well-developed early in intra-uterine life, but the Lutheran and Xg systems develop more slowly, though they are present at birth. The absorbed serum antigens of the Lewis group (Le^a/Le^b) are incompletely expressed because of lack of receptor sites on the membrane. However, within 10 days of birth, many infants become Le^+ and red cells containing the *i* antigen are usually not detectable at a year of age. Isoagglutinins to A and B groups are usually found by 6 months, although adult titres will not usually be reached until 2 years of age.

Red cell metabolism

Numerous studies of the Embden–Meyerhof pathway have demonstrated that phosphoglycerate kinase (PGK) and enolase activities are very high in the newborn, even when young cell age is taken into account. Phosphofructokinase (PFK) is a rate-limiting enzyme in this pathway, and it has been found to be consistently lower in neonates; this probably reflects decay of an unstable enzyme which contains the 'liver' homotetramer. Isoenzyme abnormalities of enolase, guanylate kinase, lactate dehydrogenase (LDH), nucleoside phosphorylase, hexokinase and PFK have also been demonstrated.

The rate of glucose consumption by the red cells in the neonatal period is less than would be expected for cells of similar age. It seems likely that the relative deficiency of PFK is responsible.

2,3-Diphosphoglycerate (2,3DPG) is unstable in neonatal red cells, which reflects increased breakdown of the compound. However, the mechanism of this increased hydrolysis is unknown.

Red cells from newborn infants are more susceptible to oxidant injury, but the mechanism is complex and is not completely understood. It is manifest by increased glutathione instability, Heinz body formation and the development of methaemoglobinaemia on oxidant stress.

Haemoglobin denaturation and precipitation (Heinz bodies) can result from an intrinsic abnormality of haemoglobin. HbF is in fact more prone than HbA to denaturation but there is no correlation between its level and the tendency to form Heinz bodies. Another mechanism would be a defect in hydrogen peroxide detoxification. This depends on NADPH generation from the hexose monophosphate (HMP) shunt, glutathione production and catalase production. Cells will be more susceptible to lipid peroxidation if there is a reduction in sulphydryl groups, increased peroxidizable membrane substrates, decreased membrane substrates or decreased membrane antioxidents (e.g. vitamin E) relative to the content of polyunsaturated fatty acids (PUFA).

In fact, the HMP shunt functions normally and can be shown to respond to oxidant stress. Glutathione peroxidase is reduced compared with that in adult cells, but *in vitro* studies have not shown a convincing relationship with oxidant vulnerability. The proposed explanation is that relative deficiencies of glutathione peroxidase, methaemoglobin reductase and catalase, along with reduced levels of membrane -SH groups and decreased levels of membrane antioxidants, work with unidentified factors to produce the defect.

Carbonic anhydrase (CA) is the second most abundant protein in adult red cells after haemoglobin, but in early fetal life the levels of the two isoenzymes (CAI and CAII) are very low, only increasing from 32 weeks' gestation. At birth, CDAI activity is 5–15% of adult red cell levels and CDA II 20–30%. However, these levels seem adequate to maintain normal function. Acetyl cholinesterase and adenylate kinase are also reported to exist at lower levels in cord blood.

Red cell life span

Despite using different methods, a number of studies have come to broadly similar conclusions on red cell lifespan in the neonate. In brief, in full-term babies it is shorter than in adults, and this is more marked in pre-term babies — the more premature they are the shorter the red cell lifespan. The methods used have included differential agglutination [^{32}P]diisopropyl fluorophosphate labelling, radio-iron incorporation and disappearance, and endogenous carbon monoxide production. The simplest method is ^{51}Cr labelling of red cells, and most studies have used this approach. The mean red cell half-life determined in full-term infants is 23.3 days (range 13–35) and in pre-term infants 16.6 days (range 9–26), compared with 26–35 days in adults. The actual lifespan is approximately 60–70 days in full-term babies, compared with 35–50 days pre-term. The reason for the shortened survival of red cells produced in the fetus is uncertain, but in one study it correlated with red cell rigidity and consequent abnormal filtrability. The assumption is that altered membrane function is the culprit.

Free plasma haemoglobin and haptoglobin

The presence of excess plasma haemoglobin represents haemolysis *in vivo* or a poor sample that has become haemolysed on blood taking. The level is not elevated in cord samples but it rises after birth to a peak of about 3 mg dl^{-1} on the third day. In full-term babies, adult levels (0.37 mg dl^{-1}) are achieved on the fifth day, but premature babies have elevated levels for longer. Haptoglobin is the α-2-glycoprotein that binds plasma haemoglobin. Low free haptoglobin levels thus usually correlate with haemolysis but, in the newborn period, low levels are the norm due to impaired synthesis. At birth the levels vary between zero and 24 mg dl^{-1}, but thereafter the value increases to reach 30–160 mg dl^{-1} at the end of the first month. Higher levels frequently represent a response to infection, as haptoglobin is an acute-phase reactant.

OXYGEN TRANSPORT AND DELIVERY

Red cells function as efficient oxygen carriers, with delivery to the tissues as the ultimate goal. The ability of blood to perform this delivery depends upon the cardiac output, the haemoglobin concentration, the delivery of oxygen to blood via the lungs and the characteristic of oxygen binding and release by haemoglobin (the oxygen-haemoglobin dissociation curve).

In the neonate, the most important factors influencing haemoglobin's oxygen affinity are the HbF and 2,3DPG concentration. A shift to the right of the oxygen dissociation curve produces reduced affinity and more oxygen release to the tissues. Conversely, a shift to the left means that oxygen tension has to fall to relatively lower values before haemoglobin releases an equivalent amount of oxygen to the tissues. Acidosis and pyrexia will cause

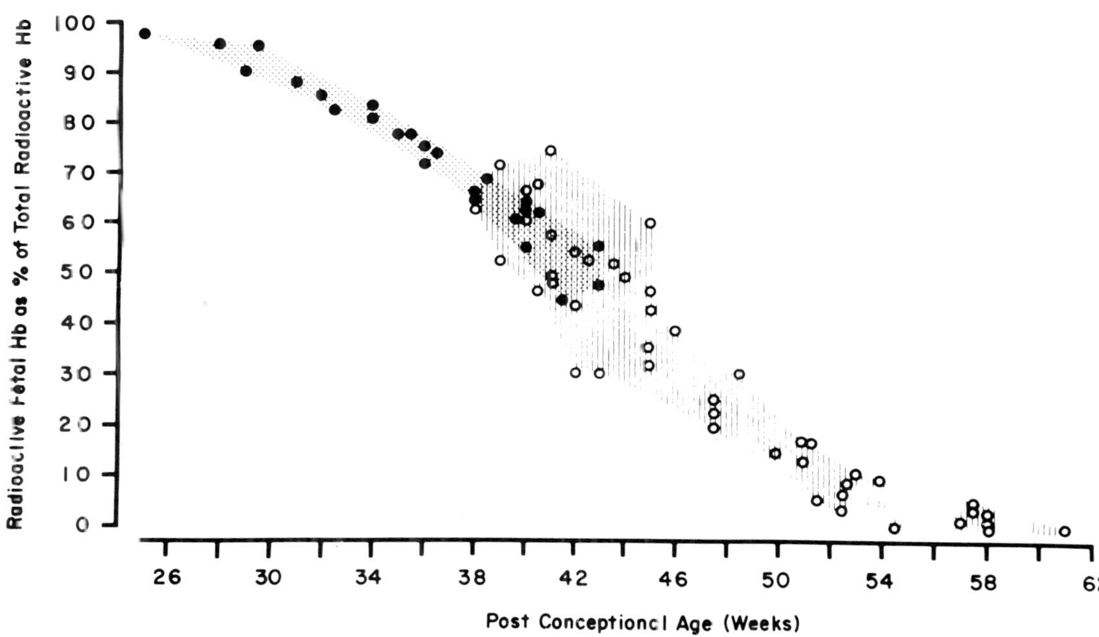

Figure 2.4 Decline in fetal haemoglobin synthesis as a function of gestational age. ●, Cord samples from pre-term babies; ○, Cord samples from full-term babies. (Reproduced from Bard, 1975, *Journal of Clinical Investigation*, *55*: 395, by copyright permission of the American Society for Clinical Investigation.)

a shift to the right, as will an increase in 2,3DPG. The latter occurs with hypoxia, anaemia and decreased red cell mass. Decreased P_{50} (the oxygen tension at 50% oxygen saturation of haemoglobin) and shift to the left (increased affinity, decreased tissue oxygen release) occur with reduced 2,3DPG, which is associated with sepsis, severe acidosis and RDS. High-affinity abnormal haemoglobins (e.g. Chesapeake, Philly) decrease oxygen availability and lead to polycythaemia. Low affinity haemoglobins (Hammersmith, Kansas) are associated with increased oxygen availability.

As stated in Chapter 1, the level of HbF in neonates is a function of the gestational age (Figure 2.4), although chronic intra-uterine hypoxia may result in an elevation. It can be clearly seen that there is a rapid fall during the third trimester, but premature babies have significantly higher levels than term babies and this affects oxygen availability. Many studies of the interaction of 2,3DPG and HbF have looked at this increased affinity compared with the adult red cell (P_{50} 8 mm Hg lower). The problem would seem to lie with deficient binding of 2,3DPG and HbF at the serine site at position 143 compared with more efficient binding at the histidine site at position 143 on the β chain.

The 2,3DPG level gradually increases with gestation to levels at term comparable with adult levels. The level then falls transiently before rising towards the end of the first week to a level that is much higher than at birth. The previously mentioned rapid rise of 2,3DPG with hypoxia is markedly diminished in neonates, and the compound is also less stable at this time.

The oxygen dissociation curve in the neonate gradually shifts to the right (Figure 2.5). The P_{50} reaches the adult mean value of approximately 27 mm Hg at about 4–6 months of age. During the first week of life there is a significant rise in the P_{50}, with consequent improved tissue oxygen delivery. However, premature babies will have a higher HbF and also a lower 2,3DPG, but the increase in oxygen affinity does not precisely correlate with the decline in HbF level. During the first week in premature newborns there is a 1 mm Hg rise in P_{50} despite a minimal change in HbF at this stage. In babies, the P_{50} is a function of the percentage of adult haemoglobin and the red cell 2,3DPG — the 'functioning 2,3-DPG fraction'. An additional factor at this time is the decline in haemoglobin, which causes a decline in oxygen carrying capacity, the product of arterial oxygen saturation and haemoglobin × 1.36 ml O_2 per gram of haemoglobin. In fact, the haemoglobin fall is more than compensated for by the right shift in the oxygen dissociation curve, with consequent improvement in oxygen delivered to tissues over the first few weeks of life (Figure 2.6). It should be remembered, however, that this will not be the case if hypoxia or acidosis occur, and in severe RDS there is a profound decrease in 2,3DPG; this effect is most marked where severe acidosis exists and is independent of the Böhr effect.

THE WHITE CELL BLOOD CELLS

Normal values at birth are affected by the site of sampling. The WBC count from cord blood is 72% of that taken by capillary sampling. Thereafter venous blood counts are 77% of capillary levels. Another confounding factor

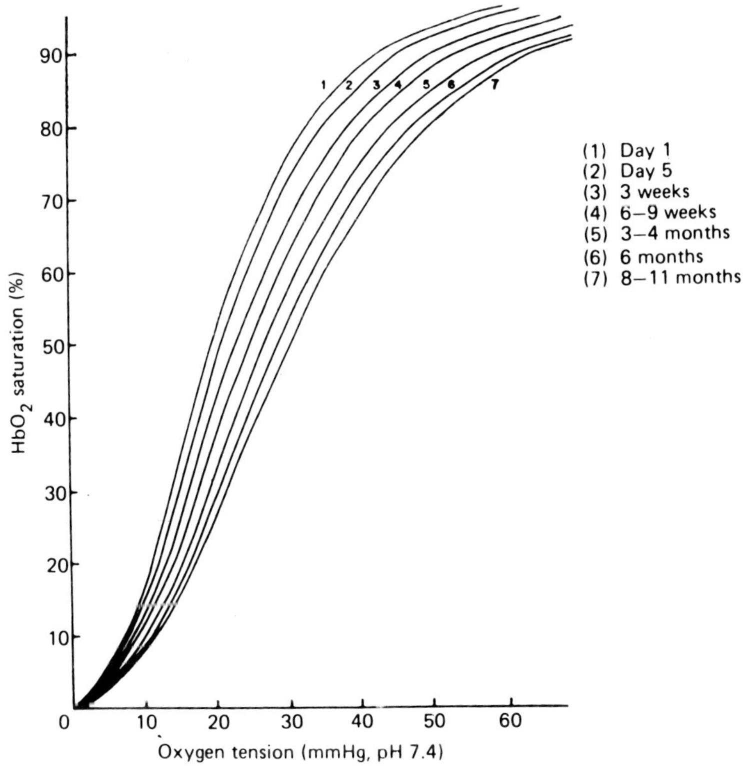

Figure 2.5 Oxygen equilibrium curves of blood from full-term infants during the first year of life. (From Oski and Delivoria-Papadopoulos, 1970, *Journal of Paediatrics*, *77*: 941, with permission of C.V. Mosby Publ.)

is that babies sampled after vigorous crying have approximately 50% higher values and a morphological 'shift to the left'. Moderate exercise, in the form of chest physiotherapy, puts up the count by 13%.

Neutrophils

The neutrophil count rises for the first 12 h of life and then declines to a plateau at 4 days in both term and premature babies (Figure 2.7, Tables 2.5 and 2.6). It can be seen that the total WBC count is lower in premature babies. Figure 2.7 and Table 2.6 also reveal the preponderance of neutrophils in the first 3 days of life, with the lymphocyte count being greater at about the fourth to seventh days. There is a morphological shift to the left, and occasionally even promyelocytes and myelocytes are present. The shift is more marked in premature babies and when there is an infection. In this situation, rare blast cells may be seen but they do not denote any primary haematological abnormality. Figure 2.8 shows the work of Manroe *et al.* (1979) in which values for immature neutrophils are recorded in a group of term babies during the first 60 h of life. The same

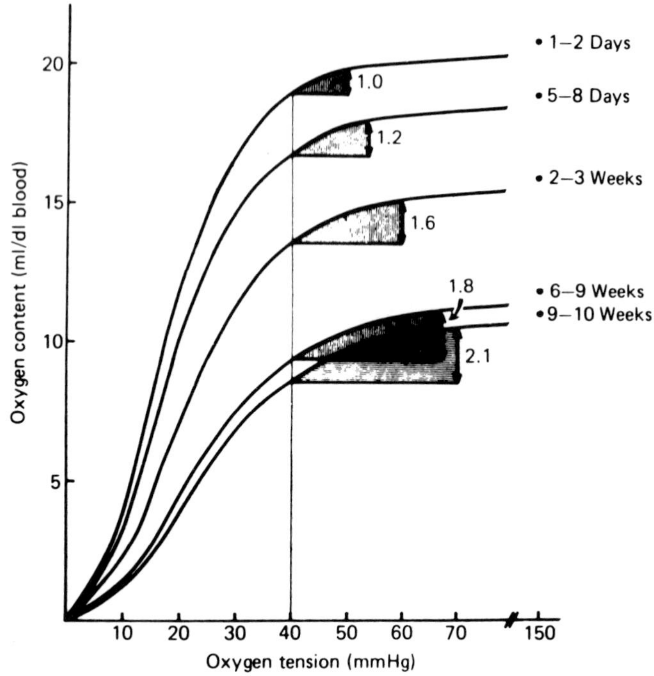

Figure 2.6 Oxygen content curve from premature babies weighing 1000–1500 g. The double arrows represent the oxygen-unloading capacity between a given arterial and venous P_{O_2}. (From Delivoria-Papadopoulos *et al.*, 1971, *Paediatric Research*, *5*: 235.

Table 2.5 Neutrophil counts in healthy full-term babies ($\times 10^9$ per litre).*

Age	5th Centile	Median	95th Centile
Birth	4.12	7.75	14.6
6 h	6.64	12.5	23.5
12 h	6.64	12.5	23.5
18 h	6.37	11.0	20.7
24 h	4.83	9.1	17.1
36 h	3.82	7.2	13.4
48 h	3.08	5.8	10.9
3 days	2.55	4.8	9.4
4 days	2.26	4.25	8.0
5 days	2.04	3.85	7.25
7 days	1.80	3.40	6.4
10 days	1.73	3.25	6.12
14 days	1.70	3.20	6.02
3–4 weeks	1.65	3.10	5.84

* From Gregory and Hey (1972).

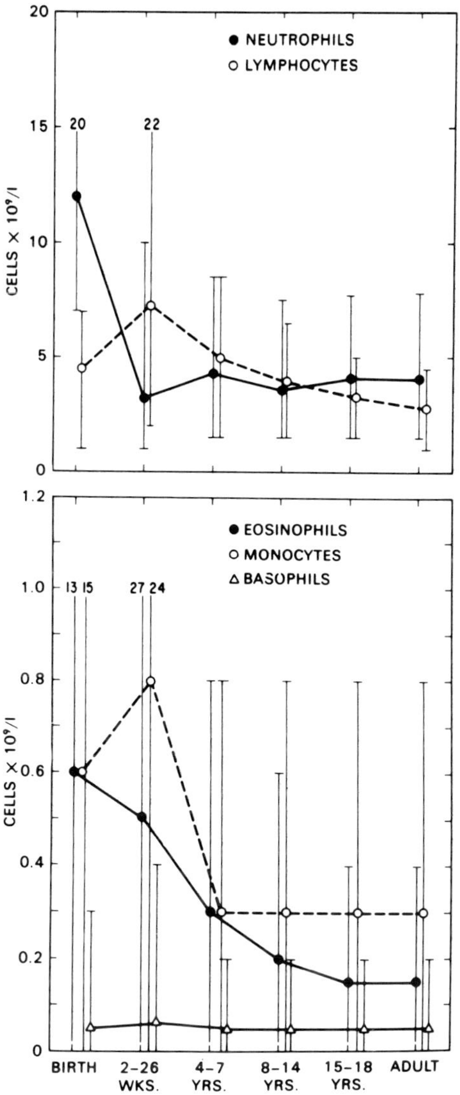

Figure 2.7 White cell numbers during childhood. (From Wintrobe MM, 1981, *Clinical Haematology* 8th edn, with permission of Lea & Febiger Publ.)

workers could find no relationship between the neutrophil count on the first 3 days of life and the following factors: birth weight, gestational age, sex, race, maternal diabetes, route of delivery, prolonged ruptured membranes, fetal bradycardia, meconium staining not associated with lung disease, transient neonatal tachypnoea, phototherapy, prophylactic antibodies and uncomplicated hyaline membrane disease. Maternal hypertension often caused a lower neutrophil count. Intraventricular haemorrhage and haemolysis were associated with higher counts. After the third day, changes in

Table 2.6 White blood cell counts in term and pre-term infants ($\times 10^9$ per litre).*

	Age (h)	Total WBC	Neutrophils	Bands/ Metamyelocytes	Lymphocytes	Monocytes	Eosinophils
Full-term	0	10–26	5–13	0.4–1.8	3.5–8.5	0.7–1.5	0.2–1.0
	12	13.5–31.0	9–18	0.4–2.0	3–7	1–2	0.2–2.0
	72	5–14.5	2–7	0.2–0.4	2–5	0.5–1.0	0.2–1.0
	144	6–14.5	2–6	0.2–0.5	3–6	0.7–1.2	0.2–0.8
Pre-term	0	5–19	2–9	0.2–2.4	2.5–6.0	0.3–1.0	0.1–0.7
	12	5–21	3–11	0.2–2.4	1.5–5.0	0.3–1.3	0.1–1.1
	72	5–14	3–7	0.2–0.6	1.5–4.0	0.3–1.2	0.2–1.1
	144	5.5–17.5	2–7	0.2–0.5	2.5–7.5	0.5–1.5	0.3–1.2

* From Xanthou (1970) and Glader (1977).

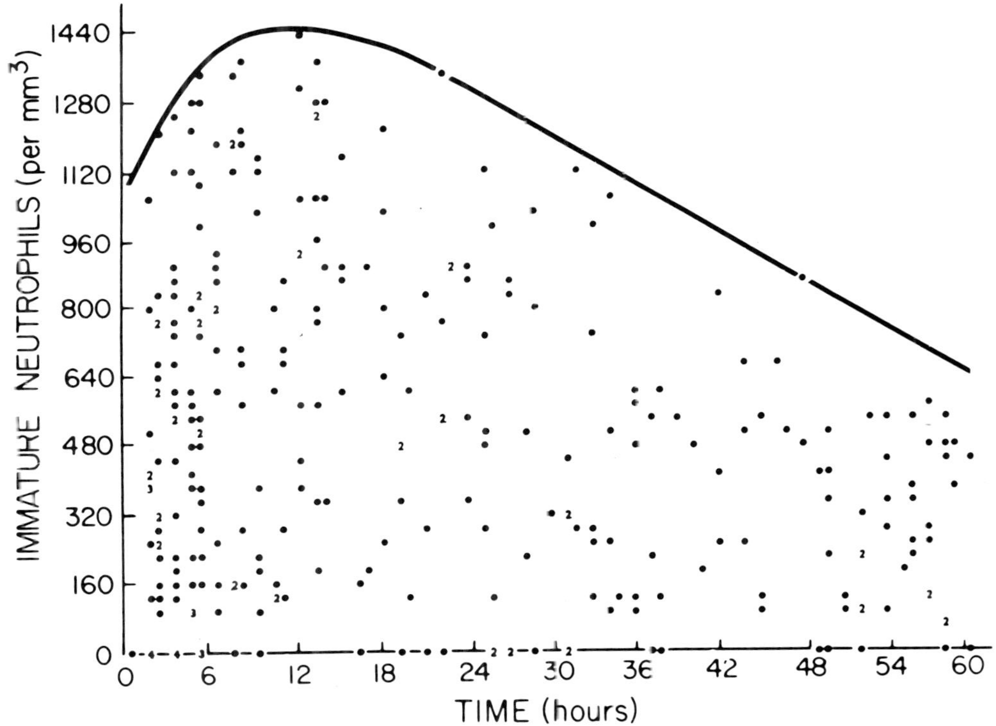

Figure 2.8 Immature neutrophil levels in normal infants during the first 60 hours of life. ●, Single values; 2, 3, 4, the number of values at the same point. (From Manroe *et al.* 1979, *J. Pediatr.*, *95*: 89.)

neutrophil and band counts are more easily interpreted as potential signals of infection.

A number of studies have shown that full-term newborn babies have normal phagocytic and bactericidal capacity. Both full-term and pre-term newborns have normal rates of superoxide anion production and normal times for activation in response to phorbolmyristate acetate. However, in pre-term infants there is a significant impairment of bactericidal capacity even though other parameters were normal (Gahr *et al.*, 1985). This parallels the defect in neutrophil killing capacity, which had been previously demonstrated in stressed full-term babies. A study by Krause *et al.* (1984), using a monoclonal antibody (31D8) that binds to highly motile neutrophils, showed that neonates had decreased neutrophil chemotaxis and a smaller subpopulation of $CD18^+$ highly motile cells. Presumably these defects may help to explain the susceptibility of these babies to bacterial infections.

Lymphocytes

As can be seen from Figure 2.7 lymphocyte counts are high during the first year, with a wide range of normality. Rises to values as high as 22×10^9 per litre occur in some apparently healthy infants and there is only a very gradual decline thereafter, with teenagers still often having higher levels than adults. These elevated levels may be physiological or they may be the consequence of frequent clinical and sub-clinical viral infections and immunizations.

Monocytes

Monocyte levels are high at birth and rise to a mean level of about 0.8×10^9 per litre in the second and third weeks, falling to a mean level of about 0.3×10^9 per litre thereafter.

Eosinophils and basophils

In the full-term infant the mean eosinophil count during the first 12 h is 0.27×10^9 per litre, with a range of $0.19–0.85 \times 10^9$ per litre. The count usually rises during the first 5 days, with a wide range from 0.1×10^9 to 2.5×10^9 per litre. The eosinophil count has been noted to fall rapidly in one study of bacterial infections in neonates. Premature babies of less than 2000 g may often have very low eosinophil counts at birth, but a progressive rise occurs and levels of greater than 0.7×10^9 per litre are frequent. Eosinophilia of greater than 1×10^9 per litre has been found to occur in up to a third of ill neonates.

Basophil counts at birth are at a mean of about 0.1×10^9 per litre and no significant relation of age to the count has been detected.

REFERENCES

Alexandre P, Andre E and Streiff F (1975) Etude sur sang. *Archives Francaises de Pediatrie* **32**: 417.

Bard H (1975) The postnatal decline of HbF synthesis in normal full-time infants. *J. Clin. Invest.* **55**: 395.

Bratteby LE (1968) *Acta Paediatrica* **57**: 132.

Delivoria-Papadopoulos *et al.* (1971) *Paediatric Research* **5**: 235.

Fogel BJ, Arias D and Kung F (1968) Platelet counts in healthy premature infants. *Journal of Pediatrics* **73**: 108.

Gahr M, Blanke R and Spear C (1985) Polymorphonuclear function in term and preterm newborn infants. *Biol Neonate* **48**: 15–20.

Gairdner D, Marks J and Roscoe JD (1952a) Blood formation in infancy: normal erythropoesis. *Archives of Disease in Childhood* **27**: 124.

Gairdner D, Marks J and Roscoe JD (1952b) Normal bone marrow *Archives of Disease in Childhood* **27**: 128.

Gairdner D (1958) *Recent Advances in Paediatrics*, ch. 2. Boston: Little Brown and Co.

Glader B (1977) Neonatal leukocyte disorders. In *Diseases of the Newborn* Shaffer AJ and Avery M (eds) 4th edn, p 587. Philadelphia: W.B. Saunders.

Gregory J and Hey E (1972) Blood neturophil response to bacterial infection in the first month of life. *Archives of Disease in Childhood* **47**: 747.

Holroyde CP, Oski FA and Gardner FH (1969) The 'pocked' erythrocyte. *New England Journal of Medicine* **281**: 516.

Kato K (1935) Leukocytes in infancy and childhood. A statistical analysis of 1,081 total and differential counts from birth to 15 years. *J. Oaediatr.* **7**: 7.

Krause PJ, Malech HL, Kristie J *et al.* (1984) Polymorphonuclear leukocyte heterogeneity in neonates and adults. *Blood* **68**: 200–204.

Manroe BL *et al.* (1979) The neonatal blood count in health and disease. *Journal of Pediatrics* **95**: 89.

Mathoth Y, Zaizov R and Varsano I (1971) Postnatal changes in some red cell parameters. *Acta Paediatricia Scandinavica* **60**: 317–320.

Moe PJ (1967) Umbilical cord blood and capillary blood in the evaluation of anaemia in erythroblastosis fetalis. *Acta Paediatricia Scandinavica* **56**: 391.

Nathan D and Oski FA (1981) Haematologic disorders of the fetus and newborn. In *Haematology of Infancy and Childhood*, 2nd edn, pp 17–50. W.B. Saunders.

Osgood EE *et al.* (1939) Total, differential and absolute leucocyte counts and sedimentation rates of healthy children from 4 to 7 years of age. *Am. J. Child.* **58**: 61.

Oski and Delivoria-Papadopoulos (1970). *Journal of Paediatrics* **77**: 941.

Sell EJ and Corrigan JJ (1973) Platelet counts, fibrinogen concentration etc in healthy infants according to gestational age. *Journal of Pediatrics* **82**: 1028.

Stockman JA and Oski FA (1980) RBC values in low birth weight infants during the first seven weeks of life. *American Journal of Diseases of Children* **134**: 945.

Stockman JA (1982) Neonatal erythropoiesis: changes in oxygen transport and delivery. In *Haematology and Oncology*. Butterworths International Medical Reviews, pp 196–223.

Stockman JA *et al.* (1984) Anaemia of Prematurity: determinants of erythropoietin response. *Journal of Pediatrics* **105**: 786.

Stockman JA *et al.* (1977). *New England Journal of Medicine* **296**: 647.

Thurlbeck SM and McIntosh N (1987) Preterm blood counts vary with sampling site. *Archives of Disease in Childhood* **62**: 74–87.

Washburn AH (1935) Blood cells in healthy young infants. III a study of 608 differential leukıcyte counts. *American Journal of Diseases of Children* **50**: 413.

Wintrobe MM (1981) *Clinical Haematology*, 8th edition. Lea & Febiger Publishers.

Williams ME, Shott RJ, O'Neal PL and Oski FA (1975) Role of dietary iron and fat on Vit E deficiency anaemia of infancy. *New England Journal of Medicine* **292**: 887–890.
Xanthou M (1970) Leucocyte blood picture in healthy full-term and premature babies during the neonatal period. *Archives of Disease in Childhood* **45**: 242.
Yao AC, Moinian M and Luid J (1969) Distribution of blood between infant and placenta after birth. *The Lancet* **2**: 891.
Zipursky A (1977) Erythrocyte morphology in newborn infants. A new look. *Pediatric Research* **11**: 843.

3

Anaemia in the neonate

E.A. Letsky
Queen Charlotte's Maternity Hospital, London

Throughout gestation and in the first few weeks of life there are dynamic changes occurring in the composition of the circulating blood of the human fetus and neonate (see Chapters 1 and 2). By approximately 6 months of age a relatively stable population of so-called adult red cells is established. There are marked physical, metabolic and antigenic differences between the fetal red cell and the adult red cell. Throughout childhood, adolescence and into old age, the responses to haematological stimuli are in essence similar. It is only the changing susceptibility to various disease processes at different times of life that creates broad separations between the clinical practice of paediatric and adult haematology. In contrast, the blood of the neonate has unique characteristics. It is changing from day to day and these changes differ in magnitude and quality depending on the gestational age at birth. In addition, interactions between fetal and maternal circulations have to be considered in the differential diagnosis of any haematological abnormality. For example, a common cause of anaemia in the neonate is blood loss, but this loss often occurs into the maternal circulation and there will be no overt signs of bleeding; haemolytic disease of the newborn may be caused by antibodies from the maternal circulation directed against antigens on the fetal red cells, but it could be due to innate membrane defects or enzyme deficiencies of the fetal red cells themselves.

This chapter deals with the acquired causes of anaemia in the neonatal period; for genetic causes see Chapter 8.

As understanding, prevention and management of haemolytic disease of the newborn due to blood-group incompatibilities between mother and fetus have undergone dramatic changes in the last decade, Chapter 5 is devoted to this topic.

HAEMATOLOGICAL CHANGES AFTER BIRTH

In the same way that it is necessary to have some knowledge of developmental changes in haemotopoiesis *in utero*, in order to understand the physiological normal ranges of haematological parameters at birth (see Chapters 1 and 2), it is also advisable to have some understanding of the haematological changes which occur in the infant beyond the neonatal period. The way in which the delivery of the newborn is managed may have far-reaching effects on blood production, extending well beyond the neonatal period. Birth, regardless of gestation, is just a single event occurring on a background of haematological changes that appear to be set in motion from the time of conception.

Term neonate

The transient changes immediately after birth, in haemoglobin, haematocrit and red cell count, are followed by a gradual steady reduction in these parameters until 7–9 weeks. At this stage the haemoglobin level has fallen to 9.5–11.0 g dl^{-1}, the haematocrit to 30–33%, and the red cell count to about $3.4 \times 10^9\ l^{-1}$. The reticulocyte count falls rapidly from birth and remains at less than 1% from the end of the first week until around 6 weeks postnatally. Erythroblasts in the bone marrow decline sharply during the first week. The sharp fall in erythropoietin activity after birth is considered to be a physiological reaction to the greater availability of oxygen. Together with the shortened red cell lifespan and increasing haemodilution accompanying growth, the fall in haemoglobin concentration is easily accounted for. The neonate is still capable of responding to increased demand during the first few weeks of life. Hypoxic and anaemic infants do not show the decrease in erythroid activity observed in the healthy newborn and they continue to produce erythropoietin. The initial cord-blood haemoglobin concentration has no effect on the level to which the haemoglobin falls. Recovery begins when a level of about 10–11 g dl^{-1} is reached.

The erythroid activity in the bone marrow starts to increase after 3–4 weeks, but there is a delay in recovery of the haemoglobin level because the rate of red cell destruction still exceeds production and continued rapid growth results in expansion of the blood volume and haemodilution. By 6 months of age a mean haemoglobin level of about 12.5 g dl^{-1} is achieved in normal infants in whom there is no evidence of iron deficiency (Siimes, 1981). This level is maintained until 2 years of age, when there is a gradual increase up to puberty (Dallman, 1987).

Racial differences must be borne in mind in determining normal haemoglobin values during childhood. It has been shown that Negro children show mean haemoglobin levels 0.5–1.0 g dl^{-1} lower than Oriental and Caucasian children throughout childhood, which do not depend on social or nutritional factors (Dallman, 1987).

Premature infants

The fall in haemoglobin and red cell count tends to occur more rapidly and earlier in pre-term infants, reaching levels of 6.5–9.0 g dl^{-1} by 4–8 weeks of age (Stockman and Oski, 1978). The premature newborn may well be able to respond appropriately to the decreased levels of haemoglobin by producing erythropoietin (Stockman *et al.*, 1984), but clinical manifestations of the anaemia may develop, particularly in those infants born before 32 weeks gestation.

The role of iron, folic acid, Vitamin B_{12} and, particularly, Vitamin E in neonatal anaemia are discussed below.

There is controversy and active debate over the reason for the greater fall in haemoglobin in premature infants compared with term neonates. Measurements of oxygen consumption related to the respiratory quotient and metabolic rate have produced contradictory results, some investigators finding reduced oxygen consumption while others have observed higher levels of oxygen consumption in pre-term infants. The debate is unresolved and the reasons for the greater fall in haemoglobin are still not clear.

THE ANAEMIA OF PREMATURITY

All newborn infants will experience a fall in haemoglobin concentration in the first few weeks of life, but the magnitude of the fall in pre-term infants is greater than in infants born at term and is seen earlier. The rapidity and extent of fall may be so great as to initiate consideration of the necessity for blood transfusion (see Chapter 7). The indications for transfusion in the special care baby unit are not well defined. Some infants tolerate very low levels of haemoglobin, with none of the accepted signs of tissue anoxia, while others suffer considerable overt clinical difficulties. More often than not this true anaemia will have a multifactorial basis, resulting from a combination of iatrogenic blood sampling and varying oxygen availability and requirements, together with a variety of medical and surgical problems. As pre-term infants have become viable *extra utero* at much earlier gestation over recent years, the anaemia of prematurity has become more complex.

To establish whether true anaemia is present and whether transfusion is indicated, some knowlege of the normal physiology and the potential of the adaptive processes in the very small pre-term infant is required.

True anaemia at any time in life is present when the oxygen demand of tissues, in order to maintain normal metabolism, exceeds the ability to delivery oxygen to the tissues. Tissue oxygenation depends on:

(1) concentration of oxygen in inspired air,
(2) pulmonary function,
(3) pulmonary–alveolar exchange of oxygen,
(4) cardiac output,
(5) concentration and composition of haemoglobin(s), and
(6) position of the haemoglobin–oxygen dissociation curve.

In the newborn baby, tissue oxygenation is different from that in the adult in several fundamental aspects. The differences are most marked in pre-term infants. Tissue oxygenation in the small pre-term infant is designed to function optimally *in utero* and is ill-adapted for postnatal life (Holland and Wardrop, 1988).

The pathophysiology of anaemia of prematurity

Erythropoietin

Maternal erythropoietin does not cross the placenta. Fetal erythropoiesis is endogenously controlled by fetally produced erythropoietin and high concentrations have been observed in the amniotic fluid and fetal blood (Thomas *et al.*, 1983) of pregnancies complicated by severe erythroblastosis fetalis. Elevated levels of erythropoietin have been demonstrated in cord blood of babies who have undergone stressful delivery or have suffered hypoxia *in utero*. However the fetal response to hypoxia or anaemia is poor compared with that of the mature infant or the adult. This reduced sensitivity to the stimulus of erythropoietin probably prevents accelerated erythropoiesis and hyperviscosity of the blood in the healthy fetus (Dallman, 1984).

The pre-term infant retains its *in utero* hyporesponsiveness to hypoxic stimuli *extra utero*. Although term infants tend to respond appropriately to falls in haemoglobin concentration by increasing erythropoietin production, the limited response in the pre-term infant leads to an inappropriately impaired erythropoietic response to hypoxic stimuli (Stockman, 1988). This together with the greatly shortened red cell lifespan is the basis of the refractory anaemia of the pre-term infant even in the face of adequate haematinics.

The degree of immaturity is a major factor in determining the erythropoietin response — the least mature having the lowest levels of erythropoietin (Brown *et al.*, 1984) in spite of low haemoglobin concentration, high haemoglobin oxygen-affinity and clinical evidence of hypoxia.

Very low birth-weight infants appear to have an inadequate haemopoietic response to anaemia-related tissue hypoxia, and this may be associated with a shift in the site of erythropoietin production (Dallman, 1984). In many of the mammalian species studied, erythropoietin is produced in the liver in fetal life and there is a gradual shift to renal production of erythropoietin in the perinatal period. Fetal, mainly liver, erythropoietin production is much less sensitive to tissue hypoxia than production in the kidney, and this may well be a contributing factor to the inadequate response of the very immature infant to the effects of severe anaemia, although this has not been confirmed in the human fetus and human adult renal and hepatic erythropoietins have been shown to be structurally identical (Jacobs *et al.*, 1985).

Recent work has confirmed that the amount of oxygen available to the tissues is diminished in the anaemia of prematurity, but the response in terms of erythropoietin production is inadequte, by adult standards. Erythropoietin levels are still related to the degree of hypoxia, the highest levels being seen in those infants with the lowest haemoglobin concentration. This had led to speculation that the cells committed to erythropoiesis in pre-term infants may be peculiarly sensitive to the effects of erythropoietin and that low levels are therefore physiologically appropriate (Stockman *et al.*, 1984), or that there are transiently reduced numbers of erythroid progenitors capable of responding to the effects of erythropoietin in infants of very low birth-weight. These contentions have recently been refuted by Shannon *et al.* (1987) who have shown that progenitor cells committed to erythroid differentiation are present during the anaemia of prematurity and that the intrinsic responsiveness of the burst forming unit–erythroid (BFU-E) pool to erythropoietin *in vitro* is normal. These results lead to the conclusion that the anaemia of prematurity results from inadequate erythropoietin production. Another exciting spin-off from this most recent work is the possibility it raises of using erythropoietin in a clinical therapeutic trial (Rhondeau *et al.*, 1988). Recombinant erythropoietin has been shown to stimulate erythroid proliferation *in vitro* (Sieff *et al.*, 1986) and has already been used to produce a reticulocyte response and to treat the anaemia of chronic renal failure (Anon., 1989). Recombinant erythropoietin might provide a therapeutic alternative to transfusion in the management of the anaemia of prematurity (Shannon *et al.*, 1987).

Pre-term infants have low erythropoietin concentrations but responsive erythroid precursors in the face of severe anaemia and could therefore be candidates for treatment. The cost is such that, in the United Kingdom, presumably central, funding would be needed. Nevertheless, compared with its use in nephrology, the administration of recombinant human erythropoietin (r-Hu Epo) in the management of anaemia of prematurity would be relatively short-term and the quantity required small so that the question of cost would be less likely to preclude its use (Anon 1989).

Of greater importance, before any widespread clinical trials can be undertaken, is predicting and defining any possible adverse effects. It was feared that administration of erythropoietin might deplete the marrow of progenitor cells, but this has not been observed in adults; however, it remains to be evaluated in neonates, who probably have a smaller pool of pluripotent stem cells per kilogram body weight. A second concern is that because stem cells are pluripotent, producing erythrocytes, granulocytes and platelets, if there is stimulation of erythropoiesis then there will be a reduction in production of white cells and platelets. *In vitro* investigations have shown that fetal progenitors exposed to large concentrations of erythropoietin produce less granulocytes and macrophages as erythroid production increases (Christensen, 1989).

The application of haematopoietic growth factors, made available by recent advances in molecular biology, to the management of anaemia in the neonate is only just beginning. At the time of writing there are already some preliminary pilot trials underway, and it is likely that treatment of the anaemia of the pre-term infant and other neonatal cytopenias will undergo profound changes.

The results of a small pilot study of the use of rHu Epo in infants with the anaemia of prematurity have recently been published (Halperin *et al.* 1990).

Seven infants were treated with rHu Epo in doses of 75 to 300 units kg^{-1} $week^{-1}$ for four weeks. The treatment was well tolerated. The number of reticulocytes increased and correction or stabilization of anaemia was observed in six of the seven infants. In three of the responders a secondary fall in haematocrit was noted either during or after discontinuation of therapy. Serum iron and ferritin levels fell rapidly following institution of rHu Epo therapy, suggesting that response to erythropoietin may be limited by the availability of iron. In most cases transient early thrombocytosis and late neutropenia were observed.

What is needed now are some double blind placebo controlled studies of use of rHu Epo and one such at least is underway (Shannon 1990). It is obvious that if treatment with rHu Epo leads to a substantial reduction in blood transfusions given to premature infants this will be a major therapeutic advance. The progress and prospects of the use of rHu Epo in pre-term infants is discussed in a recent review (Shannon 1990).

Availability of oxygen and special problems of demand and supply in the small pre-term infant

Tissue oxygen availability depends ultimately on arterial oxygen saturation, the concentration of haemoglobin and the position of the haemoglobin–oxygen dissociation curve. In small pre-term infants all of these parameters show significant differences from those observed in the term neonate.

Arterial oxygen saturation is dependent on pulmonary function and exchange at the arteriolar pulmonary vascular interface, but the amount of oxygen taken up by the blood in the lungs is partly dependent on the oxygen affinity of the circulating haemoglobin (see below).

The concentration of haemoglobin is influenced to a certain extent by erythropoietin, as discussed above, but the stimulus to erythropoietin production and the amount produced differs in the small pre-term infant from that in the more mature, and there is still active debate about whether the adaptive changes are appropriate to the need for oxygen in these immature neonates (Stockman, 1986; Shannon *et al.*, 1987).

Developmental changes in haemoglobins

With the establishment of erythropoiesis there is production of a series of different haemoglobins (Hb). These are embryonic, fetal and adult haemoglobins. There are three embryonic haemoglobins — Hb, Gower 1 and 2 and Hb Portland. They disappear by 12 weeks' gestation and it is thought that they are restricted to the primitive red cells produced in the yolk sac. Fetal haemoglobin HbF ($\alpha_2\gamma_2$) can be detected in the blood from embryos of 6–12 weeks' gestation (see Chapters 1 and 2).

From the time when hepatic erythropoiesis is established, HbF forms the major respiratory pigment, but from as early as 8–10 weeks' gestation it is possible to detect about 5–10% of adult haemoglobin — HbA ($\alpha_2\beta_2$). Between 32 and 36 weeks' gestation the production of HbA increases coincident with a sharp decline in HbF production. The decrease in HbF results in a level of HbF of less than 10% at 3 months of age and the adult level of HbF less than 1%, by 6 months to 1 year in the vast majority of infants.

The decline of fetal haemoglobin in the newborn period appears to be strictly regulated. The switch from HbF to HbA synthesis occurs around 32 weeks' gestation (Stamatoyannopoulos and Neinhuis, 1978) and it is important to realize that this is not related to birth but it is based on post-conception age. It follows, then, that the relative concentrations of HbF and HbA in cord blood will depend on gestation, babies born at 32–34 weeks having a mean of 90% HbF while those born at term will have around 70–80% HbF.

The molecular basis of this changeover from fetal to adult haemoglobin is at the centre of current investigation and has excited much interest in recent years (Wood 1982). In spite of this, studies have failed to produce a clear picture of events at the cellular level during the haemoglobin 'switch' (Stamatoyannopoulos and Nienhuis, 1989).

The efficiency of oxygen delivery to the tissues is directly related to the interactions of haemoglobin with 2,3 diphosphoglycerate (2,3DPG). High concentrations of 2,3DPG push the oxygen dissociation curve to the right and facilitate oxygen delivery to the tissues. The reduction in the oxygen affinity of HbF by interaction with 2,3DPG is only a fraction of that produced by the same concentration of 2,3DPG with HbA. The effect of this reduced reaction of HbF with 2,3DPG ensures that the oxygen affinity of fetal blood does not drop below that of its mother. This facilitates binding of oxygen from the maternal circulation in the placenta villi. More than half of the oxygen bound in the placenta by the fetal blood can be released to fetal tissue because the tissue oxygen levels in the fetus are much lower than those in the maternal tissues.

In the first few weeks of extra-uterine life there is a progressive increase in the delivery of oxygen to the tissues. This is brought about by the interactions of several factors. There is a gradual replacement of HbF by HbA, an increase in 2,3DPG levels which shifts the oxygen dissociation curve to the right, and, of course, increased availability of oxygen. The net result of these changes is that although the haemoglobin level in the term infant falls from 17 to 11 g dl^{-1} in the first 12 weeks of life, the oxygen delivery to the tissues at 3 months is greater than that in the newborn infant.

However, the baby under 1000 g, even one who is small for gestational age, is unlikely to have reached 32 weeks post-conception and therefore the switch to predominant β globin chain production has not even begun and it may be some weeks post-delivery before significant amounts of HbA are produced (Bard and Prosmanne, 1982). This will compromise delivery of oxygen to the tissues by preventing the shift of the oxygen dissociation curve to the right. This observation, however, does not explain why the nadir of haemoglobin concentration in the infant weighing less than 1000 g can be 2–3 g dl^{-1} lower than for infants born at term, before there is resumption of active erythropoiesis (Oski, 1979).

In summary the major respiratory pigment *in utero* is fetal haemoglobin ($\alpha_2\gamma_2$). The switch from predominantly γ- to predominantly β-chain synthesis ocurs at approximately 32 weeks' gestation and is a strictly post-conceptional event not affected by environment or brought forward by pre-term delivery.

Fetal haemoglobin has a high affinity for oxygen and is advantageous *in utero* in facilitating transplacental uptake of oxygen, ensuring that the oxygen affinity for the haemoglobin in the fetus is always higher than that of the mother' haemoglobin. *Extra utero* the pre-term infant is at a disadvantage in that, although there is greater availability of oxygen in the lungs and possibly oxygen uptake is facilitated, this benefit is far outweighed by the fact that the high oxygen affinity of fetal haemoglobin impairs delivery of oxygen in the microcirculation to the tissues by up to 30% compared with adult haemoglobin.

The term baby with normal development will replace fetal haemoglobin by adult haemoglobin in a matter of weeks and has already been in the process of doing so for some 8 weeks, but the very small pre-term infant will not begin the process until it has reached 32 weeks post conception, whenever it is born.

Haemoglobin concentration

Cord haemoglobin values for pre-term infants (17.5 ± 1.6 g dl^{-1}) do not vary significantly from those observed at term (see Chapter 2). Dependent upon the amount of placental transfusion and transient haemoconcentration due to poor oral fluid intake, a brief rise in haemoglobin may be seen during the first 24 hours of life. The haemoglobin returns to the original concentration of birth by the end of the first week (Chapter 2). Then a progressive fall occurs over the following 4–12 weeks. The rapidity of fall and the nadir of haemoglobin concentration vary inversely with gestational age. This fall in haemoglobin is the result, for the most part, of an absolute reduction in the red cell mass and not from the haemodilutional effect of a greater plasma volume. The red cell lifespan, already short by adult standards in the term infant, is even shorter in the pre-term baby and there is a marked reticulocytopenia, reflecting a decrease in marrow erythroid activity. Another complicating factor in the pre-term infant is particularly high oxygen requirements, both at rest and on exertion.

Even term newborns have elevated oxygen requirements because of a high proportion of lean tissue with increased metabolic activity and because of rapid growth, and these demands are exaggerated in the pre-term infant. The balance of oxygen supply and demand is at a critical level in the healthy newborn and the balance is much more difficult to maintain in the sick pre-term infant (Holland and Wardrop, 1990). Hypoxia at a tissue level will result in anaerobic metabolism and metabolic acidosis.

From the foregoing discussion it is clear that the supply of oxygen to the tissues of the healthy newborn is only just adequate. In the pre-term infant this marginal oxygen supply often fails. Superimposed on the multiple causes of anaemia in the pre-term infant are blood losses from the sampling that is essential for the monitoring and intensive management of such low birth-weight babies. This iatrogenic blood letting is probably the major cause of anaemia in such infants (Blanchette and Zipursky, 1984). Prevention and correction of true anaemia is vital in these very small pre-term infants (Roberton, 1987). Decisions regarding transfusion cannot be made on haemoglobin concentration alone.

Until more precise guidelines are available concerning the expression of true anaemia in the premature infant, the physician caring for infants will have to make decisions based on clinical judgments about the need for blood transfusions. Certain simple measurements should be instituted which will avoid unnecessary blood administration and result in only essential transfusions being given:

(1) All blood taken should be carefully recorded, and if 5–10% of the baby's blood volume is removed over a short space of time, it should be replaced with packed red cells.

(2) The haemoglobin should be measured on entry to the nursery and at regular, at least weekly, intervals thereafter. The haemoglobin will drop about 1 g dl^{-1} per week. A transfusion should never be given on the basis of haemoglobin level alone; although haemoglobin values of 7.0 g dl^{-1} or less require explanation, they may not need correction.

(3) Evaluation should include:
- (a) weight gain,
- (b) fatigue while feeding,
- (c) tachypnoea and tachycardia,
- (d) hypoxia, reflected by elevated levels of lactic and pyruvic acid.

(4) Infants with cardiac or pulmonary disease with a reduced arterial oxygen saturation may need to have the haemoglobin maintained in the range of 16–17 g dl^{-1} to ensure sufficient differential between arterial and venous oxygen tension.

One important aspect of management in these very small babies is the anticipation, prophylaxis and correction of haematinic deficiencies.

Haematinics

The pre-term infant is more prone to develop nutritional deficiencies than the term infant because of rapid growth and diminished resources. Factors that can augment the anaemia of prematurity are iron, folate, vitamin B_{12} and, possibly vitamin E deficiency.

Iron

Although iron transport to the fetus is unidirectional with ratio of maternal:fetal serum ferritin concentrations of 1:2 to 1:4, and although there are adequate fetal iron stores even in cases of maternal iron deficiency, there is some evidence that there is a reduced red cell mass in the offspring of iron-deficient mothers and that iron stores, although high by adult standards, are reduced in these infants compared with those born to iron-replete mothers (Fenton *et al.*, 1977). The fetus *in utero* normally recruits 75 ng iron per kilogram of body weight, so that iron status will be related to birth weight and maturity (Holland and Wardrop, 1990).

The role of iron in the pathogenesis of the anaemia of prematurity has excited interest for almost 50 years. As a result of innumerable investigations a clearer picture has emerged from the initial confusion. Iron deficiency is not likely to play a part in the early anaemia of prematurity unless there has been perinatal blood loss or unless repeated blood sampling has been performed for laboratory investigations (Lundstrom *et al.*, 1977). It follows, then, that the administration of medicinal iron will not prevent the initial fall in haemoglobin. However, unless the premature infant is given iron supplements some time in the first 2–4 months of life, an anaemia — the so-called late anaemia of prematurity — will inevitably develop due to iron deficiency (Stockman and Oski, 1978). The timing of the anaemia will depend on the initial haemoglobin level and the rate of growth. In general, infants with normal haemoglobin levels at birth will have depleted their iron stores and therefore limit the rate of haemoglobin synthesis by the time they have doubled their birth weight (Siimes, 1981). Approximately 75% of the infant's total body iron is contained in the haemoglobin of the circulating and developing red cells. Infants who are anaemic at birth and have a decreased red cell mass will have reduced iron reserves (Dallman, 1987).

There is now a concensus of opinion that all premature infants, and particularly those weighing less than 1500 g at birth, require supplemental iron to prevent the development of late anaemia due to iron deficiency. Cord-blood haemoglobin level, birth weight and blood-letting in the first weeks of life will determine the timing of the development of iron deficiency.

Iron supplements in low birth weight infants should be given as follows (Siimes, 1981), starting on the 15th day of life:

2 mg kg^{-1} per day for infants of 1500–2500 g birth weight,
3 mg kg^{-1} per day for infants of 1000–1500 g birth weight,
4 mg kg^{-1} per day for those of less than 1000 g birth weight,

and these supplements should be continued for at least 1 year to 15 months after birth (Oski, 1979). If the infant is receiving adequate vitamin E in relation to polyunsaturated fat in the diet, then the early introduction of supplemental iron will cause no adverse effects (see below).

Copper

More than 90% of the copper normally present in plasma is bound to ceruloplasmin. Ceruloplasmin also facilitates the absorption of iron and the release of iron from body stores. Copper is also necessary for iron metabolism within erythroid precursors. Copper deficiency mimics iron deficiency, with the production of a hypochromic microcytic anaemia, but also produces neutropenia. The term infant has abundant hepatic copper stores, sufficient to maintain him through the first 6 months of life. These stores are accumulated in the last 12 weeks of fetal life. The premature infant is born with marginal copper stores (Sutton *et al.*, 1985), and severe symptomatic copper deficiency may develop by 2–3 months in those infants fed cows' milk products with inadequate copper content. It is recommended that the infant receive 80 μg of copper per kilogram per day, and most infant formulas have been supplemented appropriately.

The diagnosis of copper deficiency anaemia is made by the demonstration of low serum copper (less than 40 μg dl^{-1}) or low ceruloplasmin values (less than 15 mg dl^{-1}), together with vacuolated erythroid precursors and maturation arrest in the granulocyte series. Anaemia and neutropenia due to nutritional copper deficiency will respond promptly to the administration of 400–600 μg of copper per day in a 1% copper sulphate solution (Oski, 1979).

Zinc

The exact role of zinc in haemopoiesis is not well understood. Deficiency is associated with diarrhoea and paranasal, perioral and perineal crusting, and dermatitis with bullae on feet and hands. Most of the zinc is acquired during the last trimester of pregnancy, therefore deficiencies will develop in the pre-term infant if sufficient quantities are not given in postnatal life. Intestinal interactions between copper and zinc may impair absorption of the former but a zinc concentration of 12.5 ng l^{-1} of formula will prevent this (Tyrala, 1986). The Committee on Nutrition of the American Academy of Pediatrics (1985) recommends an intake of 0.5 mg zinc per 100 kcal.

Vitamin E

α-Tocopherol (vitamin E) is a fat-soluble dietary factor first shown to be required for successful reproduction in rats and now known to be an essential nutrient for all animals, including man. Vitamin E has been the subject of extensive investigations over the past 40 years or so and, in animals, the signs and symptoms of vitamin E deficiency, including effects on the reproductive system, have been the subject of many reviews. Effects of deficiency of vitamin E do not readily occur in the adult human, presumably because tissues do not easily become depleted and there is a wide distribution of α-tocopherol in foodstuffs. Vitamin E deficiency syndromes have been described in neonates and particularly in premature neonates (Ehrenkranz, 1980). The reason for this is that all newborn infants are in a state of relative tocopherol deficiency and the smaller the infant at birth the greater the lack of vitamin E.

For a time it was fashionable to diagnose any unexplained anaemia in the pre-term infant as being due to haemolysis associated with vitamin E deficiency. This was easy to substantiate as all pre-term babies are vitamin E deficient by adult standards and have a shortened red blood cell lifespan whether anaemic or not.

A mother at term has a vitamin E level around 0.9 mg per 100 ml, on average, whereas her newborn baby's value is considerably lower at 0.2 mg per 100 ml. Term infants with a birthweight of 3500 g have vitamin E body stores of 20 mg, while babies with a birthweight of 1000 g will have stores amounting only to 3 mg. There is a direct relationship between the maternal level of vitamin E and that of her infant, but a newborn baby never has a value in excess of 0.6 mg per 100 ml, which is considered to be the lowest limit of normal for older children and adults.

Vitamin E is a potent anti-peroxidant at the cellular level. Deficiency of this vitamin results in an increased rate of cell-membrane lipid peroxidation which, in the case of the red cell, could theoretically lead to a shortening of the red cell lifespan and a haemolytic anaemia. Haemolytic anaemia due to vitamin E deficiency in the newborn has now been shown to be an iatrogenic invention arising from both inappropriate medication and interpretation of findings. However the story is an object lesson in the care of the newborn infant and is worth an account.

It has been shown that the dietary requirement for vitamin E increases when the intake of polyunsaturated fatty acids (PUFA) increases. Although the breast-fed infant will quickly attain normal adult levels of vitamin E, there is considerable variability in achieving normal vitamin E status in the artificially fed infant. This results in part from the PUFA content of the artificial formulas. Most infant formulas contain quantities of linoleic acid, an 18 C fatty acid with two unsaturated double bonds, far in excess of the quantities found in breast milk.

The first reports of the association of vitamin E deficiency with haemolytic anaemia in the premature neonate came from the United States of America in the late 1960s (Hassan *et al.*, 1966, Oski and Barness, 1967). These infants were aged 6–10 weeks and had been fed proprietary formulas with a high PUFA content. The administration of vitamin E to affected infants resulted in a prompt increase in the haemoglobin level and a fall in the reticulocyte count. It is clear that the severity of the haemolysis in the premature infant was related to the level of vitamin E and the PUFA content of the diet (E:PUFA ratio). The lack of reports from the United Kingdom is probably a reflection of the lower PUFA content of our proprietary formulas at that time and hence higher E:PUFA ratio. It became evident through the passage of time that it was not just the high PUFA and low vitamin E content of the diet that were predisposing factors to haemolysis in the premature infant. It has become common practice to supplement infant feeding with iron to prevent the development of late anaemia (see above). Iron acts as a catalyst in the non-enzymatic auto-oxidation of unsaturated fatty acids and can result in the peroxidation of red cell membrane lipids. It has been shown that iron-fortified formulas can trigger a haemolytic anaemia in the infant who receives large quantities of PUFA with inadequate amounts of vitamin E (Melhorn *et al.*, 1971).

There are therefore three important variables in the diet which affect the development of haemolytic anaemia associated with lack of vitamin E in the premature infant:

(1) polyunsaturated fatty acid composition,
(2) presence of added iron,
(3) vitamin E content.

The interactions of these equally important factors may help to explain the marked variability from nursery to nursery in the incidence of vitamin E deficiency haemolytic anaemia and the virtual lack of a problem in the United Kingdom. It should be appreciated that vitamin E deficiency may contribute to the magnitude of the physiological anaemia in all non-supplemented premature infants. The commercial formulas have, for the most part, corrected the potential problem by reducing the content of linoleic acid and increasing the concentration of vitamin E. Breast milk has a very low content of linoleic acid.

The problem of the triad of factors (iron, PUFA and vitamin E levels) contributing to anaemia in the premature infants is now well recognized and haemolysis can be prevented in one or more of three ways:

(1) the introduction of iron should be delayed;
(2) a water-soluble form of vitamin E can be administered to overcome the malabsorption of the natural vitamins;
(3) formulas with a low PUFA content or human milk can be fed to small premature infants.

The removal or correction of just one of the contributing triad will prevent any significant haemolysis or anaemia in the premature neonate (Zipursky, 1984).

More recently Zipursky *et al.* (1987) have shown that there is no haematological difference between infants supplemented with 0.2 i.u. oral vitamin E daily and a control group receiving no supplements. The wheel has now turned full-circle, and it would appear that in standard neonatal care the hazard of vitamin E deficiency contributing to anaemia is negligible.

It has been suggested, however, that vitamin E supplements may reduce the incidence of two serious complications of oxygen administration in the premature infant, namely retrolental fibroplasia (RLF; Curran and Cantolino, 1978) and bronchopulmonary dysplasia (BPD; Ehrenkrantz, 1980). These suggestions are based on a large number of animal experiments that have demonstrated that vitamin E deficient animals suffer more oxygen-induced damage to their lungs, and to the CNS as well as the red cells, than animals fed on a controlled vitamin E supplemented diet.

Reports of a reduction in incidence, severity and duration of RLF in the human neonate associated with vitamin E supplementation have appeared in recent years (see Ehrenkrantz, 1980). Preliminary studies suggest that the intramuscular administration of a water-dispersible preparation of DL α-tocopheral during the acute phase of therapy for respiratory distress syndrome prevents the development and modifies the severity of BPD. These findings still await confirmation from large combined studies.

Intraventricular haemorrhage and vitamin E. About 40% of newborn babies under 32 weeks' gestation develop ultrasound evidence of periventricular haemorrhage within the first 3 days of life. This bleeding may be confined to the subepidural region where it originates or it may rupture into the ventricles or brain parenchyma.

It has been suggested by a group in Manchester that vitamin E given intramuscularly to pre-term babies may protect against intraventricular haemorrhage in very pre-term infants (Sinha *et al.*, 1987). The situation is complicated by the different vitamin E preparations available, their route of administration, their ability to raise plasma vitamin E levels and their reported toxicity. There have been no properly controlled studies of the role that vitamin E may play in the prevention of intraventricular haemorrhage. Oral vitamin E, 2000 mg kg^{-1} daily, has been associated with an increased incidence of necrotizing enterocolitis (NEC) in one report (Finer *et al.*, 1984).

Although the intravenous route produces the most rapid response in vitamin E plasma levels, this method of administration cannot be recommended until concern about associated toxic effects has been resolved.

Folic acid

Serum and red cell folate levels are higher in the newborn than in the normal adult regardless of birth weight or gestation, but they fall quickly to levels which are often below the normal adult levels within several weeks of birth. This fall occurs more rapidly in the premature than in the term infant since subnormal levels are reached within the first few weeks of life, whereas low levels do not develop in the term infant until after 6 months of age. Controlled studies however have failed to demonstrate any alteration in the early anaemia of prematurity by giving routine folate supplementation. The normal premature infant absorbs folic acid easily, and although there is no general recommendations for the prophylactic use of folic acid in newborn (Stockman and Oski, 1978), a dietary provision of 20–50 μg per day would ensure sufficiency.

There is an increased risk of megaloblastic anaemia occurring in the neonate of a folate-deficient mother, especially if delivery is pre-term. The pathogenesis of development of such an anaemia is shown in Figure 4.1. The young infant's requirement for folate has been estimated at 20–50 μg per day (four to ten times the adult requirement) on a weight basis. Serum and red cell folates are consistently higher in cord than in maternal blood, but the premature infant is in severe negative folate balance because of high growth rate and reduced intake. The usual fall in serum and red cell folate in the premature neonate, and even in the absence of other complicating factors, may result in megaloblastic anaemia. This can be prevented by giving supplements of 50 μg per day (Haworth and Evans, 1981). In those

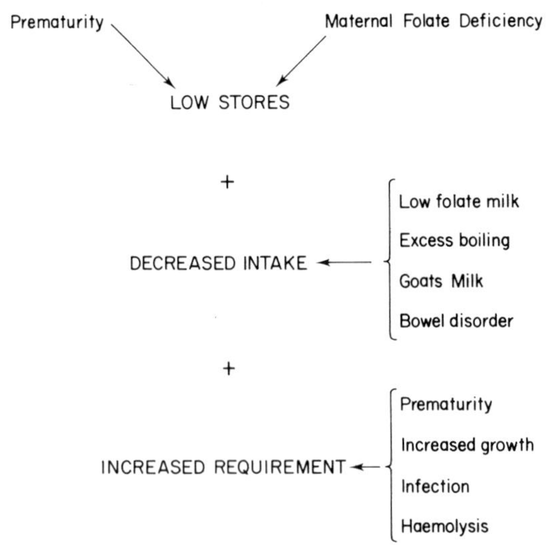

Figure 3.1 Factors contributing to the development of megaloblastic anaemia due to folate deficiency in infancy.

infants whose dietary intake would be predictably poor, such as the very immature or those with chronic diarrhoea or recurrent infections, it would appear wise to give parenteral folic acid at periodic intervals.

Vitamin B_{12}

Serum B_{12} levels in all neonates are generally higher than in maternal serum. This is the result of active transfer of vitamin B_{12} across the placenta to the fetus, at the expense of maintaining maternal vitamin B_{12} serum levels. This makes little impact on her own reserves because adult stores are of the order of 3000 μg or more and vitamin B_{12} stores in the newborn infant are about 50 μg (Roberts *et al.*, 1973). Because of these low storage reserves and because of poor dietary intake of vitamin B_{12} during the period of rapid growth, most premature infants will end up with lower than normal adult levels by the fourth or fifth month of life. There is probably no significant relationship between deficiency of vitamin B_{12} and the early anaemia of prematurity (cf. folic acid and iron deficiency).

The haemoglobin, red cell counts and haematocrit are similar in deficient and replete premature infants. Any supplements of these essential nutrients that are given to premature infants in the first few weeks of life are to prevent the late anaemia due to deficiencies that would inevitably develop by the fourth or fifth month of life.

Protein

Protein synthesis and turnover are increased in pre-term infants because of their very high metabolic rates. Adequate protein is necessary for healthy haemopoiesis and therefore dietary requirements for protein must be increased in these immature babies.

It has been shown (Ronnholm and Siimes, 1985) that human milk proteins promote general growth and erythropoiesis in very low birthweight infants. The beneficial effect particularly on erythropoiesis promoting higher haemoglobin concentration in the early weeks of life appears to be dependent on the human origin of this protein, and an uptake of 4 g kg^{-1} daily which is double the usual intake.

PATHOLOGICAL ANAEMIA IN THE NEONATE

Anaemia in the neonate can result from haemorrhage, haemolysis, or failure of red cell production (Table 4.1). Significant anaemia at birth is usually due to severe immune haemolysis or haemorrhage (Smith and Benjamin, 1968). Anaemia that becomes apparent after 24 hours is most often due to internal or external haemorrhage or non-immune haemolytic disorders. Infants with impaired red cell production do not usually develop anaemia until after 3

Table 3.1 Aetiology of anaemia in the newborn period.

Blood loss	Occult haemorrhage Obstetric accidents Internal haemorrhage Iatrogenic
Increased destruction	Immune haemolytic anaemia Infection Red cell enzyme and membrane disorders Haemoglobinopathies
Decreased production	Congenital red cell aplasia Infection Nutritional deficiencies Congenital leukaemia

weeks (Lubin and Vichinsky, 1979; Oski and Naiman, 1982). Reference red cell values for healthy term infants in the first week of life are given in Chapter 2. The rise in haemoglobin in the first 24 hours is due to shift of fluid from the intravascular to extravascular space (see above). An infant with a capillary haemoglobin below 14.5 g dl^{-1} in the first postnatal week should be regarded as anaemic. The site, and timing of samples taken is important, and reference to normal values at each stage of development is essential if data are to be interpreted correctly (see Chapter 2).

Anaemia resulting from haemorrhage

The causes of anaemia due to blood loss in the early neonatal period can be divided into three broad categories: haemorrhage due to obstetric accidents; occult blood loss and internal bleeding (Table 4.2).

Obstetric accidents

Umbilical vessels. Rupture of a normal umbilical cord may occur in an unattended precipitous delivery. Anaemia in the infant can result from haemorrhage from the cord and from internal bleeding due to trauma. The cord can also rupture in a normal delivery if there are vascular abnormalities such as an aneurysm, or if the cord is abnormally short or entangled around the fetus. Traction with forceps can result in rupture of the normal cord (Kirkman and Riley, 1959).

Haematomas of the cord, although rare, may contain large volumes of blood. A fetal mortality of over 47% has been reported associated with such blood loss (Irani, 1964).

Velamentous insertion of the umbilical cord has been reported to occur in 1% of all pregnancies (Earn, 1951). The umbilical vessels insert into the edge of the placenta — the vessels may rupture spontaneously or during labour, but most velamentous insertions of the cord do not rupture (Oski and

Table 3.2 Conditions associated with anaemia due to blood loss in the newborn.

Obstetric accidents	Rupture of normal umbilical cord Haematoma of cord or placenta Incision of placenta during caesarean section Placenta previa Abruptio placentae
Malformations of placenta and cord	Rupture of anomolous vessels Rupture of abnormal umbilical cord Velamentous insertion Vasa previa
Occult haemorrhage	Before birth or during delivery Fetomaternal: spontaneous traumatic amniocentesis external cephalic version Fetoplacental Twin to twin
Internal hacmorrhage	Intracranial Cephalhaematoma Retroperitoneal Ruptured liver Ruptured spleen Pulmonary
latrogenic blood loss	

Naiman, 1982). The incidence of fetal blood loss is estimated at 1–2% (Lubin, 1978). The condition is more common in twin than in singleton pregnancy, and where there is a low lying placenta.

The perinatal mortality rate, if the abnormal vessels do rupture, is high, many such infants being still-born in the past (Kirkman and Riley, 1959).

Placenta. Massive fetal haemorrhage can be associated with accidental incision of the placenta at caesarean section, placenta praevia or abruptio placentae. Lower segment caesarean section with anterior placentae can result in direct placental injury (Neligan and Russell, 1954). The placenta and membranes should always be examined for damage from the fetal side, following ceasarean section. Should such evidence be found, the haemoglobin of the infant should be estimated at birth and again 12–24 h later, because the initial haemoglobin may be normal. These estimations should also be carried out on all neonates born to mothers with unusual vaginal bleeding, placenta praevia or abruptio placentae. Placenta praevia is associated with anaemia in approximately 10% of the offspring (Novak, 1953) and, although abruptio placenta usually results in intra-uterine death, anaemia may well be present in surviving infants. Multilobed placentae may be associated with anomolous vessels crossing the internal os termed vaso praevia. The infant is in double jeopardy with vaso praevia, for the vessels may well be compressed as well as lacerated during the second stage of labour. The perinatal death rate ranges from 58 to 80% in these cases, the majority of infants being still-born (Kirkman and Riley, 1959). In the minority born alive, death often occurs during the first 24 hours because of unrecognized severe anaemia.

Occult haemorrhage before and during delivery

Occult loss before birth may be due to fetomaternal haemorrhage, twin-to-twin transfusion or fetoplacental haemorrhage.

Fetomaternal haemorrhage. Small numbers of fetal erythrocytes commonly enter the maternal circulation at some time during pregnancy. Occasionally these losses are of such magnitude as to cause anaemia, shock and, rarely, still-birth. This mode of occult blood loss is probably the commonest cause of anaemia in the newborn (Oski and Naiman, 1982).

Since Chown (1954) first demonstrated fetal erythrocytes in the maternal circulation by differential agglutination, many cases of fetomaternal bleeding have been reported. With improved methods of detecting fetal erythrocytes in the maternal circulation, it has been possible to identify losses of 0.5–40.0 ml of fetal blood into the maternal circulation (Cohen *et al.*, 1964). The acid elution technique of Kleihauer and Betke, for demonstration of fetal cells in a mixture containing maternal blood, is the simplest and most commonly used method. It depends on the fact that at low pH fetal haemoglobin resists acid elution whereas adult cells lose their haemoglobin leaving, after appropriate staining, a small number of deeply pigmented fetal cells in a sea of maternal ghost cells (Letsky and Sheerman-Chase, 1989). In adults, only 1% of the total haemoglobin is HbF. This small amount is restricted to approximately 8% of the total red cells. These cells are termed F cells — they contain very small amounts of HbF for the most part. Very occasionally, a maternal cell may contain up to 30% haemoglobin (Boyer *et al.*, 1975), but even a rare cell such as this is unlikely to cause confusion with a fetal cell, which will contain 60–80% fetal haemoglobin at term and stain deeply in a Kleihauer preparation. A rough quantitation of the volume of fetal blood lost, if small, can be made by comparing the number of fetal cells counted over a fixed period of time, with standard films made of known volumes of fetal blood mixed with adult blood. If the loss is large enough to figure as a percentage of the maternal cells, then a rough quantitation of the volume can be made using the fact that a fetal red cell count of 1% in the maternal circulation is indicative of a haemorrhage from the fetus in the range of 50 ml.

The identification of fetal cells by the acid elution method is limited in some situations. Where there is ABO blood group incompatibility between maternal and fetal red cells, the fetal cells may be rapidly removed from the maternal circulation by maternal antibody (Goodall *et al.*, 1958). Examination of the maternal buffy coat for erythrophagocytosis, and evidence of a rise in maternal immune anti-A or -B antibody in the weeks following delivery, provide presumptive evidence that a fetal blood loss occurred (Lubin, 1978). Genetic conditions that result in raised levels of fetal haemoglobin in the mother, such as hereditary persistence of fetal haemoglobin, sickle cell disease and heterozygous β thalassaemia, may give rise to difficulty in interpreting the results of the acid elution technique, and methods based on differential agglutination should be used.

The physiological increase in maternal haemoglobin of from 1.5 to 5.7% during pregnancy (Pembrey *et al.*, 1973) gives rise to a faint positive stain in red cells — not easily confused with fetal cells, which contain 60–80% fetal haemoglobin and stain intensely (Zipursky *et al.*, 1962). Fetal haemoglobin is relatively stable and, as well as resisting acid elution, the basis of the Kleihauer technique, it also resists alkali denaturation (Singer *et al.*, 1951). Strong alkali is added to a sample of the blood and the time it takes to denature to methaemoglobin (brown) compared with a similarly treated sample of adult blood. The alkali denaturation technique is not, however, as sensitive as the acid elution technique, and it cannot be used in the same way to quantitate fetomaternal bleeds because this would involve estimation of the total alkali resistant haemoglobin in the maternal circulation. A blood of 50 ml would raise the total fetal haemoglobin in the maternal circulation by only 1%. On the other hand, this technique, unlike the Kleihauer, is a rapid valuable bedside method of identifying the source of vaginal blood losses.

Although spontaneous fetomaternal bleeding usually occurs in the last trimester and there is an increased incidence during labour and delivery, transplacental fetal blood losses have been identified as early as 4–8 weeks' gestation (Zipursky *et al.*, 1963), and there may be chronic small blood losses throughout pregnancy as well as acute losses at or near parturition. The mechanism of passage of fetal cells into the maternal circulation is not fully understood. Erosions in the placental villi through which the cells could pass (Kline, 1948) and a correlation between occult placental haemorrhages and fetal red cells in the circulation (Wentworth, 1964) have been demonstrated. Occult fetal haemorrhages are associated with trauma incurred at amniocentesis, prenatal diagnostic fetal blood sampling, intra-uterine transfusions and external version of the fetus.

Fetomaternal transfusions during pregnancy may sensitize the mother if there are differences between fetal and maternal red cell antigens. In the case of possible Rhesus D [Rh(D)] incompatibility, the mother should be given an appropriate dose of Rh(D) immune globulin to prevent such sensitization (see Chapter 5). Usually such invasion of her circulation has no immediate adverse effect on the mother, but maternal transfusion reactions to the fetal blood have been described (Chown, 1954) and in one case led to acute renal failure (Pasternack *et al.*, 1966).

Fetoplacental haemorrhage. In some instances the blood lost from the fetus may not pass into the maternal circulation but may accumulate in the substances of the placenta (Chown, 1955) or retroplacentally (Kevy, 1962). Approximately 20% of the infant's blood volume may be lost into the placenta when there is a tight nuchal cord (Cashore and Usher, 1973). Holding the infant above the placenta before clamping the cord at delivery will result in continual loss of blood into the placenta. Decreased blood volumes in infants delivered by caesarean section, compared with those delivered vaginally, have been shown (Yao *et al.*, 1967; Kleinberg *et al.*,

1973), presumably due to holding the infant above the placenta. It has also been demonstrated in fetal lambs that, although intra-uterine asphyxia had little effect on neonatal blood volume, maternal hypotension immediately before delivery could lead to hypovolaemia in the neonate due to loss of blood into the placenta (Kitterman and Schleuter, 1974).

Twin-to-twin transfusion. In multiple pregnancy with dichorionic placentae, vascular anastamosis is uncommon. With monozygotic twins, a monochorial placenta is present in 70% of cases and twin-to-twin anastamosis occurs in almost every instance. It has been estimated that significant twin-to-twin transfusion occurs in 15% or more of all monochorial twins (Rausen *et al.*, 1965). The twin transfusion syndrome results in anaemia in the donor and polycythaemia in the recipient; there is significant morbidity and mortality in both (Fisk *et al.*, 1990). In a large series of multiple pregnancies studied by Rausen *et al.* (1965), two-thirds of all the twins known to have the twin transfusion syndrome did not survive the perinatal period. Significant anaemia at birth was not found in any of those that survived. The condition should be suspected in any pair of identical twins in whom the haemoglobin difference is greater than 5 g dl^{-1} at birth (Oski and Naiman, 1982).

The donor twin's haemoglobin may range from 3.7 to 18 g dl^{-1}, while haemoglobin values as high as 20–30 g dl^{-1} have been recorded in the recipient twin. If there has been chronic haemorrhage from one twin to the other there will be marked difference in birth-weight and organ size as well as haemoglobin levels. There may be hydramnios in the polycythaemic twin's sac and oligohydramnios in the donor sac. Disseminated intravascular coagulation has been described in the liveborn of sets of twins with a macerated still-born sibling (Moore *et al.*, 1969). The anaemic twin may develop congestive cardiac failure, whereas the plethoric twin may suffer from hyperviscosity and hyperbilirubinaemia. Kernicterus has been described (Bosma, 1954; Sacks, 1959). Polycythaemia may be seen in the neonate in the absence of twin-to-twin transfusion. It has been described as the result of maternal to fetal transfusion, in situations where no sensible explanation can be found, and in association with congenital adrenal hyperplasia (Oski and Naiman, 1982; see Chapter 4).

Internal haemorrhage

Damage to organs during traumatic delivery is the usual cause of internal bleeding in the neonate. The common sites of major haemorrhage are the subaponeurotic and subperiosteal spaces in the cranium, cerebral ventricles and subarachnoid space, liver, spleen, kidneys and lungs. Typical clinical signs of internal bleeding occur 24–72 h after birth, although problems can occur immediately after delivery (Lubin, 1978; Lubin and Vichinsky, Oski and Naiman, 1982).

Blood loss into the subaponeurotic space can be much greater than into the subperiosteum because it is not confined by periosteal attachments and can spread over the whole calvarium, but both forms of bleeding into the scalp can result in severe anaemia. Neonatal exsanguination has been described (Barrow and Peters, 1968; Robinson and Rossiter, 1968). On recovery from these enclosed haemorrhages, jaundice usually develops and may be severe enough to warrant exchange transfusion.

Life-threatening complications result from bleeding into the ventricles and subarachnoid space, particularly in the premature infant, and the outcome in terms of permanent damage in the surviving infant is unpredictable. The clinical manifestations of an intracranial haemorrhage include changes in vital signs, seizures, hypothermia, apnoea, a bulging fontanelle and anaemia. The quantity of blood loss into the spinal fluid may amount to as much as 15% of the infant's blood volume (Korobkin and Guilleminault, 1979). The diagnosis of subarachnoid haemorrhage in premature infants is difficult because of the frequency of traumatic taps (Lubin, 1978).

Rupture of the liver probably occurs more often than is clinically appreciated after traumatic delivery. In still-births and neonatal deaths an incidence of from 1.2 to 9.6% has been estimated (Brown, 1957). If the haemorrhage remains confined within the capsule of the liver, although there may be abdominal swelling decreased blood volume and anaemia, the haematoma may subside and the baby recover without complications. Should the capsule rupture, usually at 24–48 h but occasionally up to 4 days post-delivery (Lubin, 1978), the infant goes into shock coincident with the escape of blood into the peritoneal cavity. On examination, upper abdominal distension and shifting dullness will be found, and straight X-rays of the abdomen may reveal free fluid. The prognosis is poor, but some infants have survived with prompt surgical repair and blood transfusion (Lubin, 1978; Oski and Naiman, 1982).

Splenic rupture is unusal in the newborn infant but can occur after a difficult delivery or during exchange transfusion, most commonly in association with an enlarged spleen due to erythroblastosis fetalis (Philipsborn *et al.*, 1955). The condition has been described occasionally in large, healthy infants after an apparently normal delivery (Delta *et al.*, 1968).

Traumatic, particularly breech, deliveries are also associated with haemorrhages into the kidneys, adrenals and retroperitoneal space. Adrenal haemorrhage, like splenic rupture, has been described following the normal delivery of a large infant. Such haemorrhage will be accompanied by signs of renal insufficiency. Bluish discolouration of the skin of the flank, overlying a palpable mass, will suggest retroperitoneal haemorrhage, and

Table 3.3 Pallor in the newborn — differential diagnosis *

Acute blood loss	Asphyxia	Haemolytic disease
Blood pressure down	Response to oxygen	Hepatosplenamegaly
Tachycardia	Bradycardia	
Rapid shallow respiration	Recession	
Acyanotic	Cyanosis	Jaundice
No Jaundice	Moribund appearance	Positive direct antiglobulin (Coombs') test
Drop in haemoglobin	Stable haemoglobin	Anaemia

* Derived from Kirkman and Riley (1959).

should be differentiated from a solid tumour such as neuroblastoma. Bleeding into the retroperitoneal space can also be caused by perforation or rupture of an umbilical artery by catheterization (Van Leeuwen and Patney, 1969).

Premature infants on ventilation support may haemorrhage into the lungs and develop profound anaemia, often accompanied by disseminated intravascular coagulation (Cole *et al.*, 1973). Respiratory distress increases with impairment of perfusion and ventilation. Prognosis is poor and mortality is high.

Management of acute and chronic blood loss

The main differential diagnoses of pallor in the newborn and their clinical signs are listed in Table 3.3. It is essential to have a planned programme of management on delivery of a pale, distressed infant. Kirkman and Riley (1959) recommend a sensible routine, which has been modified for optimum management today.

(1) Maintain the airway and administer oxygen if necessary.

(2) Insert an umbilical catheter and take blood for haemoglobin estimation, grouping, bilirubin, Coomb's test cross-matching, blood gases and pH assessment.

(3) Promptly administer a plasma expander to maintain blood volume. Albumin 4.5% is the product of choice until suitable red cell replacement is available; it is sterile, rapidly available (cf. fresh frozen plasma) and is effective in small volume (cf. normal saline, with additional electrolyte problems).

(4) If the arterial and venous pressure have not returned to normal, repeat the procedure with red cell preparations of the appropriate group, correcting acidosis as required.

(5) Search for the cause of haemorrhage: carefully examine the infant, examine the placenta and cord, and check the maternal blood Kleihauer.

Infants who have suffered chronic blood loss *in utero* vary in their clinical state at delivery, from a hydropic infant with severe anaemia, requiring immediate resuscitation, to an asymptomatic, mildly anaemic, thriving neonate who will require only oral iron supplements, to raise the haemoglobin and replenish iron stores.

In summary, anaemia due to blood loss in the newborn infant may result from haemorrhage before, during or after delivery. Acute blood loss is poorly tolerated by the neonate and prompt diagnosis and treatment are essential for survival. Acute, severe blood loss during delivery results in a pale, shocked, hypovolaemic infant at birth, with a hemoglobin that is normal initially but falls rapidly within 6–8 hours. Jaundice and cyanosis are absent and the baby will respond to plasma volume expanders. The newborn infant who suffers internal haemorrhage following traumatic delivery rapidly deteriorates in hypovolaemic shock, 24–72 hours following delivery.

Special care and precautions should be taken when events known to be associated with, or to cause, fetal bleeding during pregnancy have occurred. For example, an unexpected maternal history suggestive of a transfusion reaction indicates loss of incompatible fetal cells into her circulation. Other conditions associated with fetal blood loss include twin pregnancies, abruptio placentae, vaso praevia, placenta previa and aminocentesis.

Anaemia due to haemolysis in the neonate

The essential feature of a haemolytic process is a shortening of the normal adult red cell (RBC) lifespan of 120 days. By this definition, virtually all term (RBC lifespan 80–100 days) and all premature (RBC lifespan 60–80 days) infants suffer from haemolysis.

In the adult, the classical triad of anaemia, reticulocytosis and hyperbilirubinaemia are the usual basic laboratory findings in any haemolytic process. In the newborn, however, features of haemolysis are more variable and, in particular, anaemia is not usually the presenting feature. Usually a haemolytic process is first detected in the investigation of jaundice occurring during the first week of life. To make the situation even more confusing, so-called physiological jaundice regularly occurs in the newborn period because of transient impaired hepatic bilirubin conjugation and increased bilirubin production. In the absence of haemolysis, bilirubin levels in term neonates are 205 $\mu mol\ l^{-1}$, with a peak at 4 days, and in premature infants 255 $\mu mol\ l^{-1}$ with a peak at 7 days (Glader and Platt, 1978). In the presence of haemolysis these levels are exceeded and clinical jaundice usually appears before 36 hours of age. In the newborn period jaundice due to haemolysis can occur despite minimal changes in the haemoglobin level, and without reticulocytosis, so that occasionally hyperbilirubinaemia is the only manifestation of neonatal haemolytic disease. Haemolysis is common in the newborn period and has multiple aetiologies, which can be broadly grouped into three large categories; iso-immunization, congenital defects of the red cell and acquired defects. In most parts of the world, the most important cause of haemolytic disease of the newborn is the production of maternal red cell antibodies against incompatible red cell antigens of the fetus; these are dealt with in Chapter 5.

Congenital defects of the red cell are discussed in Chapter 8. The acquired causes of haemolysis in the neonate are discussed below.

Anaemia associated with infection

Both intra-uterine and postnatal aquired infections are associated with anaemia and other haematological abnormalities in the neonatal period. Although these changes are sometimes produced by marrow suppression, severe neonatal infection is usually accompanied by haemolysis. Sometimes, particularly in acquired bacterial sepsis, the haemolytic process develops because of infection induced small vessel damage and resulting disseminated intravascular coagulation (DIC). This is a common complication of neonatal infection. DIC is always secondary to some other pathological process and, in the newborn, is commonly associated with asphyxia, respiratory distress syndrome, hypovolaemia and hypothermia, as well as with infection. Infants with DIC are very sick. Anaemia is only one of the many haematological and other problems arising from and associated with this process (see Chapter 6). The mainstay of management is to treat the underlying cause.

Intra-uterine infections commonly associated with haemolytic anaemia include toxoplasmosis, cytomegalovirus, congenital syphylis and rubella. The haemolytic process in these cases is thought to arise from reticulo-endothelial hyperplasia or direct injury to the red cell membrane. Occasionally an antibody produced against the infecting organism cross-reacts with an antigen on the surface of the red cell, an apparent autoantibody, which may give a positive direct anti-globulin (Coombs') test.

The clinical and haematological picture in congenital infection may resemble that seen with haemolytic disease of the newborn due to blood group incompatibility. Hepatosplenomegaly, anaemia with reticulocytosis, large numbers of circulating erythroblasts, and hyperbilirubinaemia are common features. The laboratory distinction can usually be made by finding increased IgM, a negative direct Coombs' test and antibody titres against specific infecting microorganisms, and direct harvesting of the infective agent from urine or blood. The bilirubin is usually predominantly conjugated. Clinically there are distinctive features of congenital infection such as chorioretinitis and cerebral calcification. It is not appropriate to deal with the diagnosis and investigation of all congenital neonatal infections here. The reader is referred to a recent review of perinatal infections (Freij and Sever, 1988).

Severe infection in the neonate can produce some very bizarre changes accompanying anaemia, whether the anaemia is due to haemolysis or suppression of erythropoiesis. There may be thrombocytopenia and bruising in the absence of DIC, together with leucocytosis and an increase of circulating immature white cells and even frank blasts.

In the first 24 hours of life the neutrophil count rises in both term and premature infants. Approximately 60% of the cells are granulocytes in the following few days, and the count remains relatively stable. The total count is greater than in the adult. Band forms and myelocytes are commonly seen, and occasionally promyelocytes or even blast cells are seen in the healthy term infant (see Chapter 2), although these immature forms are more frequently seen in the premature infant (Xanthou, 1970).

Somewhere between the 4th and 14th days the total count falls and the lymphocyte becomes the predominant cell, remaining so throughout early childhood (Rosse *et al.*, 1977). Under stressed conditions, neonatal neutrophils have a reduced phagocytic and bacteriocidal activity (Engle *et al.*, 1983). There is a reduced total granulocyte pool and the response to severe infection is more often neutropenia than neutrophilia. The neutrophil count is raised more frequently in the first week of life, in association with maternal hypertension, haemolytic disease, intraventricular haemorrhage and birth asphyxia (Manroe *et al.*, 1979). Consequently, it has been suggested that band forms and maturer neutrophils, expressed as a proportion of the total granulocyte cells, will give a better indication of whether the infant is infected.

In my opinion, these counts may be difficult to assess and are not useful; monocytes and degranulated band forms are often confused. The total white cell count is a much better indicator and prognostic sign, neutropenia indicating severe infection and carrying a poor prognosis. The morphology of the cells may also be helpful. 'Moth-eaten', 'shattered' vacuolated neutrophils, which are poorly granulated, are often seen in association with severe overwhelming infection. In the less acute situation, however, we are often left with a bizarre blood picture arising in an infant who is unwell and has clinical signs suggestive of infection, although the offending organism cannot be identified.

Recently, a term baby born normally to a healthy mutligravid mother at Queen Charlotte's was noted to be pale on routine second-day examination, with slight but definite splenomegaly and a few petechiae. The haemoglobin was 11.1 g dl^{-1}, the total white cell count 28 000 cm^{-3} with 30% eosinophils and 11% frank blasts; the platelet count was 30 000 cm^{-3}. The baby was sleepy and slow to feed but otherwise normal. The bone marrow aspirate contained the same proportion of blasts as the peripheral blood. The baby's haematological picture gradually improved over the next 2 weeks without treatment, as did his clinical state. At 3 months of age he was thriving and completely normal both haematologically and clinically. Extensive investigation of both mother and baby at birth and in the subsequent weeks failed to provide any clue as to the source or identity the stimulus of this transient leukaemoid reaction. In particular, no evidence for toxoplasmosis could be found (a neonatal infection in which both eosinophilia and circulating white cell blast forms have been described).

Parvovirus

Infective agents such as rubella, cytomegalovirus, toxoplasmosis, herpes simplex and vaccinia are now well-established causes of fetal damage leading to fetal loss, severe fetal or neonatal disease and congenital abnormality. More recently, reports have indicated that maternal infection with human parvovirus B19 may lead to intra-uterine infection and fetal damage (Anderson, 1987; Blacklock, 1989; Brown, 1989; Samra *et al.*, 1989). This virus deserves more detailed discussion as a cause of fetal and neonatal anaemia as it appears to have a direct effect on haematopoiesis by involving the erythron and resulting in red cell aplasia.

Although first described in patients with sickle cell disease, it is now well known that parvovirus B19 virus can induce aplastic crises in patients with a wide variety of chronic haemolytic conditions. The usual manifestation in patients without haemolysis is an exanthematous disease, mainly of schoolchildren, occurring in localized outbreaks in winter and spring. The condition is known variably as erythema infectiosum, fifth disease, slapped cheek disease or academic disease. The erythema of the facial rash gives the 'slapped cheek' appearance. There may also be a fine lacy reticular rash on legs, buttocks, neck and trunk. There may be a coryzal prodrome and gastrointestinal upset, but most children feel well. In adults, polyarthralgia is the dominant clinical expression, lasting days or weeks. However, infections may be asymptomatic in both children and adults (Smith and Ryan, 1988). Diagnosis in the adult is usually by serological methods; radioimmunoassay and enzyme linked immunoabsorbent assay are available for the detection of anti-virus specific IgM and IgG.

Early in infection there is an intense viraemia, but parvovirus B19 antigen and B19 DNA detectable by nucleic acid hybridisation are only present in the blood in the prodrome of the illness. The similarity of erythema infectiosum to rubella led investigators to look for evidence of fetal damage even before the organism had been identified. There appears to be no evidence of teratogenicity but there are increasing reports of hydrops fetalis associated with documented maternal parvovirus B19 infection, particularly if the infection occurs in the first half of pregnancy (Anderson, 1987; Anand *et al.*, 1987; Carrington *et al.*, 1987; Brown, 1989; Naides and Weiner, 1989; Samra *et al.*, 1989). The association of maternal infection with fetal hydrops is signficant, but numbers are too small to give a risk factor. However, it is clear that many infected women deliver healthy babies at term (Kinney *et al.*, 1988).

Using a recently developed molecular biological technique of *in situ* DNA hybridization it has been possible to identify specific viral DNA in fixed paraffin-embedded tissue. Four of thirteen fetuses with previously unexplained non-immunological hydrops fetalis were found to be positive using this technique with the parvovirus probe, in an Oxford study of 50 cases of non-immunological hydrops examined over the period 1974 to 1983 (Porter *et al.*, 1988). In one series of 42 women who contracted B19 infection after contact with erythema infectiosum at varying stages of gestation, three pregnancies were terminated, 29 (74%) had no fetal complications and 10 (26%) developed hydrops fetalis (Schwarz *et al.*, 1988).

At present, neither the frequency of B19 infection in pregnancy, nor the time in gestation at which the fetus is most at risk of hydrops is known. It is important, therefore, to identify those fetuses at risk so that appropriate management of the pregnancy can be planned.

The pathogenesis of hydrops fetalis associated fetal manifestations of parvovirus B19 infection was thought to be due to invasion of erythroid progenitor cells resulting in aplastic anaemia. However hybridization studies have demonstrated B19 DNA in infected fetuses in practically every organ studied, including brain, lung, spleen, kidneys, cord blood and placenta (Carrington *et al.*, 1987; Van-Elsackier-Niele *et al.*, 1989).

Maternal infection early in gestation may result in spontaneous abortion — with widespread infection of tissues or elective termination — but there has never been evidence of an embryopathy. Infection later in the first half of pregnancy may result in hydrops. Maternal infection late in gestation is not usually associated with fetal damage. These findings can be explained. Parvovirus has a prediliction for actively dividing cells and, in children and adults, the virus selectivity infects erythropoietic tissue. All tissues are dividing rapidly in the very young fetus and may therefore be infected, resulting in early fetal death. The fetus increases its red cell mass about 34-fold between the 3rd and 6th month of age, with a rapid turnover, and this may explain the predominant erythroid infection with aplastic anaemia and hydrops which is associated with infection later in gestation (Knisely *et al.*,

1988). The relative reduction in cell turnover may protect the fetus in the latter half of pregnancy (Van Elsacker Niele *et al.*, 1989).

Very recently Porter *et al.* (1990) reported the demonstration of human parvovirus in fetal tissues using combined non-isotopic *in situ* hybridization and immuno-histochemistry on routine histopathological fixed sections. They showed parvovirus DNA in macrophages–myocytes and also within myocardial fibrils, as well as in erythroblasts. This would explain the rapid development of hydrops *in utero* combining the devastating effects of profound anaemia and anoxia together with myocarditis, resulting in complete cardiac failure.

How can prenatal diagnosis of the infected fetus be established? Demonstration of IgM-specific anti-parvovirus antibody in the maternal serum will indicate recent infection. The risk to the fetus will depend on the time during gestation of maternal infection, and overall the majority will be unscathed. It has been suggested (Carrington *et al.*, 1987; Bernstein and Capeless, 1989) that maternal serum α-fetoprotein may be a marker of fetal aplastic crises during parvovirus infection. Human parvovirus is found in abundance in the liver, the site of α-fetoprotein production and also the major haemopoietic organ in the second trimester of pregnancy. Viral damage may release α-fetoprotein which is then transferred to the maternal circulation. Maternal α-fetoprotein levels might be useful in predicting outcome, by indicating the need for ultrasound screening and fetal blood sampling. Amniotic fluid analysis using hybridization techniques may identify the virus. Fetal blood sampling is useful in several respects. Effects on haemopoiesis, namely anaemia and leucopenia, will be immediately apparent. The virus may be detected and antibodies can be measured.

Therapy has only been attempted in a very few cases. Intra-uterine exchange transfusion has been performed in two hydropic fetuses, with favourable outcomes (Schwarz *et al.*, 1988), and these are now being followed up. One report (Naides and Weiner, 1988) describes a case of hydrops at 22 weeks' gestation, in which the cardiac failure appeared to be due to mycarditis and not to profound anaemia. The parvovirus was identified in ascitic fluid and in the mycardial fibrils post mortem. The fetal haemoglobin concentration was normal for gestation. The fetus was treated by direct administrations of digoxin. This was useful in palliation of fetal congestive heart failure, reduction of ascites, pericardial effusion and decreased heart rate, but it did not prevent fetal demise on the 5th day following digitalization.

Congenital malaria

Malaria remains a major health hazard in many parts of the world with at least 100–150 million cases leading to over one million deaths annually. In endemic areas, despite the greater prevalence of malaria among pregnant women, vertical transmission is thought to be rare and is not thought to play an epidemiologically important role. The rare identification of congenital malaria is accounted for by three factors — the placental barrier, the maternal immune mechanism and the composition of neonatal blood. The placenta is a preferential site of reproduction and growth for the malarial parasite. Despite a maternal blood film that may be free of parasites, asexual schizont forms may be demonstrated in enormous numbers in the intervillous spaces. The placenta is a relative and not an absolute barrier. The transmission rates, as defined by finding malarial parasites in thick films of cord blood have been quoted as ranging from 2 to 44% over the years 1932–1978 (see Meerstadt, 1986), with higher frequencies in the later reports. The parasite density in cord blood is light and may be easily missed, so the figures are likely to be an underestimation.

Maternal immunoglobulins passively acquired antenatally or during breast feeding may offer the newborn infant temporary protection. Parasites coated by immunoglobulin are rapidly cleared from the blood stream, but they are not necessarily eradicated and may lie dormant. Fetal haemoglobin has a retardant effect — maximal at birth, whatever the gestation — on the malarial parasite.

Because of these factors, if the parasites are not eradicated they may enter a latent phase. Even in non-immune individuals congenital malaria rarely presents before 3–4 weeks of age. A more prolonged latent phase would occur in infants with a high degree of passive immunity. In endemic areas, such cases presenting after several weeks or even months would be classified wrongly as acquired malaria.

Due largely to ease of travel to endemic areas and to failure of travellers to take adequate prophylactic measures, there has been an increasing number of cases of malaria both in the United Kingdom (Meerstadt, 1986) and the United States in recent years (Quinn *et al.*, 1982, Malviya and Shurin, 1984, Naeye, 1988), and reports of isolated cases of congenital malaria and reviews of the not very extensive literature. In these case reports, there is obviously no doubt about the vertical transmission of the infection.

All three species of the human malaria parasite are known to cause congenital infections. Severe fetal infection is incompatible with life, and parasites can be found in the brain, liver and spleen as well as the red cells of the still-born infant. The transfer of parasitized maternal red cells presumably often takes place at delivery so that the baby is apparently normal at birth and sometimes does not present with the maternally acquired infection until weeks or even months post-natally, unless a careful search for the offending parasite is made.

Malaria in the pregnant woman, because it is so unusual (Meerstadt, 1986), causes a great concern in the United Kingdom, but the possible transfer of infection to the fetus is not widely appreciated. Two such cases, one born at Queen Charlotte's recently, suffered life-threatening parasitaemia with profound haemolytic anaemia in the late neonatal period. In both cases the mothers were undergoing treatment for active malaria acquired abroad — one presenting in the puerperium as pyrexia of unknown origin. Signs of malaria in the newborn infant include fever and irritability. Hepatosplenamegaly and IgM antibodies in the cord blood may be found, but not always, if the infection has been acquired prenatally. The placenta and cord blood of any baby born to a mother known to have or to have had active malaria should be examined carefully. Parasitized cells tend to concentrate in the placental bed and asexual forms in the intervillous spaces, and they are sometimes found when the mother is apparently clear of infection at delivery. Treatment should be instituted immediately if there is any suggestion that there has been transfer of maternal parasites. In any case, there should be careful supervision of the infant for at least 2 months post-delivery. One infant reported in the United States had a haematocrit of 12.1% at 7 weeks of age with a 10.0% reticulocytosis (Malviya and Shurin, 1984).

Most cases of congenital malaria in non-endemic areas are initially misdiagnosed because of a general lack of awareness of the disease and its non-specific clinical features. In all four cases reported by Quinn *et al.* (1982), and in those few I have knowledge of in the United Kingdom, the admitting diagnosis in the late neonatal period was sepsis, and malaria was only considered when the offending parasite was seen in large numbers when the blood film was examined in the haematology laboratory. The newborn does not usually present with the classical febrile paroxysms with chills and sweats. Non-specific symptoms, such as irritability, poor feeding, lethargy, vomiting and diarrhoea, are associated with anaemia, which is usually very severe. The diagnosis of congenital malaria requires a high index of suspicion and the ability to recognize the parasite on a suitable tissue preparation, preferably from the placental bed at delivery, when measures can be taken to eradicate it and to prevent the severe sequelae.

Haemolytic anaemia due to maternal auto-immune disease

The rare combination of auto-immune haemolytic anaemia (AIHA) and pregnancy carries great risks to both the woman herself and the fetus. The degree of haemolysis in the fetus depends mainly on the amount and avidity of the transferred antibody for the fetal red cells. Although pregnancy may result in exacerbation of disseminated lupus erythematosis (DLE), up to 50% of women with this condition are reported to improve during pregnancy, especially in the third trimester. Haemolytic anaemia, leukopenia and thrombocytopenia have all been observed in infants of women with active disease, presumably due to IgG antibody, involved in the disease process, crossing the placenta. Administration of prednisone, 2 mg kg^{-1} per day, to the mother with prenatally active AIHA may both reduce maternal haemolysis and reduce neonatal morbidity. Management of the newborn, as in other cases of neonatal haemolysis, is directed primarily to anticipating and treating hyperbilirubinaemia to prevent kernicterus (see Chapter 5).

Rarely immune maternal antibody associated with drug administration may cause haemolysis in the newborn. The most likely situation in which this can occur is if the mother has immune IgG penicillin antibody and it has crossed the placenta, and her new-born baby is treated with penicillin. Penicillin forms a hapten with red cell membranes. The newborn red cell is damaged when the penicillin and maternally-derived penicillin antibody react. One such case is reported in the literature. Haemolysis ceases when administration of the drug is stopped.

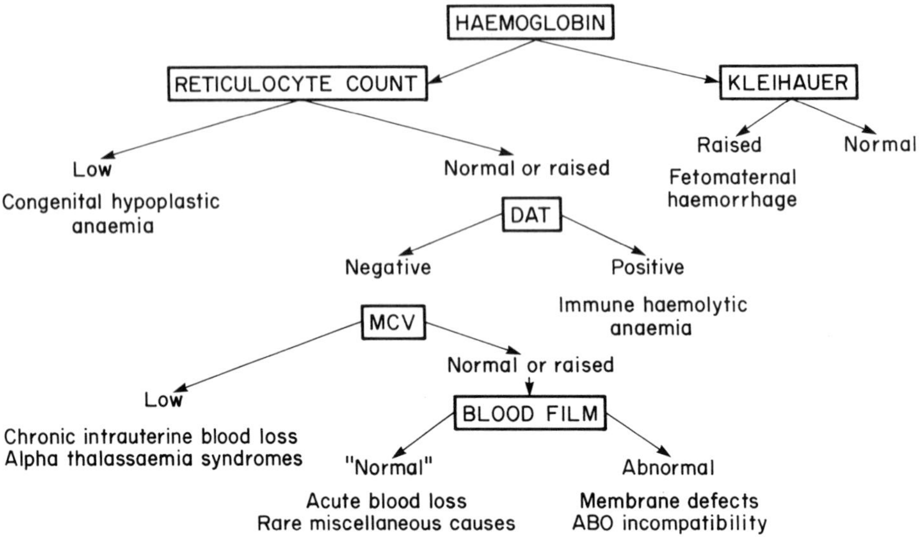

Figure 3.2 Practical approach to differential diagnosis of anaemia in the neonate.

Auto-immune haemolytic anaemia (AIHA)

AIHA has been reported in association with a variety of clinical conditions other than those already referred to. Neoplastic conditions include chronic lymphatic leukaemia, malignant lymphoma and teratoma. It may also occur in the course of both infectious mononucleosis and mycoplasma pneumonia. The diagnosis rests on the demonstration of auto-antibodies directed against red cell surface antigens. In practice this is detected by a positive direct antiglobulin (Coombs') test. Most of these antibodies detected at 37°C are of the IgG subclass. A major concern is the possibility of severe fetal haemolysis resulting from passage of maternal IgG antibodies across the placenta. It has been suggested that fetal outcome is a reflection of the severity of the maternal illness, but a review of published cases (Sacks *et al.*, 1981) showed no such relationship. In this respect the condition seems to resemble maternal autoimmune thrombocytopenia. Fetal and neonatal deaths have been reported in association both with severe maternal autohaemolysis and with mild controlled anaemia.

Because of the unpredictable risk of severe haemolysis in the fetus in association with maternal IgG antibody serial ultrasound examinations should be undertaken with amniocentesis. If there is any doubt about the severity of fetal haemolysis fetal blood sampling should be undertaken and appropriate therapy instituted if indicated. This may include maternally administered steroids, both maternal or fetal administration of intravascular immunoglobulin or, in certain cases, fetal blood transfusion. Prior to planned delivery, blood which is the least incompatible with the maternal antibody should be available both to replace maternal blood loss and for neonatal exchange transfusion should this prove necessary. The neonate should be monitored carefully for haemolysis, jaundice and persistence of maternal antibody (Sacks *et al.*, 1981).

REFERENCES

Anand A, Gray ES, Brown T, Clewley JP and Cohen BJ (1987) Human parvovirus infection in pregnancy and hydrops fetalis. *New England Journal of Medicine* **316**: 183–186.

Anderson LJ (1987) Role of parvovirus B19 in human disease. *Pediatric Infectious Diseases Journal* **6**: 711–718.

Anderson LJ and Torok TJ (1989) Human parvovirus B19. *New England Journal of Medicine* **321**: 536–538.

Anon. (1989) Erythropoietin reaches the pharmacy. *The Lancet* **ii**: 1252–1254.

Bard H and Prosmann J (1982) Postnatal fetal and adult haemoglobin synthesis in preterm infants whose birthweight was less than 1,000 grams. *Journal of Clinical Investigation* **70**: 50–52.

Barrow E and Peters RL (1968) Exsanguinating haemorrhage into the scalp in newborn infants. *South African Medical Journal* **42**: 265–267.

Bernstein IM and Capeless EL (1989) Elevated maternal serum alpha-fetoprotein and hydrops fetalis in association with fetal parvovirus B-19 infection. *Obstetrics and Gynecology 73*: 456–457.

Blacklock H (1989) Human parvovirus infections — a haematological perspective: any relevance to New Zealand Health? *New Zealand Medical Journal* **102**: 436–437.

Blanchette VS and Zipursky A (1984) Assessment of anaemia in newborn infants. *Clinics in Perinatology* **11**: 489–510.

Bosma JH (1954) Autotransfusion between two twins. *American Journal of Diseases in Children* **88**: 509.

Boyer SH, Belding TK, Margolet L and Noyes AN (1975) Fetal haemoglobin restriction to a few erythrocytes (F cells) in normal human adults. *Science* **188**: 361–363.

Brown JJM (1957) Hepatic haemorrhage in the newborn. *Archives of Disease in Childhood* **32**: 480–483.

Brown JE (1989) What threat is human parvovirus B19 to the fetus? A review. *British Journal of Obstetrics and Gynaecology* **96**: 764–767.

Brown MS, Garcia JF, Phibbs RH and Dallman PR (1984) Decreased response to plasma immunoreactive erythropoietin to 'available oxygen' in anaemia of prematurity. *Journal of Pediatrics* **105**: 793–798.

Carrington D, Gilmore DH, Whittle MJ *et al.*, (1987) Maternal serum α fetoprotein — a marker of fetal aplastic crisis during intrauterine human parvovirus infection. *The Lancet* **i**: 433–435.

Cashore WJ and Usher RH (1973) Hypovolaemia resulting from a tight nuchal cord at birth. *Pediatric Research* **7**: 399.

Chown B (1954) Anaemia from bleeding of the fetus into the mother's circulation. *The Lancet* **i**: 1213–1215.

Chown B (1955) The fetus can bleed. *American Journal of Obstetrics and Gynecology* **70**: 1298–1308.

Christensen RD (1989) Recombinant erythropoietic growth factors as an alternative to erythrocyte transfusion for patients with 'anaemia of prematurity'. *Pediatrics* **83**: 793–796.

Cohen F, Zuelzer WW, Gustafson DC and Evans MM (1964) Mechanism of isoimmunisation. I. The transplacental passage of fetal erythrocytes in homospecific pregnancies. *Blood* **23**: 621–646.

Cole VA, Norman ICS, Reynolds EOR and Rivers RPA (1973) Pathogenesis of hemorrhagic pulmonary edema and massive pulmonary hemorrhage in the newborn. *Pediatrics* **51**: 175–187.

Committee on Nutrition, American Academy of Pediatrics (1985) Nutritional needs of low birthweight infants. *Pediatrics* **75**: 976–986.

Curran JS and Cantolino SJ (1978) Vitamin E (injectable) administration in the prevention of retinopathy in prematurity: Evaluation with fluorescein angiography and fundus photography. *Pediatric Research* **12**: 404 (Abstr.)

Dallman PR (1977) In *Pediatrics* (Rudolph AM, ed.), 16th edn, p 1178. New York: Appleton-Century-Crofts.

Dallman PR (1984) Erythropoietin and the anemia of prematurity. *Journal of Pediatrics* **105**: 756–757.

Dallman PR (1987) Iron deficiency and related nutritional anaemias. In *Hematology of Infancy and Childhood* (Nathan D and Oski FA, eds) pp 274–314. Philadelphia: W.B. Saunders Co.

Davenport M (1986) Neonatal malaria and obstructive jaundice. *Archives of Disease in Childhood* **61**: 515–517.

Delta BG, Eisenstein EM and Rothenberg AM (1968) Rupture of a normal spleen in the newborn: report of a survival and review of the literature. *Clinical Pediatrics* **7**: 373–376.

Earn AA (1951) Placental anomalies. *Canadian Medical Association Journal* **134**: 1157–1166.

Ehrenkranz RA (1980) Vitamin E and the neonate. *American Journal of Disease in Children* **134**: 1157–1166.

Engle WA, Schreiner RL, Baehner RL (1983) Neonatal white blood cell disorders. *Seminars in Perinatology* **7**: 184–200.

Fenton V, Cavill I and Fisher J (1977) Iron stores in pregnancy. *British Journal of Haematology* **37**: 145–149.

Finer NN, Peters KL, Hayek K and Merkel Cl (1984) Vitamin E and necrotizing enterocolitis. *Pediatrics* **73**: 387–393.

Fisk NM, Borrell A, Hubinont C, Tannirandorn Y, Nicolini U and Rodeck CH (1990) Feto-fetal transfusion syndrome: do the neonatal criteria apply *in utero*? *Archives of Disease in Childhood*, in press.

Freij BJ and Sever JL (eds) (1988) Infectious complications of pregnancy, *Clinics in Perinatology* **15**(2).

Glader BE and Platt O (1978) Haemolytic disorders of infancy. *Clinics in Haematology* **7**: 35–61.

Goodall HB, Frances S, Graham FS, Miller MD and Cameron C (1958) Transplacental bleeding from the fetus. *Journal of Clinical Pathology* **11**: 251–260.

Grose C, Itani O and Weiner CP (1989) Prenatal diagnosis of fetal infection; advances from amniocentesis of cardocentesis — congenital toxoplasmosis, rubella, cytomegalovirus, varicella virus, parvovirus and human immunodeficiency virus. *Pediatric Infectious Diseases Journal* **8**: 459–468.

Hassan H, Hashim SA, Van Itallis TB and Sebrell WH (1966) Syndrome in premature infants associated with low plasma vitamin E levels and high polyunsaturated fatty acid diet. *American Journal of Clinical Nutrition* **19**: 147–157.

Halperin DS, Wacker P, Lacourt G *et al.* (1990) Effects of recombinant human erythropoietin in infants with the anaemia of prematurity; a pilot study. *Journal of Pediatrics* **9**: 779–786.

Haworth C and Evans DIK (1981) Nutritional aspects of blood disorders in the newborn. *Journal of Human Nutrition* **35**: 323–334.

Holland BM and Wardrop CA (1990) in (Arander J, Harvey D and Rylance G, eds) *Pharmacology of Newborn Infant Oxygen Transport by the Blood — Haematinics and Blood Cell Component Therapy in the Neonate*. Butterworth, London.

Irani PK (1964) Haematoma of the umbilical cord. *British Medical Journal* **2**: 1436–1437.

Jacobs K, Shoemaker C, Rudersdorf R *et al.* (1975) Isolation and characterization of genomic and DNA clones of human erythropoietin. *Nature* **313**: 806–810.

Kevy S (1962) Clinical pathologic conference. *Journal of Pediatrics* **60**: 304–314.

Kinney JS, Anderson LJ, Farrar J, *et al.* (1988) Risk of adverse outcomes of pregnancy after human parvovirus B19 infection. *Journal of Infectious Diseases* **157**: 663–667.

Kirkman HN and Riley HD (1959) Post-hemorrhagic anemia and shock in the newborn: a review. *Pediatrics* **24**: 97–105.

Kitterman JA and Schleuter MA (1974) Effects of intrauterine asphyxia on neonatal blood volume (Abstract). *Pediatric Research* **8**: 447.

Kleinberg E, Phibbs R and Dong L (1973) Lack of placenta to infant transfusion with delayed cord clamping after Caesarean section delivery (Abstract). *Pediatric Research* **7**: 403.

Kline BS (1948) Microscopic observations of the placental barrier in transplacental erythroblastosis fetalis in normal pregnancy. *American Journal of Obstetrics and Gynecology* **56**: 226–237.

Knisely AS, O'Shea PA, McMillan P, Singer DB and Magid MS (1988) Electron microscopic identification of parvovirus virions in erythroid-line cells in fetal hydrops fetalis. *Pediatric Pathology* **8**: 163–170.

Korobkin R and Guilleminault C (eds) (1979) *Advances in Perinatal Neurology*, vol 1. London: SP Medical and Scientific Books.

Letsky EA and Sheerman-Chase J (1989) Kleihauer. In *Laboratory Haematology*. (Chanarin I, ed.) pp 161–165. Churchill Livingstone, Edinburgh.

Lubin BH (1978) Neonatal anaemia secondary to blood loss. *Clinics in Haematology* **7**: 19–34.

Lubin B and Vichinsky E (1979) Anemia in the Newborn Period. *Pediatric Annals* **8**: 416–434.

Lundstrom L, Siimes MA and Dallman PR (1977) At what age does iron supplementation become necessary in low birthweight infants? *Journal of Pediatrics* **91**: 878–883.

Malviya S and Shurin SJB (1984) Congenital malaria. Case report and review. Clinical Pediatrics **23**: 516–517.

Manroe BL, Weinburg AG, Rosenfeld CR and Browne R (1979) The neonatal blood count in health and disease. I. Reference values for neutrophilic cells. *Journal of Pediatrics* **95**: 89–98.

Meerstadt PW (1986) Congenital malaria. Review article. *Clinical and Experimental Obstetrics and Gynecology* **13**: 78–82.

Melhorn DK, Gross S and Childers G (1971) Vitamin E-dependent anaemia in the premature infant. I. Effects of large doses of medicinal iron. *Journal of Pediatrics* **79**: 569–580.

Moore CM, McAdams AJ and Sutherland JM (1969) Intrauterine disseminated Intravascular coagulation: a syndrome of multiple pregnancy with a dead twin fetus. *Journal of Paediatrics* **74**: 523–528.

Naeye RL (1988) Antenatal malarial infections. Review article. *Progress in Clinical and Biological Research* **281**: 165–173.

Naides SJ and Weiner CP (1989) Antenatal diagnosis and palliative treatment of non-immune hydrops fetalis secondary to fetal parvovirus B19 infection. *Prenatal Diagnosis* **9**: 105–114.

Neligan GA and Russell JK (1954) Blood loss from the foetal circulation, a hazard of lower segment Caesarian section in cases of placenta previa. *Journal of Obstetrics and Gynaecology of the British Empire* **61**: 206–212.

Novak F (1953) Post-haemorrhagic shock in newborns during labor and after delivery. *Acta Medica Jugoslavica* **7**: 280–292.

Oski FA (1979) Nutritional Anaemias. *Seminars in Perinatology* **3**: 381–395.

Oski FA and Barness LA (1967) Vitamin E deficiency: A previously unrecognised cause of hemolytic anemia in the premature infant. *Journal of Pediatrics* **70**: 211–220.

Oski FA and Naiman JL (1982) *Hematologic Problems in the Newborn*, 3rd edn. WB Saunders and Co., Philadelphia.

Pasternack A, Furuhjelm V, Von Knoring J, Skrefvars B and Kuhlback B (1966) Acute renal failure after haemolysis probably due to foeto-maternal transfusion. *Acta Medica Scandinavica* **180**: 13–15.

Pembrey ME, Weatherall DJ and Clegg JB (1973) Maternal Synthesis of Haemoglobin F in pregnancy. *The Lancet* **i**: 1350–1355.

Philipsborn HJ Jr., Traisman HS, Greer D Jr. (1955) Rupture of the Spleen: A complication of erythroblastosis fetalis. *New England Journal of Medicine* **252**: 159–162.

Phillips HM, Holland BM, Jones JG, Abdel-Moiz AL, Turner TL, Wardrop CAJ (1988) Definitive estimate of rate of haemoglobin switching: measurement of percent hemoglobin F in neonatal reticulocytes. *Pediatric Research* **23**: 595–597.

Playfair JHL, Wolfendale MR and Kay HEM (1963) The leucocytes of peripheral blood in the human fetus. *British Journal of Haematology* **9**: 336–344.

Porter HJ, Khong TY, Evans MF, Chan VT-W and Fleming KA (1988) parvovirus as a cause of hydrops fetalis: detection by in situ DNA hybridisation. *Journal of Clinical Pathology* **41**: 381–383.

Porter HJ, Heryet A, Quantrill AM and Fleming KA (1990) Combined non-isotopic in situ hybridisation and immunohistochemistry on routine paraffin wax embedded tissue: identification of cell type infected by human parvovirus and demonstration of cytomegalovirus DNA and antigen in renal infection. *Journal of Clinical Pathology* **43**: 129–132.

Quinn TC, Jacobs RF, Mertz GJ, Hook EW III and Locksley RM (1982) Congenital malaria: A report of four cases and a review. *Journal of Pediatrics* **2**: 229–232.

Rausen R, Seki M and Strauss L (1965) Twin transfusion syndrome. *Journal of Pediatrics* **66**: 613–628.

Rhondeau SM, Christensen RD, Ross MP, Rothstein G and Simmons MA (1988) Responsiveness to recombinant human erythropoietin of marrow erythroid progenitors from infants with the 'anaemia of prematurity'. *Journal of Pediatrics* **112**: 935–940.

Roberts PD, James H, Petrie A, Morgan JO and Hoffbrand AV (1973) Vitamin B_{12} status in pregnancy among immigrants to Britain. *British Medical Journal* **iii**: 67–72.

Robinson RJ and Rossiter MA (1968) Massive subaponeurotic haemorrhage in babies of African origin. *Archives of Disease in Childhood* **43**: 684–687.

Ronnholm KAR and Siimes MA (1985) Haemoglobin concentration depends on protein intake in small preterm infants fed human milk. *Archives of Disease in Childhood* **60**: 99–104.

Rosse C, Kraemer MJ, Dillon TL, McFarland R and Smith NJ (1977) Bone marrow cell population of normal infants: the predominance of lymphocytes. *Journal of Laboratory and Clinical Medicine* **89**: 1225–1240.

Sacks MO (1959) Occurence of anemia and polycythemia in phenotypically dissimilar single ovum human twins. *Pediatrics* **24**: 604–608.

Sacks DA, Platt LD and Johnson CS (1981) Autoimmune hemolytic disease during pregnancy. *American Journal of Obstetrics and Gynecology* **140**: 942–945.

Samra JS, Obhrai MS and Constantine G (1989) Parvovirus infection in pregnancy. *Obstetrics and Gynecology* **73**: 832–834.

Schwarz TF, Roggendorf M, Hottenträger B *et al.* (1988) Human parvovirus B19 infection in pregnancy. *The Lancet* **iii**: 566–567.

Shannon KM (1990) Anemia of prematurity: progress and prospects. *American Journal of Pediatric Hematology/Oncology* **12**: 14–20.

Shannon KM, Naylor GS, Torkildson JC *et al.* (1987) Circulating erythroid progenitors in the anemia of prematurity. *New England Journal of Medicine* **317**: 728–733.

Sieff CA, Emerson SJG, Mufson A, Gesner TG and Nathan DG (1986) Dependence of highly enriched human bone marrow progenitors on hemopoietic growth factors and their response to recombinant erythropoietin. *Journal of Clinical Investigation* **77**: 74–81.

Siimes MA (1981) Pathogenesis of iron deficiency in infancy. In *Iron Nutrition Revisited — Infancy, Childhood, Adolescence. Report on the Eighty-second Conference of Pediatric Research — Columbus, Ohio* (Oski FA and Parson HA, eds) pp 96–108. Ross Laboratories. Colombus, Ohio.

Singer K, Chernoff AI and Singer L (1951) Studies on abnormal haemoglobins. I. Their demonstration in sickle chell anaemia and other haematologic disorders by means of alkali denaturation. *Blood* **6**: 413–428.

Sinha S, Toner N, Chiswick M *et al.* (1987) Vitamin E supplementation reduces frequency of periventricular haemorrhage in very preterm babies. *The Lancet* **i**: 466–471.

Smith JJ and Benjamin F (1968) Post-hemorrhagic anemia and shock in the newborn at birth. A review and etiologic classification. *Obstetrical and Gynecological Survey* **23**: 511–521.

Smith MA and Ryan ME (1988) Parvovirus infections. From benign to life-threatening. *Postgraduate Medicine* **84**: 127–128, 131–134.

Stamatoyannopoulos GI, Nienhuis AW (eds) (1979) *Cellular and molecular regulation of haemoglobin switching*. Grune and Stratton, New York.

Stamatoyannopoulos G and Nienhuis AW (eds) (1989) Haemoglobin Switching. Part B. In *Cellular and Molecular Mechanisms*. New York: AR Liss.

Stockman JA II (1988) Erythropoietin: off again, on again. *Journal of Pediatrics* **112**: 906–908.

Stockman JA and Oski FA (1978) Physiological anaemia of infancy and the anemia of prematurity. *Clinics in Haematology* **7**: 3–18.

Stockman JAS III, Graeber JE, Clark DA, McClellan K, Garcia JF and Kavey REW (1984) Anaemia of prematurity: determinants of the erythropoietin response. *Journal of Pediatrics* **105**: 786–792.

Sutton AM, Harview A, Cockburn F *et al.* (1985) Copper deficiency in the pre-term infant of very low birth weight. *Archives of Disease in Childhood* **60**: 644.

Thomas RM, Channing CE, Cotes PM *et al.* (1983) Erythropoietin and cord blood haemoglobin in the regulation human fetal erythropoiesis. *British Journal of Obstetrics and Gynaecology* **90**: 795–800.

Tyrala EE (1986) Zinc and copper balances in preterm infants. *Pediatrics* **77**: 513–517.

Van-Elsackier-Niele AM, Salimans MM, Weiland HT, Vermey-Kreers C, Anderson MJ and Versteeg J (1989) Fetal pathology in human parvovirus B19 infection. *British Journal of Obstetrics and Gynaecology* **96**: 768–775.

Van Leeuwen G and Patney M (1969) Complications of umbilical vessel catheterisation: peritoneal perforation. *Pediatrics* **44**: 1028–1030.

Wentworth P (1964) A placental lesion to account for foetal haemorrhage into the maternal circulation. *Journal of Obstetrics and Gynaecology of the British Commonwealth* **71**: 379–387.

Wood WG (1982) Developmental Haemopoiesis. In *Blood and its Disorders* (Hardisty RM, and Weatherall, DJ eds), 2nd edn, pp 75–98. Oxford: Blackwell Scientific Publications.

Xanthou M (1970) Leucocyte blood picture in healthy full-term and premature babies during neonatal period. *Archives of Disease in Childhood* **45**: 242–249.

Yao AC, Wist A and Lind J (1967) The blood volume of the newborn infant delivered by Caesarean section. *Acta Paediatrica Scandinavica* **56**: 585–592.

Zipursky A (1984) Vitamin E deficiency in newborn infants. *Clinics in Perinatology* **11**: 393–402.

Zipursky A, Neelands PJ, Chown B and Israels LG (1962) The distribution of fetal hemoglobin in the blood of normal children and adults. *Pediatrics* **30**: 262–268.

Zipursky A, Pollock J, Chown B and Israels LG (1963) Transplacental foetal haemorrhage after placental injury during delivery of amniocentesis. *The Lancet* **ii**: 493–494.

Zipursky A, Brown RT, Watts J *et al.* (1987) Oral Vitamin E supplementation for the prevention of anemia of the premature infant: a controlled trial. *Pediatrics* **79**: 61–68.

4

Polycythaemia in the newborn infant

E.A. Letsky
Queen Charlotte's Maternity Hospital, London

INTRODUCTION

Polycythaemia in the neonatal period has been recognized as a relatively common occurrence over the last 10 to 15 years. Laboratory testing of the blood as a screening procedure at birth or in the first day of life reveals many cases, only a fraction of which develop overt clinical signs attributed to hyperviscosity.

Controversies centre around the need, or otherwise, to screen all neonates within hours of birth for indications of this potential problem, and whether prophylaxis of those symptomless babies considered to be at risk has any effect on the incidence of late manifestations such as cerebral defects affecting motor co-ordination and perhaps intellectual performance.

There is confusion among clinicians about which infants are likely to suffer effects in the neonatal period and which infants, symptomatic or not, will have sequelae. The whole subject has been extensively reviewed (Mentzer, 1978; Oski and Naiman, 1982; Black and Lubchenco, 1982; Danish, 1986; Oh, 1986; Black, 1987).

DEFINITION

Polycythaemia and hyperviscosity are not synonymous terms. Three factors, the deformability of the red cells, the plasma viscosity and the haematocrit, determine the viscosity of the blood. Of these factors, the most important dependent variable affecting whole-blood viscosity in the neonate is the haematocrit (Brooks and Backes, 1981; Black, 1987). There is an almost linear relationship between viscosity and haematocrit below a haematocrit of 60–65%, but the relationship becomes exponential at higher haematocrits. Dunn (1970) used a capillary haematocrit of 75% or greater to diagnose polycythaemia. A *central* venous haematocrit of 65% or more is the generally accepted screening test today. The blood of all infants with a central venous haematocrit of 65% or more will, on *in vitro* testing, prove to be hyperviscous; in contrast, hyperviscosity is never demonstrated *in vitro* using blood of neonates with haematocrits below 60%. Blood with haematocrit values between 60 and 64% prove to be hyperviscous on *in vitro* examination in up to 23% of cases (Ramamurthy, 1979), presumably because of the other variables which affect hyperviscosity. The red blood cells of the healthy neonate are less 'filterable' than those of normal adults. At low pH or in conditions of reduced oxygen tension, the newborn red cells become even less 'filterable'. Some babies have been shown to have hyperviscous blood on the basis of marked reduction in red cell filterability (Gross and Hathaway, 1972). Increases in osmolality and lipid concentrations will also result in increased whole-blood viscosity.

INCIDENCE

The reported incidence of neonatal 'thick blood syndrome' (Wesenberg, 1978) varies considerably depending on the criteria used for diagnosing the condition. A venous haematocrit of 65% or more is the generally accepted screening test today, but the peripheral venous haematocrit is significantly higher than the umbilical venous haematocrit; the viscosity of umbilical venous blood is considerably elevated only when the haematocrit is over 65% and, therefore, if a *peripheral* venous haematocrit of over 65% is used as a diagnostic screening test of hyperviscosity, the condition will be over-diagnosed. This may account for the fact that the majority of infants *reported* to have high venous haematocrits remain asymptomatic (Ramamurthy, 1979). The overall incidence of hyperviscosity is not well established, and reported incidences vary from 4.0 down to 2.34% (Ramamurthy, 1979; Wirth *et al.*, 1979). More recently, a study of 494 healthy newborns (with weight appropriate for gestational age) found only 0.45% to have venous haematocrits above 65% (Brooks and Backes, 1981). These reported differing incidences probably depend on sampling sites, patient population and cord clamping practices.

METHOD OF HAEMATOCRIT DETERMINATION

Because viscosity determinations are not available to most physicians caring for newborn infants, venous haematocrit values are used to identify cases at risk. However if the haematocrit is determined by derivation of values obtained in an automatic electronic counter, the haematocrit is significantly lower than values obtained on the same sample by centrifugation. Inaccurate mean cell volume (MCV), resulting from poor deformability of the neonatal erythrocyte, contributes to erroneous haematocrit values.

In one study, the diagnosis of hyperviscosity would have been missed in seven out of ten infants if Coulter-count haematocrits of more than 65% from venous blood had been used (Villalta *et al.*, 1989). Coulter-count haematocrit values are lower than spun haematocrit values and are poorly correlated with hyperviscosity.

It is strongly recommended that infants with suspected hyperviscosity syndrome are screened by haematocrit values obtained by microcentrifugation.

AETIOLOGY

The aetiology of hyperviscosity syndrome in the neonatal period is multifactorial but the causes can be divided into two main groups — active and passive (Table 4.1).

Table 4.1 Neonatal polycythaemia.

Active causes (Increased intra-uterine erythropoiesis)	Passive causes (Erythrocyte transfusion)
Placental insufficiency	Maternal–fetal
Maternal diabetes	Twin-to-twin
Neonatal thyrotoxicosis	Delayed cord clamping
Congenital adrenal hyperplasia	Unattended delivery
Chromosome abnormalities	

The active form occurs in those circumstances where the fetus, in response to intra-uterine hypoxia and other stimuli, produces an increased number of red cells. The passive forms of neonatal polycythaemia refer to those circumstances in which the fetus receives a red cell transfusion. This may be either maternal or twin-to-twin in origin or result from delayed clamping of the cord (Table 4.1).

Impaired placental function with resultant intra-uterine hypoxia appears to be a major factor in many of the conditions associated with active neonatal polycythaemia, which include small size for gestational age and post-mature infants (Wirth *et al.*, 1979; Rawlings *et al.*, 1982) pre-eclampsia, severe maternal heart disease and maternal smoking (Meberg *et al.*, 1979). Maternal drugs such as propranolol have been incriminated (Gladstone *et al.*, 1975), but polycythaemia in the infant is probably due to the condition for which the mother is being treated. Hyperinsulinaemia in the fetus is associated with increased levels of erythropoietin (Widness *et al.*, 1981). Polycythaemia occurs frequently in the infants of mothers with both overt and gestational diabetes. Down's syndrome, trisomy 13 and trisomy 18 have all been associated with neonatal polycythaemia, thought to be due to increased fetal erythropoietin activity. In Down's syndrome, marked elevation of erythropoietin concentration has been reported.

Morbidity and mortality in the polycythaemic recipient twin in fetus-to-fetus transfusion is at least as high as in the anaemic donor twin. Although a difference of 5 g dl^{-1} in haemoglobin concentration post-delivery is noted with significant twin–twin transfusion syndrome, *in utero* such a difference may not be observed and diagnosis may necessitate a marker such as adult red cells to demonstrate a shared circulation (Fisk *et al.*, 1990).

In normal term infants the most frequent cause of polycythaemia is delayed clamping of the cord. Infants with polycythaemia range in gestational age from 33 to 43 weeks. The condition is characteristically associated with the more mature infant, since the haematocrit rises with gestation. There is a higher incidence among the infants small for gestational age at term and in post-mature infants compared with healthy term of appropriate birth-weight.

CLINICAL FEATURES

The standard evaluation of newborn infants in most centres would not detect the majority of those who have polycythaemia and may therefore be at risk for hyperviscosity syndrome. When quiet, these infants may not appear plethoric, and it is only when roused and active that they become very flushed or cyanosed. The signs usually become evident within the first 24 h as the haematocrit rises due to a physiological decrease in plasma volume. The most consistent findings in newborns with established hyperviscosity are lethargy and hypotonia within 6 h of birth, poor suck and vomiting, difficulty in arousal, irritability when aroused, poor response to light, tremulousness and easy 'startleability'. Some of these central nervous system (CNS) signs and symptoms may be a result of the metabolic abnormalities, hypoglycaemia and hypocalcaemia, commonly associated with polycythaemia rather than a direct result of hyperviscosity itself. Observed complications include hyperbilirubinaemia with kernicterus and heart failure, as well as the other problems due to vascular occlusion (Schmidt and Zipursky, 1984) (Figure 4.1). Respiratory distress and cyanosis

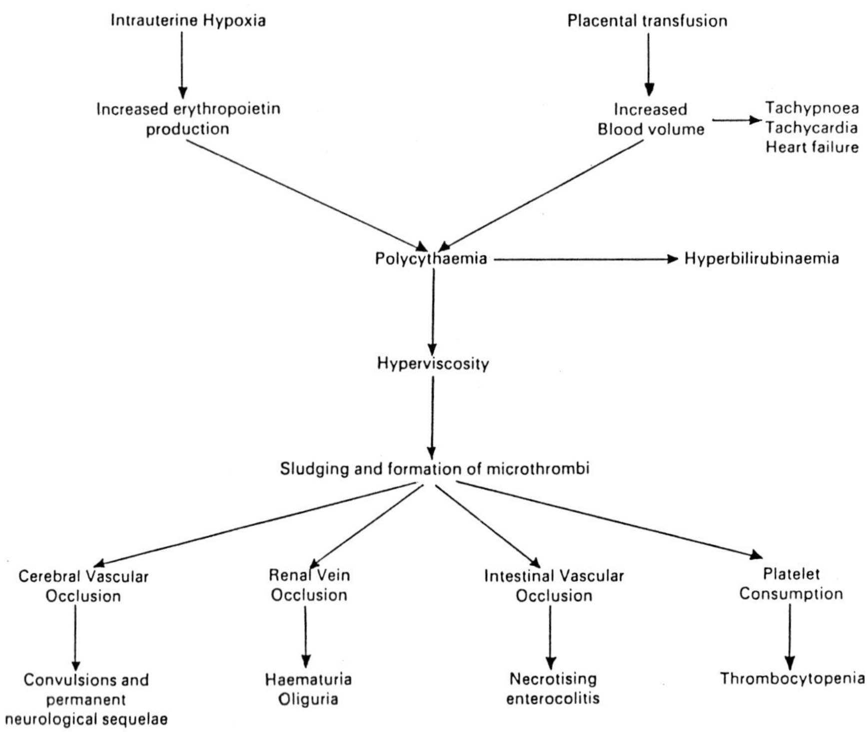

Figure 4.1 Pathogenesis of polycythaemia and clinical manifestations of hyperviscosity in the newborn infant.

together with congestive cardiac failure may be severe enough to simulate cyanotic congenital heart disease.

Hyperbilirubinaemia is attributed to an increased red cell mass leading to increased bilirubin production. Thrombocytopenia is often observed but it is not associated with laboratory evidence of disseminated intravascular coagulation (DIC) and is thought to be due to local aggregation of platelets in the sluggish peripheral circulation (Katz *et al.*, 1982). In the full-blown hyperviscosity syndrome, sludging and formation of thrombi in the peripheral circulation lead to characteristic clinical manifestations due to tissue anoxia, depending where the circulation is compromised. Seizures may occur (Allen and Chilcote, 1979), priapism and testicular infarction (Jung *et al.*, 1980), renal vein thrombosis, renal failure (Herson *et al.*, 1982), gangrene, distal bowel obstruction (Malinowski and Kleinman, 1979) and necrotizing enterocolitis have all been described (Hakanson and Oh, 1977).

Late neutrological sequelae described have included running and laughing fits (Sugimoto *et al.*, 1979), fine motor and speech abnormalities, spastic diplegia (Black *et al.*, 1982) and significant neurodevelopmental abnormalities (Goldberg *et al.*, 1976). In addition, a recent prospective control study has shown significant lower achievement in terms of IQ scores and arithmetic and reading achievement at 7 years in 49 children with hyperviscosity in the neonatal period, compared with 40 controls (Black *et al.*, 1989). However, most publications agree that in untreated neonatal polycythaemia with minor or no symptoms, significant late neurological manifestations are very rare.

MANAGEMENT

It is clear from the available literature that all symptomatic infants with hyperviscosity require treatment in order to relieve the immediate clinical symptoms and to avoid late neurological sequelae. Dramatic improvement has been observed in patients with respiratory disturbance, cardiac failure, gastrointestinal and CNS signs and symptoms. The aim is to lower the haematocrit and thereby the viscosity. Partial exchange transfusion is performed, removing whole blood and replacing it with equal volumes of fresh (frozen) plasma to achieve a haematocrit (Hct) of 55% which is considered to be a 'safe' level.

The formula used to calculate the volume to be exchanged is:

$$\text{Total blood volume} \times \frac{(\text{Observed Hct} - \text{desired Hct})}{\text{Observed Hct}}.$$

If we take the neonatal blood volume to be 85 ml kg^{-1} (Mentzer, 1978) and the desired haematocrit 0.55 in a baby weighing 2.0 kg, with a haematocrit of 0.75 the volume to be exchanged would be

$$2 \times 85 \times \frac{0.75 - 0.55}{0.75} \simeq 45 \text{ ml};$$

usually the volume approximates to 20 ml kg^{-1}. The exchange can be performed in 10 ml aliquots.

The problem of management arises in those neonates who have been identified as having significant polycythaemia with or without hyperviscosity, who are symptom free. These infants may be at risk particularly of late neutrologic sequelae. Do these patients receive 'prophylactic' exchange transfusion? Some paediatricians are in favour of universal screening and prompt treatment of any neonate with polycythaemia (Allen and Chilcote, 1979; Goldberg *et al.*, 1982). Others have been unable to demonstrate any significant benefit in babies with hyperviscosity but without symptoms who have undergone partial exchange transfusion, compared with a control untreated group (Van Der Elst *et al.*, 1980; Black *et al.*, 1982; Host and Ulrich, 1982). An increased incidence of necoritizing enterocolitis following exchange transfusion has been reported (Black and Lubchenko, 1982) but never confirmed. It is felt by some that this fact should be taken into consideration before plasma exchange becomes an accepted treatment for all patients with hyperviscosity.

Until further experience is available, the benefits of prophylactic exchange transfusion must remain speculative — the additional information available to date serves to make the problem more, not less, complex and speculation continues (Black *et al.*, 1989).

SCREENING

There is no doubt that all neonates at special risk of developing hyperviscosity should be screened within the first hours of life. Because of the changing haematocrit in the first few hours, it has been suggested that blood sampling should be delayed until 8 hours post delivery (Shohat *et al.*, 1982). Symptoms are not usually present at birth but develop during the first 24 hours when the concentration of red cells rises secondary to absorption of excess plasma. It is very unusual for symptoms to develop after the first 48 h of life (Sheftel, 1981). The infants to be screened include small and large for gestational age infants, infants of mothers with diabetes, pre-eclampsia and other placental insufficiency syndromes, and twins. The haematocrit is the preferred screening method for hyperviscosity. A capillary haematocrit of more than 65–70% is taken to indicate the need for venous haematocrit. All those infants with a venous haematocrit of more than 65% established by microcentrifugation (Villalta *et al.*, 1989) will have hyperviscous blood, as well as a small proportion of those with venous haematocrits between 60 and 65%. In laboratories with the facility, viscosity of the blood should be measured in these infants. The infants should be carefully examined for symptoms and signs of hyperviscosity. In addition, the blood sugar, calcium and bilirubin levels should be estimated. In this respect, infants of 3–4 days' gestation may develop hyperbilirubinaemia because of transient polycythaemia, but will no longer be polycythaemic at the time of identification (Ramamurthy, 1979).

Ideally all infants should be screened for polycythaemia in the first few hours of life, but it is not the practice in most units to perform a capillary or venous haematocrit on all healthy term infants of appropriate birth-weight. Where this has been performed, a variable incidence of polycythaemia in these otherwise healthy infants of between 0.45 and 4.00% has been reported (see above).

The timing of the estimation of haematocrit is crucial and the postnatal variation in haematocrit in the first 18 h of life should be taken into consideration in the diagnosis of neonatal polycythaemia and hyperviscosity (Ramamurthy and Berlanga, 1987; Merlob, 1989; Ramamurthy, 1989).

SUGGESTED PRACTICAL APPROACH

Healthy, term infants appear to be at little risk of polycythaemia and hyperviscosity and need not be routinely screened (Brooks and Backes, 1981). In units where only the babies known to be at risk of significant polycythaemia are screened, the paediatrician must remain constantly alert to early clinical signs of the condition. In those identified polycythaemic babies with mild or no symptoms of hyperviscosity, keeping the baby warm and well-hydrated is probably all that is required to prevent sludging in the peripheral circulation (Katz *et al.*, 1982). All infants with significant symptoms should undergo partial exchange with fresh frozen plasma in order to bring the haematocrit down to a safe level of 55%.

REFERENCES

Allen JP and Chilcote R (1979) Transient erythrocytosis during the neonatal period: possible neurologic complications. *Southern Medical Journal* **72**: 681–686.

Black VD (1987) Neonatal Hyperviscosity Syndromes. *Current Problems in Pediatrics* **17**: 73–130.

Black VD and Lubchenco LD (1982) Neonatal polycythemia and hyperviscosity. *Pediatric Clinics of North America* **29**: 1137–1147.

Black VD, Lubchenko LD, Luckey DIV *et al.* (1982) Developmental and neurologic sequelae of neonatal hyperviscosity syndrome. *Pediatrics* **69**: 426–431.

Black VD, Camp BW, Lubchenco LD *et al.* (1989) Neonatal hyperviscosity association with lower achievement and IQ scores at school age. *Pediatrics* **83**: 662–667.

Brooks GI and Backes CR (1981) Hyperviscosity secondary to polycythemia in the appropriate for gestational age neonate. *Journal of the American Osteopathic Association* **80**: 415–418.

Danish ED (1986) Neonatal polycythemia. In *Progress in Hematology*, vol XIV, pp 55–98. London: Grune & Stratton.

Dunn PM (1970) Neonatal polycythaemia. *Archives of Disease in Childhood* **45**: 273 (Abstr.).

Fisk NM, Borrell A, Hubinont C, Tannirandorn Y, Nicolini U and Rodeck CH (1990) Feto-fetal transfusion syndrome: do the neonatal criteria apply *in utero*? *Archives of Disease in Childhood* (in press).

Gladstone GR, Hordof A and Gersony WM (1975) Propanolol administration during pregnancy: effects on the fetus. *Journal of Pediatrics* **86**: 962–964.

Goldberg K, Wirth FH, Hathaway WE *et al.* (1982) Neonatal hyperviscosity II. Effects of partial plasma exchange transfusion. *Pediatrics* **69**: 419–425.

Gross GP and Hathaway WE (1972) Fetal erythrocyte deformability. *Pediatric Research* **6**: 593–599.

Hakanson DO and Oh W (1977) Necrotizing enterocolitis and hyperviscosity in the newborn infant. *Journal of Pediatrics* **90**: 458–461.

Herson VC, Raye JR, Rowe JC and Phillips AF (1982) Acute renal failure associated with polycythemia in a neonate. *Journal of Pediatrics* **100**: 137–139.

Host A and Ulrich M (1982) Late prognosis in untreated neonatal polycythaemia with minor or no symptoms. *Acta Paediatrica Scandinavica* **71**: 629–633.

Jung AL, McGaughey HR and Matlak ME (1980) Neonatal testicular infarctions and polycytemia. *Journal of Urology* **123**: 781–782.

Katz J, Rodriguez E, Mandani G and Branson HE (1982) Normal coagulation findings, thrombocytopenia and peripheral hemoconcentration in neonatal polycythemia. *Journal of Pediatrics* **101**: 99–102.

Malinowski BC and Kleinman LI (1979) Polycythemia in the newborn first observed as distal bowel obstruction. *American Journal of Diseases in Children* **133**: 962–963.

Meberg A, Haga P, Sande H and Foss OP (1979) Smoking during pregnancy — haematological observations in the newborn. *Acta Paediatrica Scandinavica* **68**: 731–734.

Mentzer WC (1978) Polycythemia and the hyperviscosity syndrome. *Clinics in Haematology* **7**: 63–74.

Merlob P (1989) Postnatal alteration in hematocrit and viscosity in normal infants and in those with polycythemia. *Journal of Pediatrics* **114**: 169.

Oh W (1986) Neonatal polycythemia and hyperviscosity. *Pediatric Clinics of North American* **33(3)**: 523–532.

Oski FA and Naiman JL (1982) Polycythemia and Hyperviscosity in the neonatal period. In *Hematologic Problems in the Newborn*, 3rd edn, pp 87–96. New York: WB Saunders Co.

Ramamurthy RS (1979) Neonatal polycythemia and hyperviscosity: state of the art. *Perinatology–Neonatology* **3**: 38–40.

Ramamurthy RS and Berlanga RN (1987) Postnatal alteration in hematocrit and viscosity in normal and polycythemic infants. *Journal of Pediatrics* **110**: 929–934.

Ramamurthy RS (1989) Postnatal alteration in hematocrit and viscosity in normal infants and in those with polycythemia. *Journal of Pediatrics* **114**: 169–170.

Rawlings JS, Pettett GP, Wiswell TE and Clapper J (1982) Estimated blood volumes in polycythemic neonates as a function of birth weight. *Journal of Pediatrics* **101**: 594–599.

Schmidt B and Zipursky A (1984) Thrombotic diseases in the newborn infants. *Clinics in Perinatology* **11**: 461–489.

Sheftel DN (1981) Neonatal polycythemia and the hyperviscosity syndrome. *Wisconsin Medical Journal* **80**: 39–40.

Shohat M, Merlob P and Reisner SH (1982) Neonatal polycythemia. *Pediatrics* **70**: 155–156.

Sugimoto T, Matsamura T, Sakomoto Y and Tanluchi K (1979) Running and laughing fits as the sequelae of the neonatal hyperviscosity syndrome. *Brain and Development* **1**: 323–326.

Van Der Elst CW, Molteno CD, Malan AF and de V Heese H (1980) The management of polycythaemia in the newborn infant. *Early Human Development* **4**: 393–403.

Villalta IA, Pramanik AK, Diaz-Blanco J and Herbst JJ (1989) Clinical and laboratory observations: Diagnostic errors in neonatal polycythemia based on method of hematocrit determination. *Journal of Pediatrics* **115**: 460–462.

Wesenberg RL (1978) Neonatal 'thick blood' syndrome. *Hospital Practice* **13**: 137–145.

Widness JA, Susa JB and Garcia JF (1981) Increased erythropoiesis and elevated erythropoietin in infants born to diabetic mothers and in hyperinsulinaemic rhesus fetuses. *Journal of Clinical Investigation* **67**: 637–642.

Wirth FH, Goldberg KE and Lubchenco LO (1979) Neonatal hyperviscosity I. Incidence. *Pediatrics* **63**: 833–836.

5

Haemolytic disease of the newborn

E.A. Letsky
Queen Charlotte's Maternity Hospital, London

Haemolytic disease of the newborn (HDN) is a condition in which the lifespan of the infant's red cells is shortened by the action of specific antibodies derived from the mother. The immune antibodies in the maternal plasma are small molecule immunoglobulins of the IgG subclass and therefore, unlike the naturally occurring large molecule antibodies of the ABO blood group systems (IgM), are able to cross the placenta.

Although HDN can theoretically occur in any situation where the mother lacks a paternally derived antigen that her baby carries on its red cells, there is no doubt that, prior to the introduction of the specific immunoglobulin for the prevention of Rhesus D (RhD) haemolytic disease, Rh(D) HDN was by far the most important form of HDN, in terms of clinical severity and frequency, in Caucasian populations. Since introduction of prophylaxis, the numbers of babies affected by severe HDN has fallen dramatically (Figure 5.1) and the proportion of HDN due to antibodies other than anti-D have risen, but the most severe cases are (with very rare exceptions) still caused by anti-D antibodies.

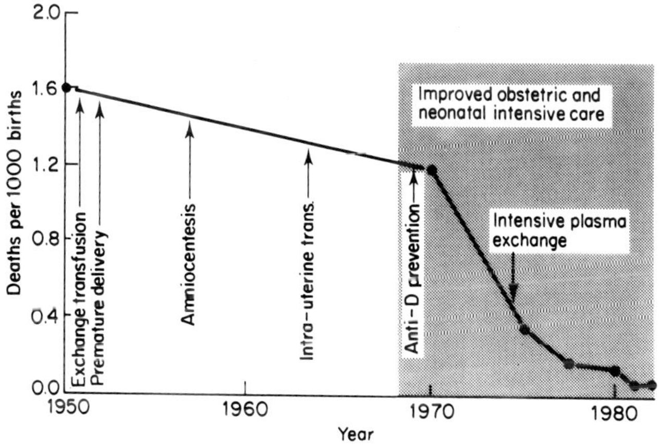

Figure 5.1 Perinatal deaths due to anti-D haemolytic disease of the newborn per 1000 births. (From Tovey, 1984 with permission)

Before embarking upon an account of the pathogenesis and management of established HDN, a short outline of the history of the development of haemolytic disease prevention in the offspring of RhD-negative women and of the changing epidemiology of this severe problem is appropriate.

HISTORY

Before the introduction of prophylaxis, 1 in 200 pregnancies were associated with the development of anti-D antibodies in the mother, and of these 20% lost their infants in the first affected pregnancy and 40% in subsequent affected pregnancies (Tovey, 1990). At Queen Charlotte's Hospital in London, between 1946 and 1949, 11 035 babies were delivered and 34 died because of Rh anti-D antibodies, a death rate of 3.2 per 1000 births. The neonatal unit had a constant occupancy of babies receiving exchange transfusions to correct anaemia and prevent kernicterus.

During 1988 at the same hospital, 4255 babies were delivered — 16 mothers presented with anti-D antibodies. Seven fetuses received intra-uterine transfusions, two had exchange transfusions and there were no intra-uterine deaths, still births or neonatal deaths.

How have these dramatic changes come about? Undoubtedly the main influence on the changing incidence has been prevention by passive administration of anti-D immunoglobulin to the Rh(D)-negative mother at times of risk when Rh(D)-positive red cells from her fetus enter her circulation (see Figure 5.1).

The discovery of this protective phenomenon and the development of successful prophylaxis programmes is an exciting and sometimes bizarre story which is eloquently recounted in a recent review article by one of the pioneers in the field (Clarke, 1989). The first step in human biological terms was the observation that there may be some mode of natural protection. Epidemiological studies showed that the incidence of haemolytic disease of the newborn in Rh(D)-negative women who carried an ABO incompatible fetus was less than expected (Levine, 1943). This led to the hypothesis that ABO incompatible matings may have a protective effect because the naturally occurring maternal anti-A or anti-B eliminated the fetal Rh(D)-positive red cells and so blocked the production of Rh antibodies (Race and Sanger, 1950). Several epidemiological studies followed, confirming the original findings and added weight to the hypothesis.

The next step was to find some way of applying the principle of this natural protection to all women at risk by using an appropriate antibody to remove the Rh(D)-positive cells from her circulation. Male Rh(D)-negative volunteers were injected with Rh(D)-positive red cells and with preparations of anti-D immunoglobulin. Attempts using administration of IgM anti-D to prevent production of anti-D antibodies failed, and after this the use of IgG anti-D was tried, with resounding success. It was necessary to clear about 95% of the Rh-positive cells to prevent immunization, and this was achieved by a pure IgG anti-D preparation administered by deep intramuscular injection within 24 hours of transfusing the Rh(D)-positive red cells to the male volunteers. The next step was to see if this method would protect

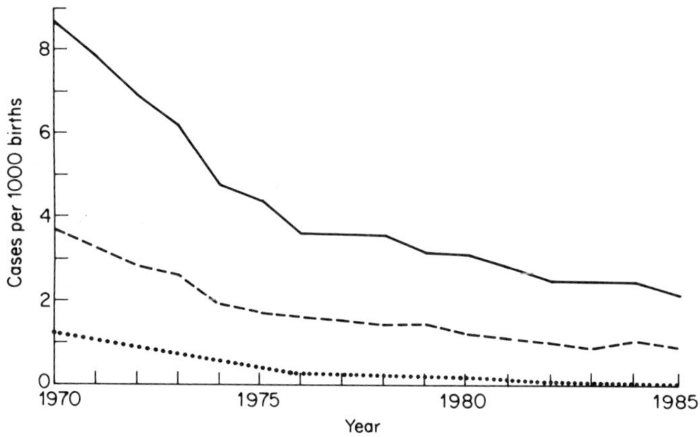

Figure 5.2 Incidence of Rh antibodies (anti-D) per 1000 births 1970 to 1985.

Rh(D)-negative women in pregnancy. Clinical trials were embarked upon in the 1960s. By 1967 collective experience from the United States, Germany and the United Kingdom showed clearly the protective effect of injection of IgG anti-D to the mother within 48 hours of delivery of Rh-positive ABO compatible fetus (see Clarke, 1989) compared with non-treated matched controls. It had taken less than 30 years for the appreciation of the pathogenesis of Rh(D) HDN to lead not only to ideas of how it may be prevented but also to the institution of programmes for prophylaxis of this devastating condition.

Over the years since the introduction of universal prophylaxis in the late 1960s, refinements have been added but the principle remains the same. Small numbers of new cases still occur annually (Figure 5.2) and an account of the total management and background follows.

RHESUS BLOOD GROUP SYSTEM

This is the most complex of the blood group systems. It is characterized by more than 30 known antigens and a much large number of complex alleles. The Rh antigens are most probably lipoprotein and they are confined to the red-cell membrane. The system was first described by Landsteiner and Wiener in 1940.

The Wiener system proposed that the Rh phenotype is determined by a single genetic locus with many alleles. The Fisher–Race System on the other hand assumes that the inheritance of the Rh antigens is determined by three pairs of allelic genes, *C–c̄, D–d, E–ē*, acting on three closely linked loci. Despite expansion over the years, the Fisher–Race System does not cover all the reactions that have been observed within the Rh system, but because the *CDE/c̄d̄ē* nomenclature is easy to use and enables practical visualization of how a given sample of cells will react with available anti-sera, the World

Health Organization has recommended that the Fisher–Race System be adopted.

A number of variants exist for each of the common Rh antigens e.g. D^u, C^w, C^x, E^w. The D^u antigen is of particular importance and is common in black populations. In most individuals, the D^u antigen differs from the normal D only in that there are fewer antigenic sites per red blood cell, and the D^u antigen will react weakly and variably with the various anti-D antisera. There are however some D^u variants that have both a qualitative and quantitative defect. Such individuals can make anti-D antibodies and should be identified at the Regional Transfusion Centre if the specific antisera are not available on site. If a structural D variant is excluded, then it is not necessary to treat the D^u individual as Rh(D)-negative for transfusion purposes. Similarly, D^u individuals with a straightforward, weakly expressed normal D antigen are not considered candidates for either antenatal or postnatal prophylaxis with passively administered anti-D immunoglobulin. If, however, there are no facilities for excluding structural D^u variants then it is safer to treat all D^u individuals as Rh(D)-negative.

Basically, therefore, there are considered to be six antigens, and the main combination of genes at the three loci are:

Rh(D)-positive	*Rh(D)-negative*
$C D \bar{e}$ or R_1	$\bar{c} d \bar{e}$ or r
$\bar{c} D E$ or R_2	$C d \bar{e}$ or r'
$C D E$ or R_z	$\bar{c} d E$ or r''
$\bar{c} D \bar{e}$ or R_o	$C d E$ or R_y

This classification follows the convention that possession of a *D* gene and antigen is termed Rh(D)-positive, whereas absence of a *D* gene and antigen is termed Rh(D)-negative.

DD homozygous *Dd* heterozygous	Rh(D)-positive
dd	Rh(D)-negative

It follows that any Rh(D)-positive offspring of an Rh(D)-negative mother has to be heterozygous *Dd* Rh(D)-positive having received a D antigen from the father but a d antigen from the mother. It also follows that if the father is homozygous Rh(D)-positive then he can only have Rh(D)-positive children. Whereas if he is heterozygous (*Dd*) Rh(D)-positive, there is a 50:50 chance of him fathering a Rh(D)-negative baby who will not be affected by maternal anti-D.

Approximately 15% of the Caucasian population of the United Kingdom are Rh(D)-negative — the remaining 85% are Rh(D) positive.

Difficulties in determining the zygosity of an Rh-positive individual arise from the fact that there is no antisera that will identify the d antigen. Probabilities of genotype are worked out from reactions with the five available antisera, which react with C-D-E and $\bar{c}$ and $\bar{e}$ antigens, and frequencies of combinations of these antigens derived from population studies. This is why the report on paternal blood for rhesus genotyping will always be preceded by the word 'probable'.

Rh(D) HAEMOLYTIC DISEASE OF THE NEWBORN

The disease begins in intra-uterine life and may result in death in utero. In live-born infants the haemolytic process is maximal at the time of birth and thereafter diminishes as the concentration of maternal antibody in the infant's circulation declines. During pregnancy the fetal and maternal circulations are separate. Red cells are not thought to cross the placental barrier in significant numbers in normal circumstances. Oxygen, nutrient and waste exchange takes place by diffusion across the intervillous space. IgG antibodies cross the placenta freely, carrying passive immunity for the fetus against infective agents to which the mother has had a healthy immune response. Following delivery of the neonate, rupture of the placental villi and connective tissue at separation allows escape of fetal blood cells into the maternal circulation prior to constriction of open-end maternal vessels. This is when, unless prevented, sensitization takes places in the majority of cases.

PROPHYLAXIS OF RHESUS HAEMOLYTIC DISEASE

The stimulus for primary induction of antibody formation has been shown to be Rh(D)-positive fetal cells entering the maternal circulation when they reach the end of their lifespan. If rhesus anti-D immune globulin is injected into the mother, the antibody coats the fetal Rh(D)-positive antigen sites and the coated cells are rapidly removed from the maternal circulation by cells of the reticulo-endothelial systems. Maternal immune system cells are prevented from producing antibody against the fetal Rh(D)-positive cells in the presence of adequate antibody.

Fetal cells in the maternal circulation can be identified and quantitated crudely using the Kleihauer technique (Letsky and Sheerman-Chase, 1989).

Basic recommendations in the United Kingdom

Anti-D immunoglobulin should be administered to any non-sensitized Rh(D)-negative woman:

(1) post delivery, if she gives birth to an Rh(D)-positive infant,
(2) post-therapeutic abortion or identified spontaneous abortion,
(3) antenatally at 28 and 34 weeks' gestation if she has no living children,
(4) to cover antenatal procedures such as amniocentesis and chorion villus sampling,
(5) if she threatens to abort or miscarry.

Post partum anti-D

All Rh(D)-negative women who give birth to an Rh(D)-positive baby, and who have produced no identifiable antibodies, should receive a standard dose of 500 i.u. anti-D within 72 hours of delivery. This is an arbitrary time, there is no magic about it. In particular, if a woman is sent home without receiving anti-D it is well worth giving the anti-D if she is identified as being at risk, certainly within the first week of delivery and probably up to 3–6 weeks post-partum. The half-life of fetal cells in the maternal circulation is approximately 40 days. A Kleihauer examination of fetal cells within the maternal circulation should be carried out to make sure that the estimated bleed is no more than 4 ml, which will be covered by the standard dose of 500 i.u. If a larger loss of fetal cells into the mother's circulation has occurred, a proportionally larger dose of anti-D immunoglobulin should be administered. In the vast majority of cases, fetal losses into the maternal circulation are less than 1.0 ml (Letsky and Sheerman-Chase, 1989).

Post-abortion anti-D

It has been reported that transplacental haemorrhage occurs in 20% of cases undergoing therapeutic abortion, 4% of which are associated with a bleed of more than 0.2 ml into the maternal circulation. The volume of fetal blood crossing into the maternal circulation following spontaneous abortion is usually less than 0.1 ml but the mothers still run the risk of being sensitized (Queenan *et al.*, 1971). In the past, many women developed antibodies following early terminations or spontaneous abortions because of the concept that sensitization could not occur in early pregnancy. The D antigen has been shown to be expressed on fetal red cells as early as 38 days post-conception (Bergstrom *et al.*, 1967), therefore all women who have a therapeutic or identified spontaneous abortion should receive a standard dose of 250 i.u. anti-D regardless of possible group of fetus or Kleihauer estimation. It is also advisable to protect the Rh(D)-negative woman who suffers an ectopic pregnancy as sensitization has been described in such women who were not given anti-D immunoglobulin.

Antenatal anti-D

It is estimated that approximately one per cent of Rh(D)-negative women may be sensitized during the antenatal period due to transplacental passage of fetal red cells in apparently non-eventful pregnancy without any invasive procedures. Ideally, all nonsensitized Rh(D)-negative women should receive antenatal prophylaxis in every pregnancy. In the United States and Canada, where supplies of anti-D are abundant, Rh(D)-negative women receive 1500 i.u. of anti-D at 28 and 34 weeks' gestation in all pregnancies. In the United Kingdom, where supplies are limited, antenatal prophylaxis is confined to those women who have no living children and the dose they receive is less, 500 i.u. at 28 and 34 weeks' gestation. It is important to repeat therapy, once instituted, at six-week intervals because it has been shown that very low levels of passively administered anti-D may enhance antibody formation in the presence of an antigenic stimulus. If an Rh(D)-positive fetus is delivered at term it is obvious that anti-D should be administered in the usual way, even if antenatal prophylaxis has been given.

Prophylaxis of antenatal procedures

Invasive procedures such as amniocentesis fetal blood sampling, which may encourage transplacental fetal red cell invasion of the maternal circulation, should be covered by passively administered anti-D. The dose to be given is 250 i.u. at up to 20 weeks gestation and 500 i.u. thereafter. External versions or breech presentations are very rarely performed nowadays, but these should be similarly covered with administration of anti-D. To this list of procedures chorion villus sampling must now be added (Warren *et al.*, 1985).

Threatened abortion or miscarriage

If a woman threatens to abort or miscarry, with external or evidence of internal bleeding, a standard dose of anti-D should be given, the amount depending on gestation; theoretically, this prophylaxis should be repeated at 6-week intervals throughout the pregnancy. The D antigen is expressed on red cells as early as 38 days' gestation, so the widely-held belief that women suffering early abortions need not be protected is not to be encouraged (see above).

Reasons for failure of prophylaxis (Figure 5.2)

Injection not given

The non-identification of the woman at risk and failure to administer prophylaxis appropriately remains the most potent cause of failure of prophylaxis.

Inadequate dosage of anti-D

There are still some centres that do not perform a routine Kleihauer to identify those women who require more than the standard 500 i.u. Mistakes can be made, and rigid quality control must be applied to all laboratories that attempt to quantitate fetal cells in the maternal circulation.

Prior sensitization

A number of women who have been antenatally sensitized but do not have any identifiable antibody at the time of delivery, even if enzyme-treated Rh(D)-positive cells are used in the test system. In this case, any passively administered anti-D will be ineffective once the maternal immune system has been primed.

Injection badly given

Unless the injection is given deeply intramuscularly it will not be absorbed appropriately and will fail to have the desired effect.

DEVELOPMENT OF SYNTHETIC ANTI-D HUMAN MONOCLONAL ANTIBODY TO RHESUS D ANTIGEN

In the United Kingdom the main limiting factor preventing administration of anti-D immunoglobulin during the antenatal period to all antibody-lacking Rh(D)-negative women in every pregnancy is lack of supply. Anti-D immunoglobulin is produced from the plasma of human Rh(D)-negative volunteers who are deliberately sensitized and bled at regular intervals, or from the very few women now who have been severely sensitized in the past by Rh(D)-positive pregnancies.

The *in vitro* production of human monoclonal antibodies has wide-ranging clinical potential. A monoclonal antibody directed against the Rh(D)-antigen can be a useful blood-typing reagent but more importantly, if safe for human administration, could be used to prevent HDN, thus replacing the immune serum from immunized male volunteers used at present.

There are two ways of making human monoclonal antibody-producing cell lines. In the first, the antibodies are produced by somatic cell hybridization. This method has been hampered by difficulty in establishing suitable human myeloma cell lines in culture. The second method involves lymphocyte transformation by Epstein–Barr (EB) virus so that the cells secrete specific antibody. Long-term production of antibody can only be achieved if the cell lines are cloned.

One of the first reports of successful production of monoclonal anti-D suitable for a laboratory reagent in blood grouping came from Crawford and colleagues (1983). They described a method for continuous *in vitro* production of a human monoclonal antibody to Rhesus D antigen by a cloned EB virus-transformed, lymphoblastoid cell line was established from peripheral blood cells from a rhesus-negative blood donor who had been immunized with rhesus D antigen. These preparations are now widely used in blood transfusion serology laboratories. However, the development of the use of monoclonal anti-D antibodies to replace polyclonal anti-serum in prophylaxis of HDN is as yet in its infancy. Almost all IgG anti-D molecules belong to the subclass IgG1 and IgG3. Although the evidence available suggests that IgG3 is the most effective of the two, it is possible that both classes will be required for effective prophylaxis.

A more important problem to be overcome before these antibodies can be used for prophylaxis is how to ensure that the final preparation is free of viruses and DNA. Preliminary trials are now underway (Hughes-Jones, 1988).

MANAGEMENT OF Rh(D)-HDN

The Rh(D)-negative pregnant woman with antibodies

All Rh(D)-negative women should be screened, at the minimum, at booking, at 28 weeks, 34 weeks and at delivery, and if no active anti-D antibody production is detected the woman receives prophylaxis as described above.

If a woman has antibodies at booking or if antibody is detected on subsequent testing, the pregnancy becomes high risk. Since the numbers of sensitized pregnancies has fallen dramatically, most peripheral centres will only see one or two women at risk per year and, while this is fortunate in general and an advance in terms of public health, it means that very few groups now have expertise in monitoring progress, instituting therapy, prime timing of delivery and in the skilled procedures of intra-uterine fetal transfusion.

It is essential that any woman at risk should, once identified, at least have her case drawn to the attention of one of the expert referral centres, so that collective experience may be applied to her case (Figure 5.3).

Disasters occur when a woman is referred for urgent treatment late in a sensitized pregnancy with a frank or incipient hydrops in utero, which

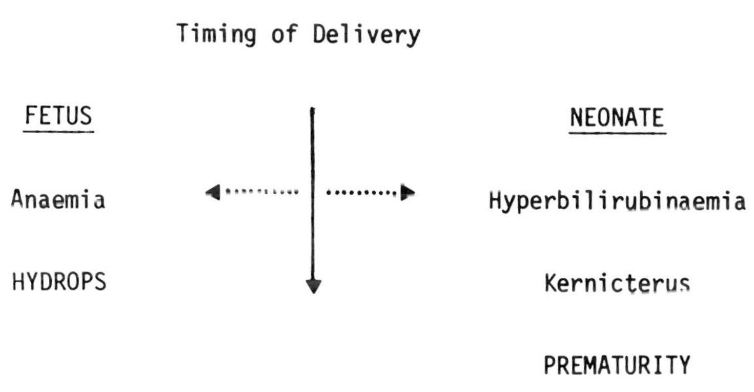

Figure 5.3 Basic problems in haemolytic disease of the newborn.

might well have been prevented by earlier intervention. Not only are most centres untutored in the techniques of intra-uterine transfusion and other fetal therapy, they are unfamiliar with interpreting the significance of a maternal antibody concentration and amniotic fluid bilirubin and with other methods of monitoring severity of disease in the fetus.

Monitoring severity of disease in the fetus

Maternal antibody quantitation

The detection of anti-D antibodies in the maternal circulation alerts the clinician to a possible problem; it does not indicate the group of the fetus or whether the fetus is at risk of severe HDN. Of more significance is whether the antibody concentration is rising. In addition, the zygosity of the father and previous history are important prognostic factors. There has been much interest recently in the method of antibody quantitation, following the introduction of a standard preparation of anti-D. Large numbers of sera can be examined at the Regional Transfusion Centre by an automated procedure. This does away with observer error in interpreting the indirect antiglobulin (Coombs') test and also with manual dilution errors, but is not really vastly superior in other ways. It is very important, however, for the units who see only relatively few cases. It has been shown that if the antibody is quantitated at less than 5 i.u. ml^{-1} (Harrison *et al.*, 1984) or 4 i.u. ml^{-2} (Bowell *et al.*, 1982), then there is no indication for further investigation or intervention. For many years at Queen Charlotte's (a referral centre), we monitored significant numbers of sensitized women using the indirect antiglobulin titre, and if the concentration was less than 1 in 16 then no further action was taken antenatally. Retrospectively, no fetuses seem to have come to any harm using this criterion.

Because techniques of antibody determination vary from laboratory to laboratory it is essential that those concerned with managing the case are familiar with the methodology and reliability of the method used in their own laboratory or referral centre. In the end, the antibody is only an indication of a potential problem and indicates the necessity or otherwise of further invasive procedures. It should be remembered that every amniocentesis, and particularly fetal blood sampling, carries the risk of stimulating increasing antibody concentration by releasing further fetal cells into maternal circulation (see below).

Amniotic fluid bilirubin

Principle and biochemical basis. In a normal pregnancy, unconjugated bilirubin is present in the amniotic fluid, the concentration decreasing toward term. This is presumed to be due to some leakage of the normal breakdown products of fetal haemoglobin in their transplacental passage to the maternal liver (which converts fetal bilirubin to the non-toxic water-

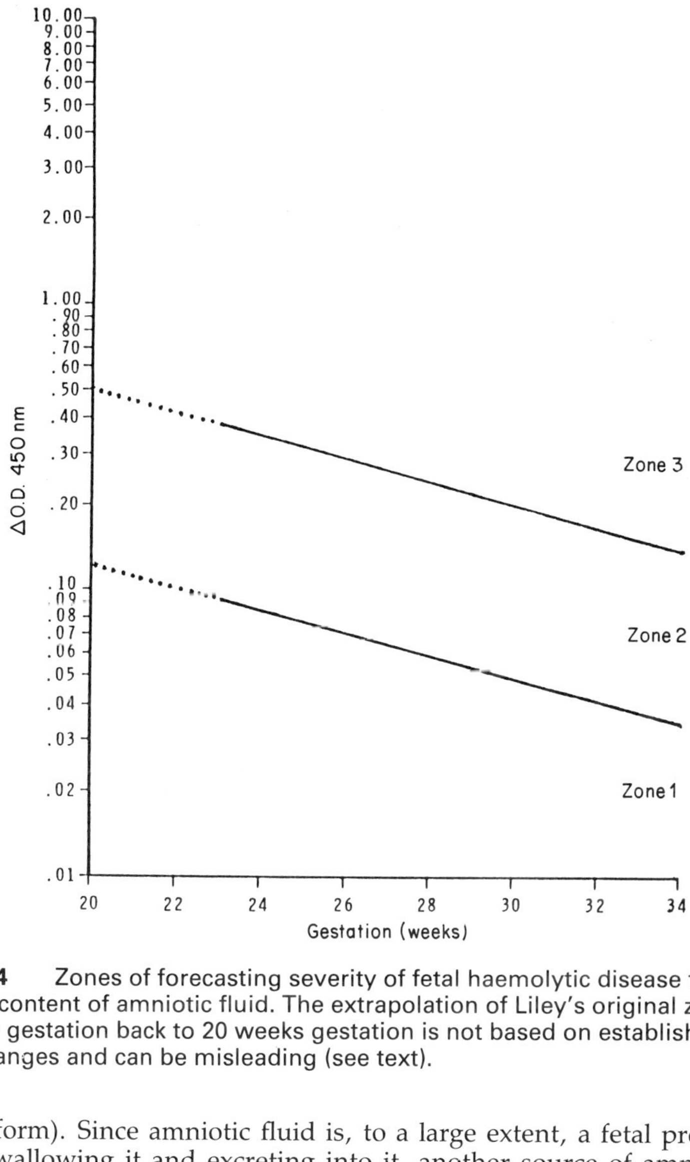

Figure 5.4 Zones of forecasting severity of fetal haemolytic disease from the bilirubin content of amniotic fluid. The extrapolation of Liley's original zones from 27 weeks gestation back to 20 weeks gestation is not based on established normal ranges and can be misleading (see text).

soluble form). Since amniotic fluid is, to a large extent, a fetal product, the infant swallowing it and excreting into it, another source of amniotic fluid bilirubin may be tracheal and pulmonary fluid. In a pregnancy complicated by fetal haemolytic disease, the bilirubin concentration in amniotic fluid rises above the known normal level for gestation (Baker and Letsky, 1989). This raised concentration of bilirubin is directly related to the severity of haemolysis. By measuring total bile pigment and the spectroscopic curve with quantitative of Δ O.D. 450 nm value it is possible to assess the severity of fetal haemolytic disease (Liley, 1961). A more accurate picture of the progress of the disease can be obtained if serial measurements are performed.

Unfortunately, normal ranges and abnormal amniotic Δ 450 nm bilirubin

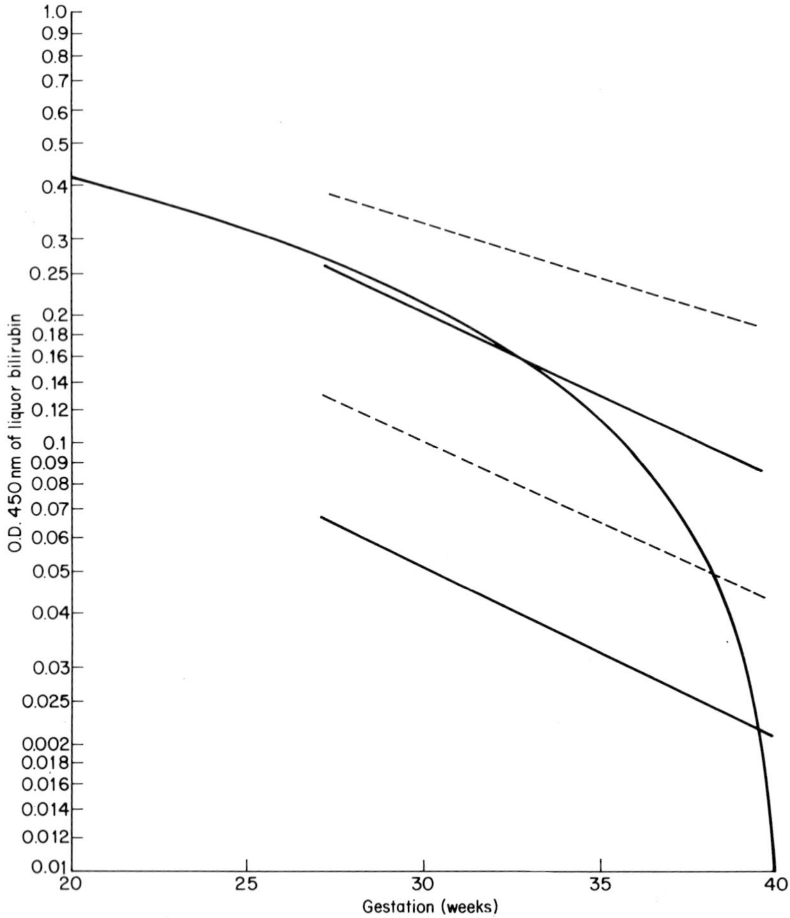

Figure 5.5 Whitfield's (1970) curved action line is super-imposed on Liley's zones of severity of fetal haemolysis based on estimations of amniotic fluid bilirubin concentration. This gives guidelines for appropriate management related to gestation i.e. intra-uterine transfusion or if the fetus is viable delivery and exchange transfusion if indicated.

values are not widely available or reliably interpretable before 24 weeks' gestation. After 34–35 weeks' gestation the amniotic fluid becomes increasingly cloudy and it is not possible to obtain reliable spectrophotometric measurements of bile pigment. False estimates of severity are made if Liley's original zones are extrapolated back from 27 weeks to 20 weeks, which is common practice (see Figure 5.4).

Amniocenteses for bilirubin content are usually carried out at two week intervals between 24 and 34 weeks' gestation. By plotting the Δ 450 nm values on a specially prepared graph, relating Liley's zones of severity to gestation age (Figure 5.4), it is possible to predict the outcome of the pregnancy and to take the appropriate measures when needed, for example intra-uterine transfusion or premature delivery of the fetus. This is facilitated by adding the so called Whitfield Action Line (Figure 5.5) and superimposing this on the Liley zones (Whitfield, 1970). The Liley zones are:

(1) Rh(D)-negative or mildly affected fetus;
(2) indeterminate, usually moderately severe disease;
(3) severe disease, impending fetal death.

Special problems. Contamination of the amniotic fluid with fresh or altered blood diminishes the accuracy of the prognosis. This may be seen directly by eye, but sometimes only from the spectral curve. For this reason the amniotic fluid should be scanned in a spectrophotometer from 320 to 700 nm to detect pigments other than bilirubin, for example, methaemoglobin or oxyhaemoglobin. Altered blood classically gives a peak at 405 nm and fresh blood (oxyhaemoglobin) at 413 nm. Later in gestation, meconium may interfere with spectrophotometric amniotic fluid examination, but after 34 weeks the bile pigment estimations tend to be unreliable anyway, because of increasing turbidity in the amniotic fluid. One of the main sources of error in assessing severity of haemolytic disease (in addition to contamination by pigments other than bile products) is incorrect gestational age (Nicolaides *et al.*, 1986a). It is therefore very important to have the gestational age checked by ultrasound in the early weeks following conception in these high-risk pregnancies.

However, until skills of safe fetal blood sampling have spread to many more obstetric centres (Bowell *et al.*, 1988), estimation of amniotic fluid bilirubin will continue to play an important part in management of haemolytic disease of the fetus (Nicolaides *et al.*, 1986a).

Ultrasound examination

The introduction of ultrasound techniques has greatly facilitated the investigation and management (Bang *et al.*, 1982) of the fetus at risk of serious HDN. The use of X-rays, with their potential hazards, can now be abandoned.

With real-time ultrasound scanning the growth of the fetus can be monitored. In particular, the abdominal circumference can be plotted on a normal-growth chart enabling detection of the first signs of abnormal abdominal swelling due to underlying hepatosplenamegaly. Early ascites and scalp oedema can also be visualized on the scanning screen. Detailed examination of the heart will detect early signs of stress and incipient failure (Chitkara *et al.*, 1988).

All the foregoing investigations give indirect and sometimes misleading information of the seriousness of the problem (Nicolaides *et al.*, 1988a). In some cases with a history of previous intra-uterine death early in gestation, or of indirect evidence of rapidly progressive disease, a direct sample of fetal blood must be taken (see below) to accurately assess the severity of disease. It is possible for a fetus to appear normal on ultrasound examination and yet have a haemoglobin of 4 g dl^{-1} or below at 20 24 weeks' gestation (Nicolaides *et al.*, 1988).

Fetal blood sampling

If other parameters (rapidly rising maternal antibody concentration, or previous intra-uterine fetal death) indicate that severe fetal haemolytic disease before 24 weeks' gestation is to be expected, earlier action may have to be taken. This would involve fetal blood sampling at 18 weeks' gestation (McKenzie *et al.*, 1988; Nicolaides *et al.*, 1986b), when the blood group — haemoglobin PCV, DAT, etc. — can be estimated (Millar *et al.*, 1985; Nicolaides *et al.*, 1985) directly and intravascular transfusion administered if indicated (Nicolaides *et al.*, 1988b). Normal haematological values have been established for fetal blood samples obtained at 18–24 weeks' gestation (Millar *et al.*, 1985).

However, sampling of fetal blood should not be carried out routinely early in gestation in patients with Rh isoimmunization, and intra-uterine transfusion should be delayed as long as possible, because the procedures lead inevitably to feto-maternal bleeding and increase in maternal antibody production (Nicolini *et al.*, 1988; Bowell *et al.*, 1988).

Management of severe disease in the fetus

The changing incidence of HDN and the improvements in fetal and neonatal therapy have resulted in many review articles on the subject in recent years, from which much of the following data has been drawn (Bowman, 1975; Urbaniak, 1985; Tovey, 1986; Clarke *et al.*, 1987; Grannum and Copel, 1988; Mollison *et al.*, 1987; Rodeck and Letsky, 1989; McClure, 1990).

The aim is to prevent hydrops *in utero* and to time delivery so that the infant has a maximal chance of survival (Figure 5.3). Over the past 10 years there have been dramatic improvements in the care of the pre-term infant, and so the old adage 'better in than out' is no longer true in many situations. Many babies delivered at 28 weeks' gestation survive, with no long-term handicap (Figure 3.6), and it is unusual for those of 32 weeks' gestation or more to present any more than routine problems for the average Special Care Baby Unit (SCBU).

Measures to suppress haemolytic disease in utero

Oral desensitization

Marked reduction of Rhesus HDN has been reported following oral administration of Rh(D)-positive red cell stroma in enteric coated capsules (Bierme *et al.*, 1979). The mechanism by which Rh(D)-positive red cell stroma interferes with maternal production of anti-D immunoglobulin and reduces the severity of Rh(D) HDN is obscure (Bierme *et al.*, 1982). The results of the original study from France await confirmation by other centres. Meanwhile, the use of Rh(D)-positive red cell stroma must be regarded as experimental (Bierme *et al.*, 1982).

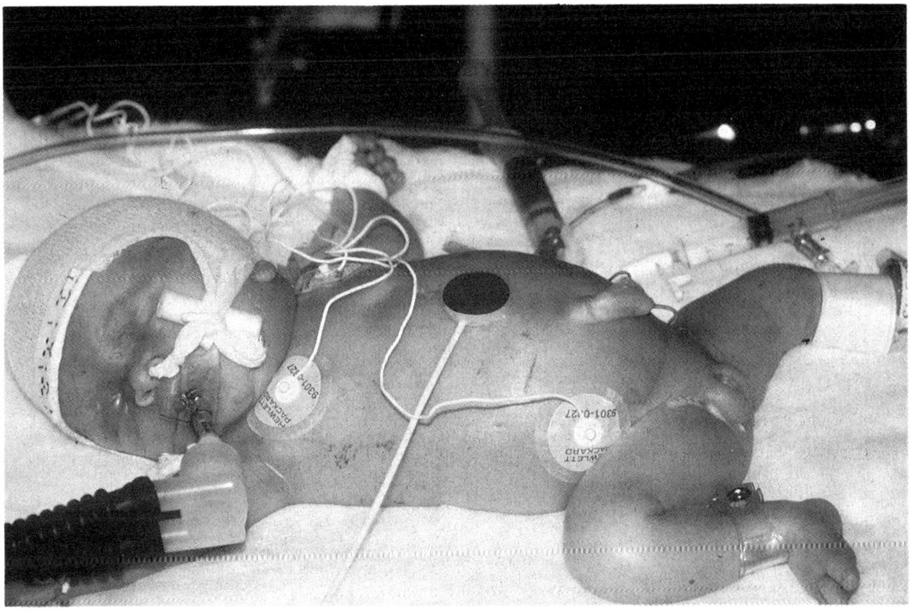

Figure 5.6 Exchange transfusion. The HDN, due to anti-D, was untreated in utero at 31 weeks' gestation. The pigmentation is due to phototherapy, and the baby is ventilated for RDS. The gestation is similar to the fresh neonatal hydrops shown in Figure 5.7. Hb = 3.8 g dl^{-1} at delivery. Three double volume exchanges were performed. The baby is now alive and well and 6 years old.

Intravascular immunoglobulin (i.v. IgG)

In common with all immune-based diseases, the effect of high dose IgG is now being investigated. The possibility of modifying fetal red cell destruction by maternal (or fetal) high dose IgG therapy is intriguing and deserves consideration. There are several pilot trials in progress and one report of apparent successful modification of disease using maternal Ig administration (Camara *et al.*, 1988).

Plasma exchange to reduce maternal antibody titre

Regular plasmapheresis two to three times weekly, from as early as 10 weeks' gestation, has been reported to reduce the severity of fetal haemolytic disease (Fraser *et al.*, 1976). Although the anti-D levels may be reduced initially, the levels rise very rapidly when the plasma exchanges are discontinued. There are many practical problems. Results from various centres are conflicting. The reports from groups who believe plasmapheresis to be beneficial are not convincing because the outcomes are not compared with any suitable control group. Indeed, overall the survival rate of infants is no better than from those centres who do not use plasmapheresis.

Intra-uterine transfusion

Death of the fetus from severe anaemia may be prevented by the introduction of compatible adult donor cells into the fetal circulation by various methods. The factors that are important in determining the need for and timing of intra-uterine transfusion are:

(1) the level and trend of bilirubin content of amniotic fluid,
(2) the gestation, and
(3) the past obstetric history.

Intra-peritoneal transfusions

Since the first description of successful intra-uterine transfusion by Liley in the early 1960s (Liley, 1961) techniques have improved considerably (Bowman, 1975; McClure, 1990). It is possible to administer the first intraperitoneal transfusion from as early as 22–23 weeks' gestation, but the outlook for fetuses developing hydropic changes at an early gestational age remains extremely poor, possibly because fetal ascites prevents adequate absorption of transfused red cells through the lymphatics (Figure 5.7).

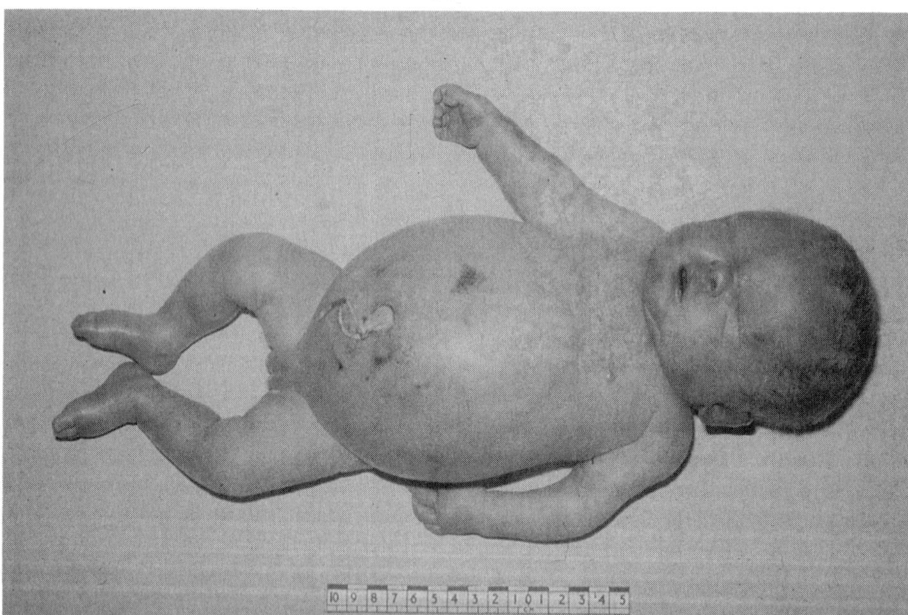

Figure 5.7 Hydrops — fresh neonatal death at 31 weeks' gestation. Unsuccessful attempts had been made to treat the anaemia with intra-peritoneal transfusions, the puncture marks are visible. Some of the ascites is undoubtedly due to unabsorbed transfused blood.

Intravascular transfusion

In 1981, Rodeck and colleagues described a technique for direct intravascular transfusion which can be performed as early as 18 weeks' gestation either by direct fetoscopic vision, as originally described (Rodeck *et al.*, 1984), or by the now preferred method using ultrasound guidance (Daffos *et al.*, 1984; Berkowitz *et al.*, 1986).

The umbilical cord is entered and a pure fetal blood sample obtained for haematological and biochemical analysis (see above). Group O Rh(D)-negative packed red cells are introduced into the lumen of the vessel at a rate of 1–3 ml min^{-1}. The quantity of blood transfused is determined by the estimated fetal blood volume, the pre-transfusion fetal haematocrit (Nicolaides *et al.*, 1988), and the concentration of donor cells (Rodeck *et al.*, 1984; Berkowitz *et al.*, 1986; Grannum and Copel, 1988).

The transfusions are started as early as 18 weeks' gestation, if indicated, and repeated at 1–3 week intervals until 32–34 weeks; delivery is planned in collaboration with expert neonatal and haematological advice.

A survival rate of 84% in a series of 50 fetuses referred before 25 weeks' gestation has been reported from a centre using these measures (Berkowtiz *et al.*, 1986). Intracardiac transfusions have also been given with success, but the fetal mortality may be unacceptably high (Westgren *et al.*, 1988).

Combination of intraperitoneal and intravascular transfusion

It is now the practice at Queen Charlotte's Maternity Hospital to combine the two techniques of intra-uterine transfusions from 22 weeks' gestation onwards (Nicolini and Rodeck, 1988). The advantage is that the interval between transfusions can be prolonged (Nicolini *et al.*, 1990). Immediate correction of anaemia is achieved by the intravascular transfusions and the haemoglobin level can be maintained by the slower absorption of intraperitoneally introduced packed red cells.

Intra-uterine exchange transfusion

Some authors have reported successes using exchange transfusion rather than 'top-up'. Protagonists argue that there is less hazard of overloading the fetal circulation and precipitating hydrops, and transfusion intervals may be longer. However each procedure takes much longer, is more complex and requires considerable skill. The outcome overall in these centres is no better than using conventional 'top-up' transfusions (Grannum *et al.*, 1986; Poissonnier *et al.*, 1989).

Few long-term follow-up studies have been made on the effect of intra-uterine transfusion on subsequent development, but there does not seem to be any obvious ill effect reported from the many centres using this therapy. One relatively early assessment of surviving children who received intra-uterine transfusions between 1965 and 1976 showed developmental achievements to be within the normal range (White *et al.*, 1978).

MANAGEMENT OF THE BABY AFTER BIRTH

Cord blood should be taken at delivery for (1) ABO Rh(D) grouping, (2) direct antiglobulin test, (3) serum bilirubin and (4) haemoglobin.

Babies who are born after a series of intra-uterine transfusions often have a normal haemoglobin at delivery, negative direct antiglobulin test and group as Rh(D)-negative because of successful replacement of fetal red cells by transfused donor blood combined with suppression of fetal marrow. These babies often require only phototherapy to control jaundice of prematurity and, maybe, a top-up transfusion to correct anaemia several weeks after delivery. The main problems are not haematological but those arising from immaturity — although many more fetuses are now kept *in utero* till 35–37 weeks' gestation.

On the other hand, those infants who have not received intra-uterine treatment may be born severely anaemic — even hydropic — and will rapidly accumulate dangerous concentrations of bilirubin if prompt measures are not taken to prevent this. The main risk to the neonate is that of kernicterus, arising from hyperbilirubinaemia (Figure 5.8). The liver of the neonate does not produce glucoronyl transferase and cannot convert bilirubin to an excretable form. Consequently bilirubin accumulates and, if not removed (by exchange transfusion), will collect in the tissues, causing jaundice and brain tissue damage (Figure 5.9). Deeply jaundiced infants often exhibit signs of damage to the central nervous system. These signs develop usually after the age of 36 hours. At any time after this, the infant who has previously behaved normally becomes increasingly lethargic and

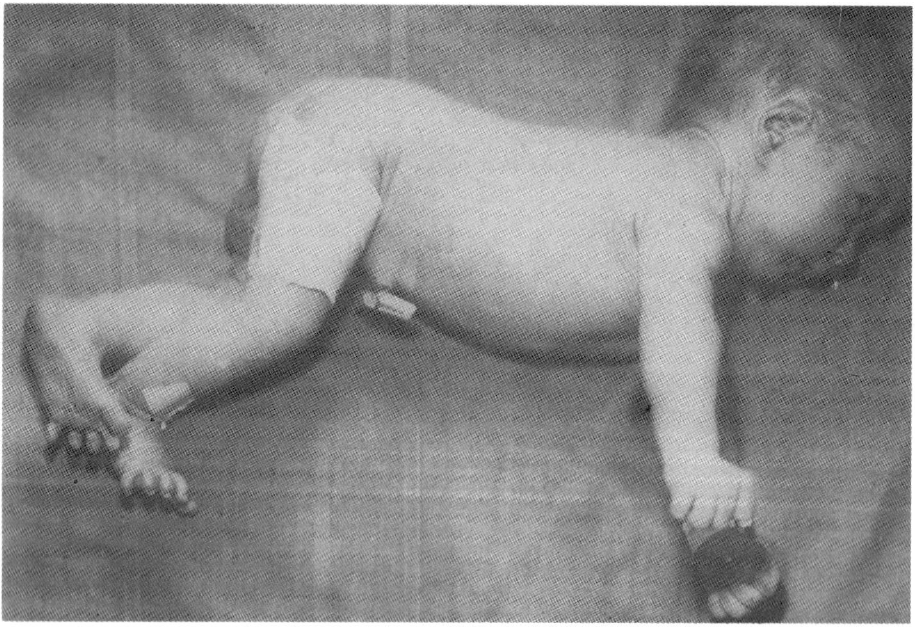

Figure 5.8 Kernicterus in a baby with HDN who eventually died.

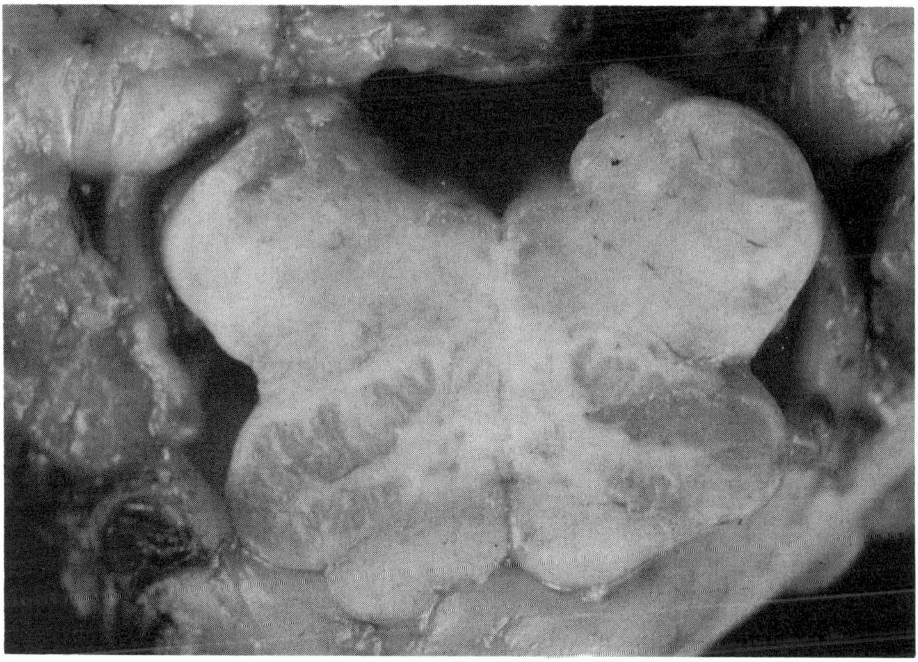

Figure 5.9 Medulla showing bilirubin staining at post mortem.

reluctant to feed and may exhibit opisthotonus and develop a high pitched cry. At this stage in 70% of cases, respiration becomes irregular and the infant grows cold and dies. Those who recover have permanent brain damage, characterized by variable deafness, visual impairment, spasticity and mental retardation.

Exchange transfusion for management and prevention of hyperbilirubinaemia

In addition to controlling existing hyperbilirubinaemia, exchange transfusion corrects anaemia and blood volume abnormalities. The first exchange transfusion also washes out about one-third of the anti-D antibody in the neonatal circulation. A two-volume exchange (170 ml kg^{-1}) will remove 85–90% of the infant's circulating Rh(D)-positive cells, which would otherwise contribute to the bilirubin pool. However, a two-volume exchange transfusion removes only 25% of the infant's total bilirubin, due in the main to the fact that a large part of the total bilirubin is in the extravascular compartment. Maximum reduction of the bilirubin is achieved by a two-volume exchange for a single procedure. There is no point in increasing the volume but, after the exchange transfusion, serum levels rapidly rebound to 70–80% of the pre-exchange values. For further details of exchange transfusion, see Chapter 7.

Other measures to reduce hyperbilirubinaemia

Enzyme induction

Phenobarbitone, 30 mg administered to the mother 3 times daily for 48–72 hours prior to delivery, reduces peak bilirubin levels in the affected neonate. Since there is a latent period of 2–3 days before adequate enzyme induction occurs, treatment is more successful if administered to the mother than if given to the baby post delivery. However, the administration of phenobarbitone makes the infant sluggish and may induce other enzymes not beneficial to the pre-term neonate, and therefore routine use of phenobarbitone is not recommended.

Phototherapy

Phototherapy is effective in reducing the serum unconjugated bilirubin concentration in newborn infants. When exposed to blue light bilirubin is readily converted into less lipophilic smaller water soluble components (Cashore and Stern, 1984). Used alone in the mildly affected baby or following exchange transfusion in the more severely affected, it will reduce peak bilirubin levels and the need for further exchange transfusion. This is a major advance in the treatment of all types of indirect hyperbilirubinaemia in the infant.

Despite initial concerns to the contrary the procedure seems to carry no major side-effects. Because there is a risk of retinal damage, all babies should have their eyes protected. Phototherapy increases evaporative water loss, therefore extra fluid should be administered to the baby undergoing this treatment.

Loose green stools are an indication of the excretion of the photobilirubin isomer. These should cause no concern unless there is bowel stasis, when the unstable isomer may be converted back to the stable toxic unconjugated isomer and reabsorbed.

Criteria for exchange transfusion

Clinical evidence of severe disease at delivery, such as pallor, petechiae or hepatosplenomegaly, are indications for immediate exchange transfusion without waiting for cord blood results. If the cord haemoglobin is less than 8.0 g dl^{-1} or the bilirubin more than 100 μmol l^{-1}, the exchange transfusion should be instituted within 1 hour of birth.

The baby who does not require immediate exchange should be monitored haematologically at regular 3–4 hour intervals, with particular reference to the bilirubin. A rapidly rising bilirubin is an indication for exchange. For all SCBU, charts are available that indicate the levels of bilirubin at which exchange should be undertaken related to the birth weight and gestation, so that kernicterus will be prevented (see Chapter 7).

Albumin administration

The binding of bilirubin to albumin is of importance in the prevention of bilirubin excephalopathy. There are no controlled trials to show that the administration of albumin reduces the number of exchange transfusions required, or the incidence of kernicterus, but administration of albumin before or during exchange transfusion significantly increases the amount of bilirubin removed and increases the albumin binding capacity of the infant's plasma after the exchange transfusion.

Albumin should not be added to blood used to exchange a severely anaemic or hydropic baby because the resulting increase in plasma colloid pressure may precipitate or augment heart failure.

OTHER CAUSES OF FETO-MATERNAL ALLOIMMUNIZATION

In theory, any fetal red cell antigen may cause alloimmunization if the mother lacks that antigen. Thus any red cell antigen which the father possesses and the mother lacks, if inherited by the fetus, can cause maternal alloimmunization. Ideally, all pregnant women should have their blood tested in the 12th, 28th and 34th weeks of pregnancy for antibodies to red cell antigens. These examinations not only alert the obstetrician to possible cases of HDN, but also identify the mother for whom there may be difficulty in providing compatible blood quickly in an obstetric emergency.

Rhesus blood group c and E

Within the Rhesus blood group system the most immunogenic antigens after D are c and E (Mollison *et al.*, 1987). These antibodies are found most usually in women who are Rh(D)-positive and lack the c and E antigens, for example those women who have the genotype *Cde*/*Cde* (R_1R_1). The management of HDN due to alloimmunization by antigens other than anti-D is the same as that for Rh(D) HDN and there is, as yet, no way of preventing these conditions. Some cases of HDN due to anti-c are as severe as anti-D HDN and may end in hydrops if intra-uterine transfusions are not given. Anti-E antibodies, in my experience (and many others), never caused severe HDN but may cause considerable difficulty in cross-matching if not identified.

Theoretically, prevention of alloimmunization to other red-cell antigens by transfusion or pregnancy could be prevented in a manner similar to that with anti-D. In practice, it would be very time-consuming and costly to Rh phenotype all women in pregnancy and to produce sufficient quantities of anti-c and anti-E from male 'volunteers' by injections of incompatible blood to produce the appropriate immunoglobulin.

Kell blood group

The Kell red cell blood group (Mollison *et al.*, 1987) is a good example of a system which occasionally causes problems. Ninety-five per cent of the British population are Kell-negative (*kk*); the remaining five per cent are Kell-positive and the majority are heterozygous *Kk*. Only one in 500 individuals are found to be homozygous *KK* positive. The antibody anti-K is usually found in patients who have had multiple transfusions, either as a large number of donations to cover a single traumatic incident or as recurrent supportive therapy over a long period. When anti-K is found in antenatal sera, the majority of patients have a history of transfusion, but the husband's blood should be tested to determine his Kell status — usually he is Kell-negative which indicates transfusion alloimmunization, providing that extramarital pregnancy can be excluded. Occasionally, the husband is Kell-positive but statistically he is likely to be heterozygous *Kk*. If he is one of the rare one in 500 *KK* homozygous Kell-positives, then all the children he fathers will be Kell-positive and at risk of HDN from maternal anti-K. There is no difficulty in finding blood for intra-uterine or exchange transfusion as 90% of the population are *kk* Kell-negative.

Kell haemolytic disease can be very severe and rapidly fatal *in utero* at relatively early gestation.

It would apear that amniotic fluid bilirubin levels are unhelpful in assessing severity of disease (Berkowitz *et al.*, 1982; Caine and Mueller-Heubach, 1986; Mollison *et al.*, 1987) and the disease process is thought to be one of erythroid hypoplasia rather than haemolytic anaemia. It is thought that the anti-Kell antibody has a disproportionate effect on erythroid precursors (compared with anti-D), causing relatively more anaemia and less jaundice. Reticulocytosis is less marked and there are few erythroblasts in the face of very severe anaemia. At Queen Charlotte's Maternity Hospital we have seen amniotic fluid bilirubin levels in the mild or unaffected Liley zone when a baby is hydropic *in utero* and has died within days of investigation. It has also been observed that severe disease is possible with low titre of maternal anti-Kell antibody.

We recommend fetal blood sampling in all cases thought to be at risk, so that Kell grouping can be established and haematocrit can be dirctly measured at a time when appropriate management can be planned. There is no doubt that, for HDN due to anti-Kell, a different approach to management has to be adopted.

ABO blood group incompatibility

Even before the striking reduction in Rh(D)-HDN due to prophylaxis, the most frequent cause of HDN was the haemolysis due to ABO incompatibility. Although the incidence in the United Kingdom and the United States has been found to be approximately 2% of all births, in only one in 3000 births does severe ABO HDN occur. Mild cases not requiring exchange transfusion are identified one in 150 births. Less than 5% of affected newborns require phototherapy, and only in the very rare case is exchange transfusion required. There is a one in three chance in marriage that the husband's red cells will be ABO incompatible with the wife's serum. However, the husband may be heterozygous in respect of the allele for the incompatible antigen, for example *AO* rather than *AA* (homozygous), so that the chance of ABO incompatibility between fetal red cells and maternal serum is one in five.

It is therefore surprising that ABO HDN is relatively uncommon. There are several factors that explain this. A- and B-like substances are widespread in vegetable and animal life. The agglutinins, anti-A and B, are often called naturally occurring antibodies, which is strictly a misnomer because they develop during the first few months of life, probably as a result of exposure to A- and B-like substances elaborated by Gram-negative bacteria that colonize the gut. Naturally occurring anti-A and anti-B are usually IgM immunoglobulins that will not cross the placenta. The maternal antibody can only cause HDN if it is of the IgG type.

Group O women who have had ABO incompatible pregnancies may develop IgG anti-A or B (immune antibody). Also group O individuals who have been vaccinated or immunized with preparations derived from hog stomach or pneumococcal vaccine which contain an A substance, may develop immune lytic IgG anti-A anti-body which can persist for some years (hog pepsin is used in the preparation of TAB and diphtheria toxoid). But even if the Group O mother has a high titre of lytic IgG anti-A or anti-B antibody, it is unlikely to cause problems for the ABO incompatible fetus *in utero* because the A and B antigens, unlike Rh antigens, are present not only on the fetal red cells but also on cells of all other tissue and body fluids. Neutralization of maternal antibody by soluble fetal antigens and by antigens carried on cells other than the red cells will help to protect the incompatible fetal red cells.

Another factor which may help to protect the fetal red cells is that the A and B antigens, although detectable in the 5-week embryo, do not have the antigenic strength of adult red cells in the neonate and therefore will not react fully with antibody that crosses the placenta.

The vast majority of cases of HDN due to ABO incompatibility occur in group O mothers with A or B infants, because group O individuals make more avid antibody and are more likely to produce immune antibody; unlike Rh disease, 40–50% of cases occur in firstborn infants and the disease does not become more severe with each subsequent pregnancy.

Although determinations of lytic IgG and anti-A and anti-B titres does not give a good indication of the severity of the likely outcome of ABO maternal–fetal incompatibility, routine serological evaluation will detect some cases of lytic anti-A and anti-B in maternal serum. If potent antibodies are found, this will alert the obstetrician to examine cord blood to enable HDN to be diagnosed as soon as possible after birth.

Apart from the occasional case with a history of other previously affected infants and/or lytic IgG in the maternal serum, screening of cord blood for ABO incompatibility is not usually performed. The diagnosis of ABO HDN is usually made in the work-up of a mature infant who develops jaundice in the first 24 hours of life. In fact, the diagnosis may be quite difficult to make because the direct antiglobulin (Coombs') test (DAT) is not always positive and there may be a very mild degree of anaemia, although such infants can develop a marked reticulocyte response and occasionally go on to develop jaundice of a severity which may lead to kernicterus. The danger is that with early discharge post-delivery, now common, the jaundice may develop at home. The confirmation of the diagnosis is made by finding IgG lytic antibody of the appropriate blood-group specificity in the maternal serum (Brouwers *et al.*, 1988). The blood film characteristically has large numbers of spherocytes. If exchange transfusion is undertaken in ABO HDN, then fresh group O donor blood of the same Rh type as the infant should be used: the plasma containing anti-A and anti-B may be removed and replaced with fresh platelet-rich group AB plasma. Alternatively, group O cells of the appropriate Rh type (recovered from a bank of frozen cells) may be used, the cells being suspended in plasma protein fraction or albumin to which bilirubin will bind (see Chapter 7).

ANTENATAL SCREENING

Serological evaluation of the mother should be carried out at approximately 16 weeks. All Rh-negative women should be screened again at 28 and 34 weeks. Ideally, all women should be screened again at these times in order to identify those who have IgG antibodies which might lead to other forms of HDN, for example, Kell, c, Duffy, Kidd, etc.

The serological investigations that should be carried out are routine grouping and an indirect Coombs' test to detect IgG antibodies in maternal serum. When these are found, they should be characterized in terms of specificity and titre by standard serological techniques (see Chapter 7).

NEONATAL SCREENING

It is very important to anticipate, identify and treat HDN, because if haemolysis and subsequent jaundice are managed effectively the prognosis is excellent. The direct antiglobulin test (Coombs' test) should be carried out routinely on all cord bloods of babies born to mothers who have an IgG blood-group antibody identified in antenatal screening. The specificity of the antibody will usually have been identified in the maternal blood by testing the serum with a mixed panel of red cells bearing a variety of antigens. Affected infants should have cord blood haemoglobin and bilirubin levels estimated and exchange transfusion should be initiated where appropriate.

Because HDN may occasionally arise unexpectedly, either because IgG antibodies were not detected in the maternal sera even late in pregnancy, or because screening was not carried out at all, and as there are difficulties in the diagnosis of some cases of HDN due to ABO sensitization, it might seem that the ideal approach to screening for HDN would be to carry out a haemoglobin, direct antiglobulin test and to estimate serum bilirubin on all newborn infants. However, this is impractical and it would certainly not be cost-effective. Hence, neonatal screening is reserved for those infants who are born of mothers known to have IgG antibodies, those with a previous history of HDN for any reason, and as part of the work-up for those who become jaundiced in the neonatal period.

REFERENCES

Bang J, Bock JE and Trolle D (1982) Ultrasound guided fetal intra-venous transfusion for severe rhesus haemolytic disease. *British Medical Journal* **284**: 373–374.

Baker SP and Letsky EA (1989) Amniotic fluid bilirubin. In *Laboratory Haematology (Chanarin I, ed.) 163–165. Edinburgh: Churchill Livingstone.*

Bergstrom H, Nilsson LA, Nilsson L and Ryttinger L (1967) Demonstration of Rh antigens in a 38-day-old fetus. *American Journal of Obstetrics and Gynecology* **99**: 130.

Berkowitz RL, Beyta Y and Sadovsky E (1982) Death in utero due to Kell sensitisation without excessive elevation of the Δ OD 45 value in amniotic fluid. *Obstetrics and Gynecology* **60**: 746–749.

Berkowitz RL, Chitkara, U, Goldberg JD, Wilkins I, Chervenak FA and Lynch L (1986) Intrauterine intravascular transfusion for severe red blood cell isoimmunisation: ultra-sound guided percutaneous approach. *American Journal of Obstetrics and Gynecology* **155**: 574–581.

Bierme SJ, Blanc M, Abbal M and Fournie A (1979) Oral Rh treatment for severely immunised mothers. *The Lancet* **i**: 604–605.

Bierme SJ, Blanc M, Fournie A, Abbal M (1982) Desensitization by Oral Antigen. In *Rh Hemolytic Disease; New Strategy for Eradication.* (Frigoletto FD Jr, Figgis Jewett J and Konugres AA, eds), pp 249–266. Boston: GK Hall.

Bowell PJ, Wainscoat JS, Peto TEA and Gunson HH (1982) Maternal anti-D concentration and outcome in rhesus haemolytic disease of the newborn. *British Medical Journal* **285**: 327–329.

Bowell PJ, Selinger M, Ferguson J, Giles J and McKenzie IZ (1988) Antenatal fetal blood sampling for alloimmunized pregnancies: effect upon maternal anti-D potency levels. *British Journal of Obstetrics and Gynaecology* **95**: 759–764.

Bowman JM (1975) Rh Erythroblastosis fetalis 1975. *Seminars in Hematology* **12**: 189–207.

Brouwers HAA, Overbeeke MAM, van Ertbruggen I, *et al.* (1988) What is the best predictor of the severity of ABO-haemolytic disease of the newborn. *The Lancet* **ii**: 641–644.

Caine ME and Mueller-Heubach MD (1986) Kell sensitisation in pregnancy. *American Journal of Obstetrics and Gynecology* **154**: 85–90.

Camara de la C, Arrieta R, Gonzalez A, Inglesias E and Omenaca F (1988) High-dose intravenous immunoglobulin as the sole prenatal treatment for severe Rh immunization. *New England Journal of Medicine* **318**: 519–529.

Cashore WJ and Stern L (1984) The management of hyperbilirubinaemia. *Clinics in Perinatology* **11**: 339–358.

Chitkara U, Wilkins I, Lynch L, Mehalek H and Berkowitz RH (1988) The role of sonography in assessing severity of fetal anaemia in Rh and Kell-isoimmunised pregnancies. *Obstetrics and Gynecology* **71**: 393–398.

Clarke CA (1989) Preventing rhesus babies: the Liverpool research and follow-up. *Archives of Disease in Childhood* **64**: 1734–1740.

Clarke CA, Whitfield AGW and Mollison PL (1987) Death from Rh haemolytic disease in England and Wales in 1984 and 1985. *British Medical Journal* **294**: 1001.

Crawford DH, Barlow MJ, Harrison JF, Winger L and Huehns ER (1983) Production of human monoclonal antibody to Rhesus D antigen. *The Lancet* **i**: 386–388.

Daffos F, Forestier F and Capella-Pavlowsky M (1984) Fetal blood sampling during the third trimester of pregnancy. *British Journal of Obstetrics and Gynaecology* **91**: 118–121.

Fraser ID, Bothamley JE, Bennett MO *et al.* (1976) Intensive antenatal plasmapheresis in severe rhesus isoimmunisation. *The Lancet* **i**: 6–9.

Grannum PAT and Copel JA (1988) Prevention of Rh isoimmunization and treatment of the compromised fetus. *Seminars in Perinatology* **12**: 324–335.

Grannum PA, Copel J, Plaxe SC, Scioscia AL and Hobbins JC (1986) In utero exchange transfusion by direct intravascular injection in severe erythroblastosis fetalis. *New England Journal of Medicine* **314**: 1431–1434.

Harrison KL, Baker JW, Popper EI and Harden PA (1984) Value of maternal anti-D concentration in predicting the outcome of Rh(D) haemolytic disease. *Australian and New Zealand Journal of Obstetrics and Gynaecology* **26**: 6–8.

Hughes-Jones NC (1988) Human monoclonal antibodies and haemolytic disease of the newborn. *British Journal of Haematology* **70**: 263–265.

Landsteiner K and Weiner AS (1940). Are agglutinable factors in human blood recognisable by immune sera for Rhesus blood. *Proc. Soc. Exp. Biol.* **43**: 223.

Letsky EA, Sheerman-Chase J (1989) Kleihauer. In *Laboratory Haematology* (Chanarin I, ed.), pp 161–163. Edinburgh: Churchill Livingstone.

Levine P (1943) Serological factors as possible causes in spontaneous abortions. *Journal of Heredity* **34**: 71–80.

Liley AW (1961) Liquor amnii analysis in the management of the pregnancy complicated by rhesus sensitisation. *American Journal of Obstetrics and Gynecology* **82**: 1359–1370.

McClure G (1990). Haemolytic disease of the newborn (Erythroblastosis Fetalis). In *Textbook of Neonatology*, 2nd edn (Roberton NRC, ed.) Edinburgh: Churchill Livingstone (in press).

McKenzie IZ, Bowell PJ, Castle BM, Selinger M and Ferguson FJ (1988) Serial fetal blood sampling for the management of pregnancies complicated by severe rhesus (D) isoimmunisation. *British Journal of Obstetrics and Gynaecology* **95**: 753–758.

Millar DS, Davis LR, Rodeck CH, Nicolaides KH and Mibashan RS (1985) Normal blood cell values in the early mid-trimester fetus. *Prenatal Diagnosis* **5**: 367–373.

Mollison PL, Engelfreit CP and Contreras M (eds.) (1987) Haemolytic disease of the newborn. In *Blood Transfusion in Clinical Medicine*. 8th edn, pp 637–687. Oxford: Blackwell Scientific Publications.

Nicolaides KH, Rodeck CH, Millar DS and Mibashan RS (1985) Fetal haematology in rhesus isoimmunisation. *British Medical Journal* **220**: 661–663.

Nicolaides KH, Rodeck CH, Mibashan RS and Kemp JR (1986a) Have Liley charts outlived their usefulness? *American Journal of Obstetrics and Gynecology* **155**: 90–94.

Nicolaides KH, Soothill PW, Rodeck CH and Campbell S (1986b) Ultrasound-guided sampling of umbilical cord and placental blood to assess fetal wellbeing. *The Lancet* **I**: 1065–1068.

Nicolaides KH, Fontanarosa M, Gabbe SG and Rodeck CH (1988) Failure of ultrasonographic parameters to predict the severity of fetal anemia in rhesus isoimmunisation. *American Journal of Obstetrics and Gynecology* **158**: 920–926.

Nicolaides KH, Soothill PW, Clewell WH, Rodeck CH, Mibashan RS and Campbell S (1988) Fetal haemoglobin measurement in the assessment of red cell isoimmunisation. *The Lancet* **i**: 1073–1075.

Nicolini U and Rodeck CH (1988) A proposed scheme for planning intra-uterine transfusion in patients with severe Rh-immunisation. *Journal of Obstetrics and Gynecology* **9**: 162–163.

Nicolini U, Kochenour NK, Greco P *et al.* (1988) Consequences of fetomaternal haemorrhage after intrauterine transfusion. *British Medical Journal* **297**: 1379–1381.

Nicolini U, Kochenour NK, Greco P, Letsky E and Rodeck CH (1990) When to perform the next intra-uterine transfusion in patients with Rh allo-immunization: combined intravascular and intraperitoneal transfusion allows longer intervals. *Fetal Therapy* **4**: 14–20.

Poissonnier MH, Brossard Y, Demedeiros N *et al.* (1989) Two hundred intrauterine exchange transfusion in severe blood incompatibilities. *American Journal of Obstetrics and Gynecology* **161**: 709–713.

Queenan JT, Gadow EL and Lopes AC (1971) Role of spontaneous abortion in Rh

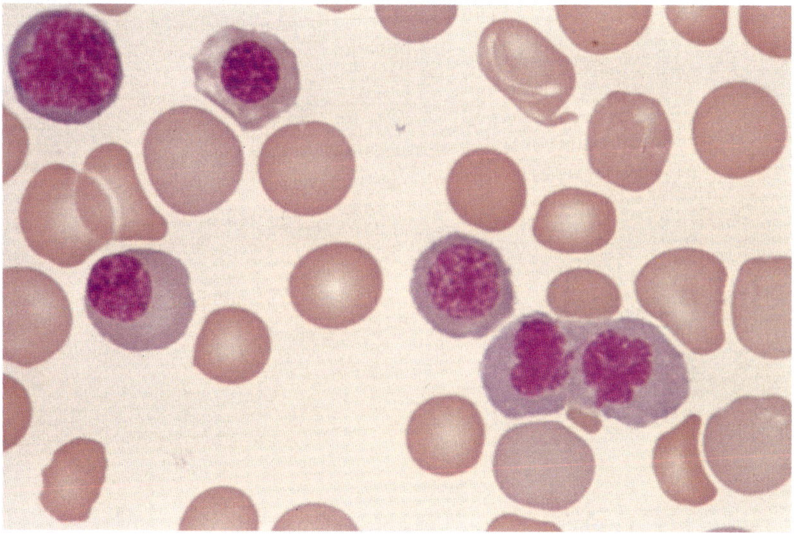

Plate 1. Rhesus D hydrops at 38 weeks showing circulating normoblasts.

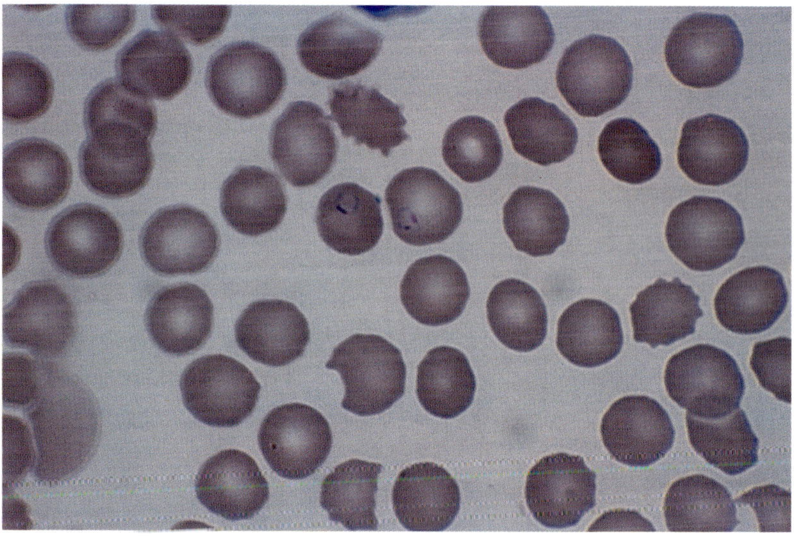

Plate 2. Neonatal malaria *P. falciparum*. Mother was treated in pregnancy and the baby presented aged 4 weeks.

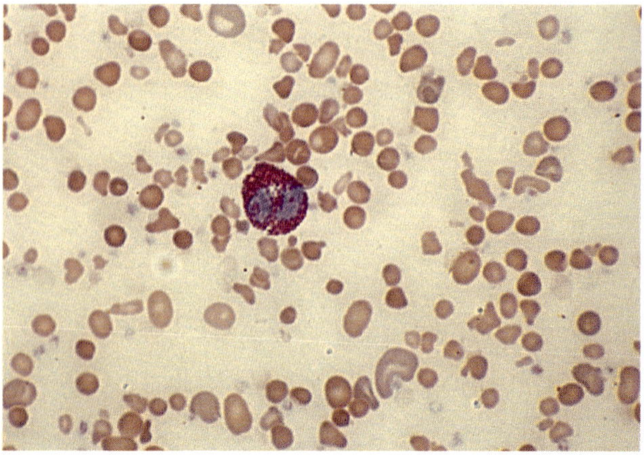

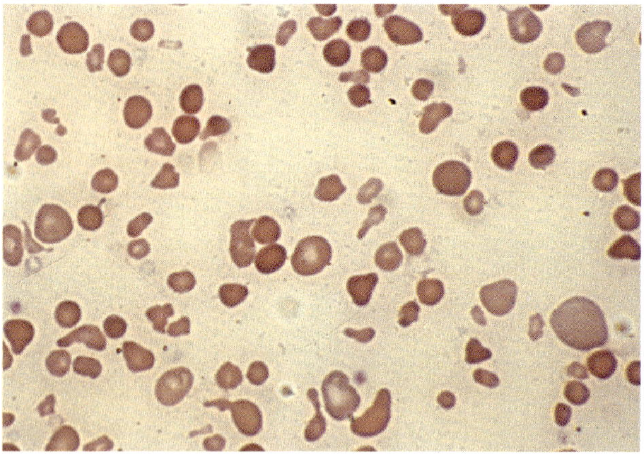

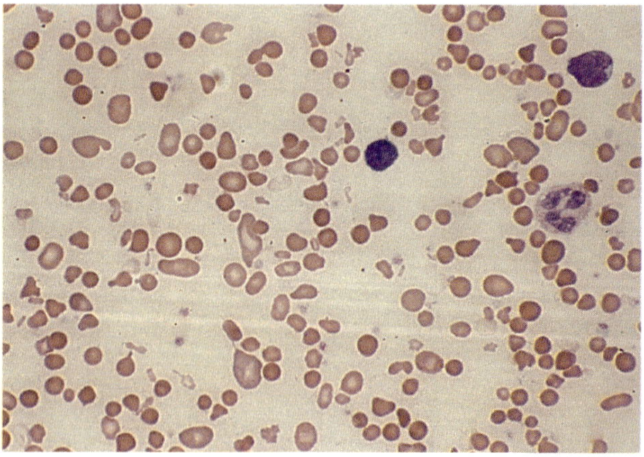

Plates 3, 4 and 5. Hereditary pyropoikilocytosis with many bizarre red cells of varying shapes and size.

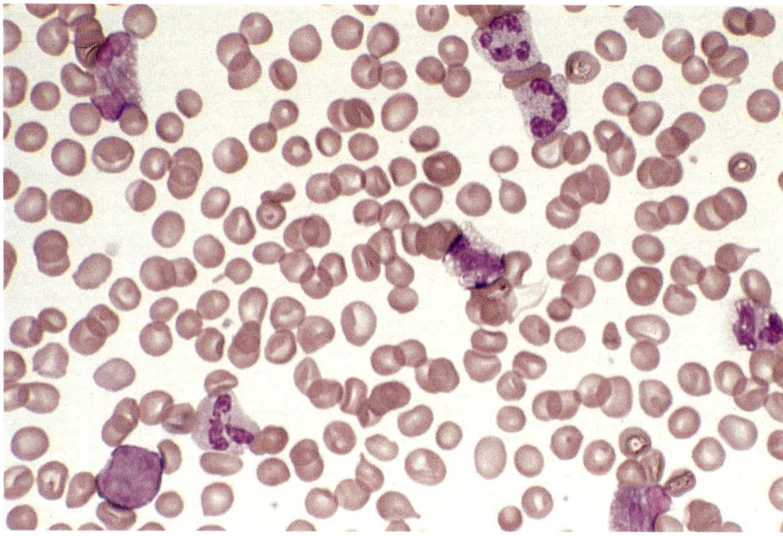

Plates 6. and 7. Congenital toxoplasmosis, showing a leukaemoid reaction with numerous neutrophils and blasts.

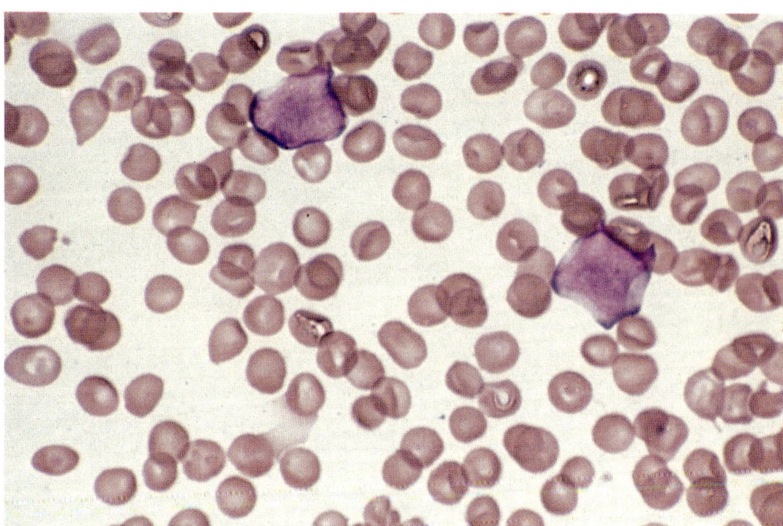

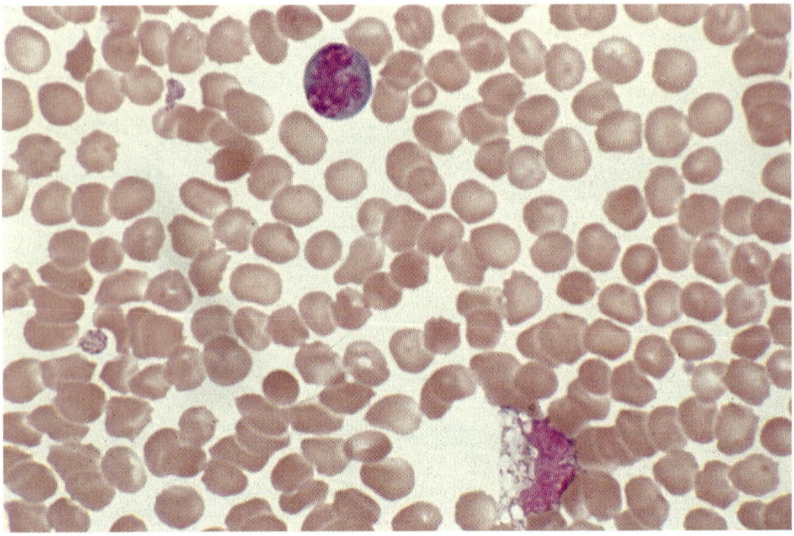

Plates 8 and 9. Fatal *herpes simplex* infection in the neonatal period. Activated lymphocytes and ragged vacuolated neutrophils are present in response to the overwhelming infection.

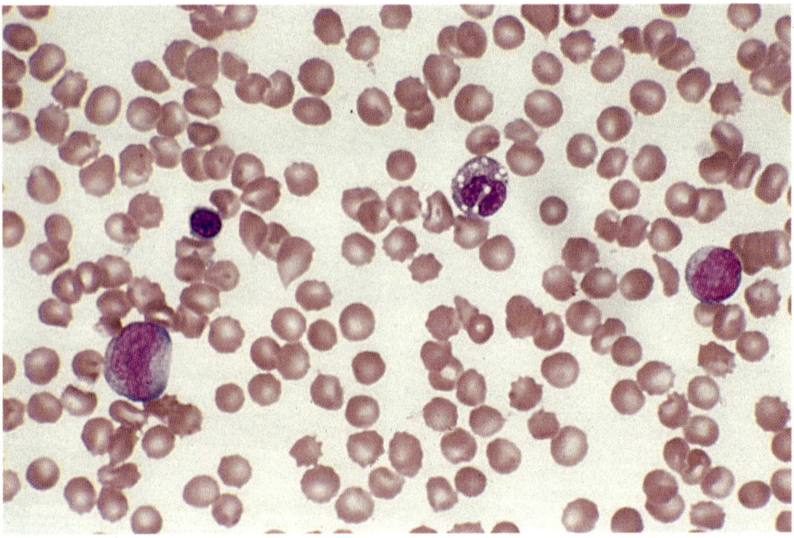

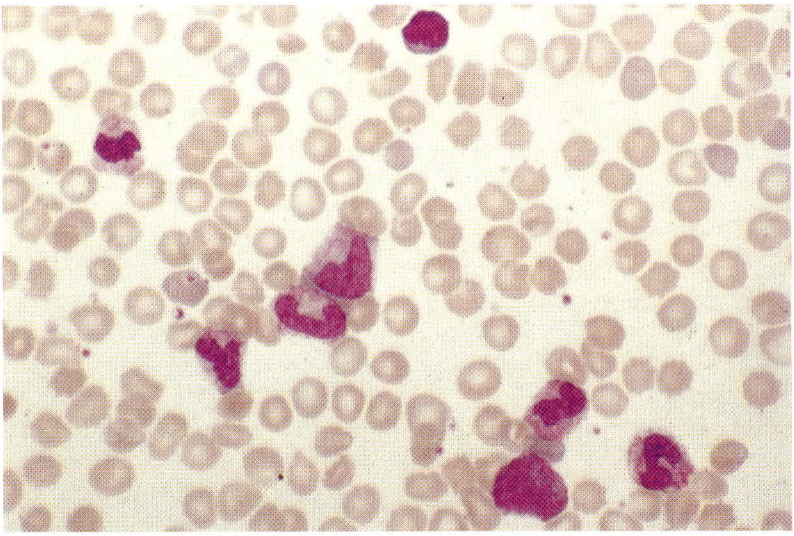

Plate 10. Blood from a 25 week gestation baby with a severe bacterial infection showing toxic and left-shifted neutrophils.

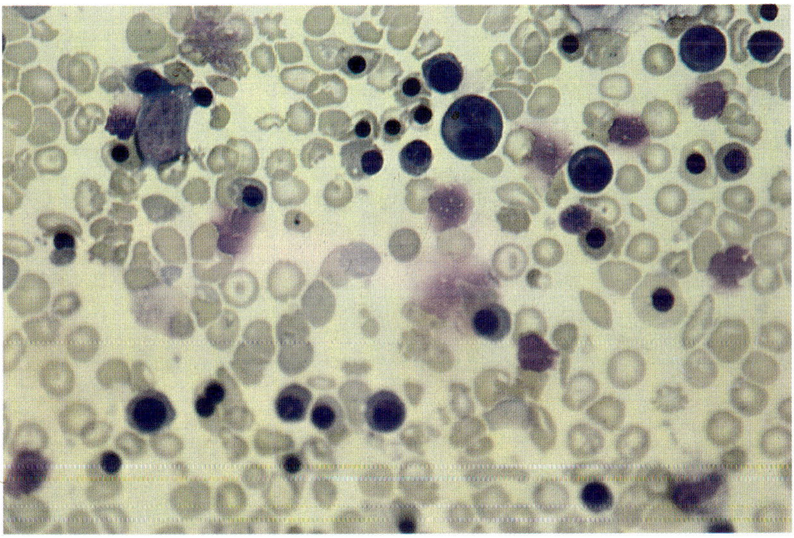

Plate 11. Bart's Hydrops cord blood. Numerous bizarre red cell precursors in a stillbirth born to a South East Asian woman at 32 weeks.

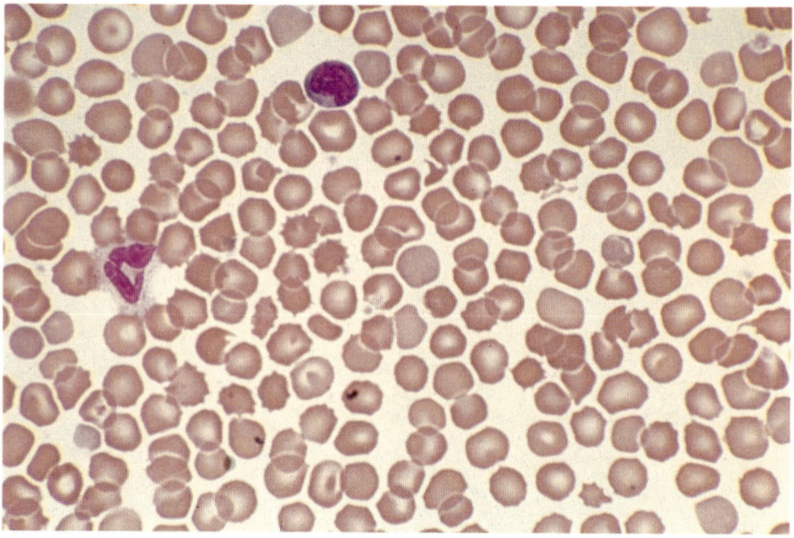

Plate 12. Normal cord blood from a healthy term baby showing the usual and normal variation in red cell shapes and sizes along with Howell-Jolly bodies.

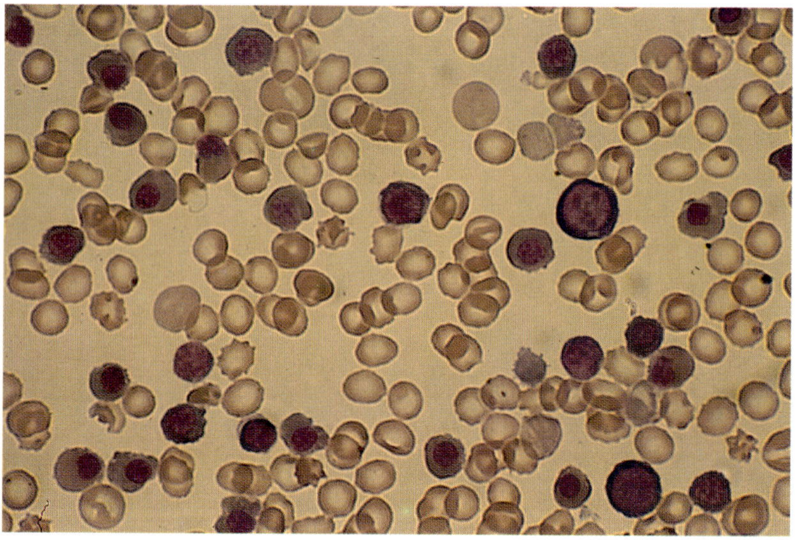

Plate 13. Severe haemolytic disease of the newborn (HDN). Blood taken in utero at 25 weeks during a fetal transfusion.

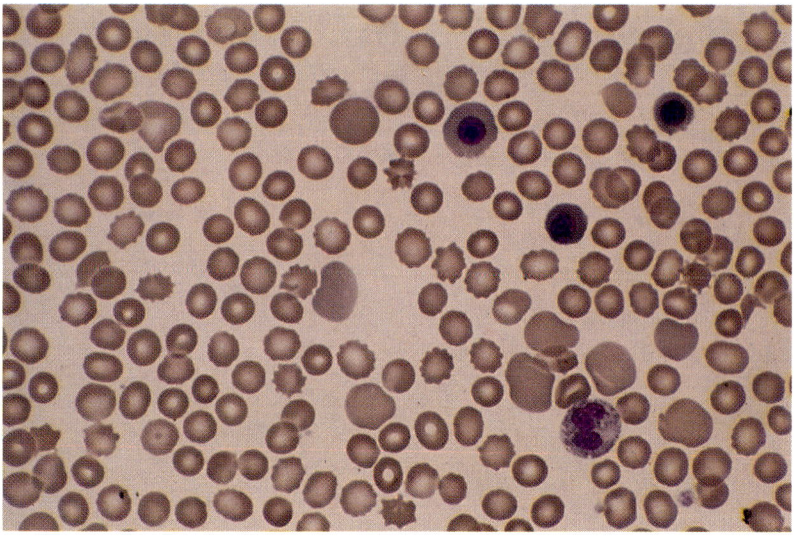

Plate 14. Severe HDN. Blood taken following an intrauterine transfusion showing a double population of red cells (donor/fetus).

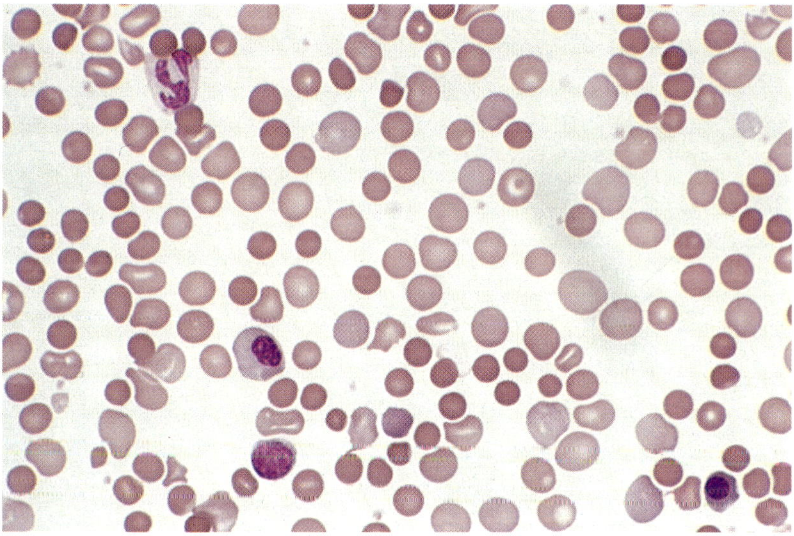

Plate 15. ABO incompatibility (mother was blood group O and baby group B). Numerous spherocytes and polychromatic macrocytes are seen.

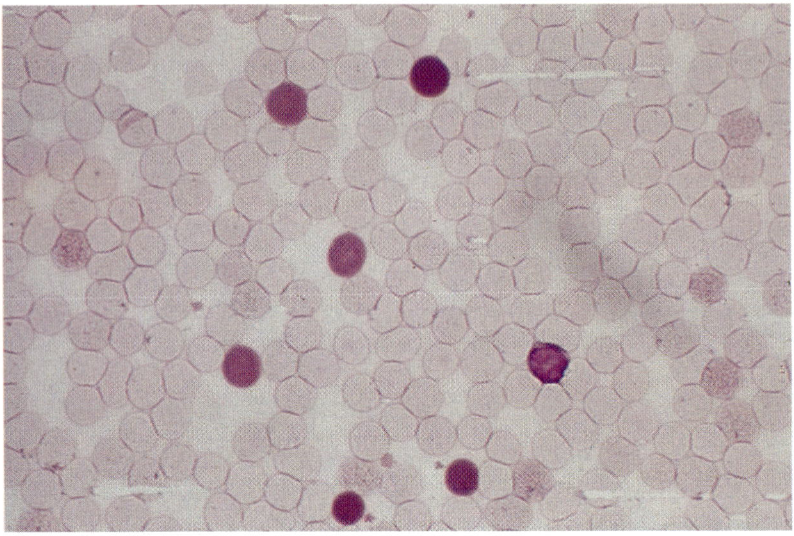
Plate 16. A Kleihauer from a mother with pink-staining "F-cells".

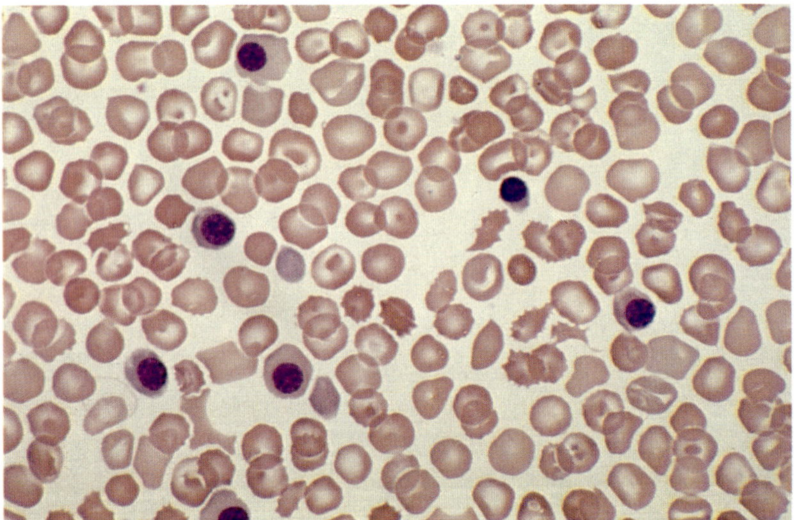
Plate 17. A normal premature baby (23 weeks) with the usual great variation in red cells and their precursors which confuses so many haematologists.

Immunisation. *American Journal of Obstetrics and Gynecology* **110**: 128.
Race RR and Sanger R (1950) *Blood Groups in Man*, pp 234–236. Oxford: Blackwell Scientific Publications.
Rodeck CH and Letsky E (1989) How the management of erythroblastosis fetalis has changed. *British Journal of Obstetrics and Gynaecology* **96**: 759–763.
Rodeck CH, Holman CA, Karnicki J, Kemp JR, Whitmore DN and Austin MA (1981) Direct intravascular fetal blood transfusion by fetoscopy in severe rhesus isoimmunisation. *The Lancet* **i**: 625–628.
Rodeck CH, Nicolaides KH, Warsof SL, Fysh WJ, Gamsu HR and Kemp JR (1984) The management of severe rhesus isoimmunisation by fetoscopic intravascular transfusion. *American Journal of Obstetric Gynecology* **150**: 749–774.
Tovey LAD (1984) The contribution of antenatal anti-D prophylaxis to the reduction of the morbidity and mortality in Rh-haemolytic disease of the newborn. *Plasma Therapy and Transfusion Technology* **5**: 99–104.
Tovey LAD (1986) Haemolytic disease of the newborn — the changing scene. *British Journal of Obstetrics and Gynaecology* **93**: 960–966.
Tovey LAD (1990) Haemolytic disease of the newborn and its prevention. *British Medical Journal* **300**: 313–3116.
Urbaniak SJ (1985) Rh (D) haemolytic disease of the newborn: the changing scene. *British Medical Journal* **291**: 4–6.
Warren RC, Butler J, Morsman JM, McKenzie C and Rodeck CH (1985) Does chorionic villus sampling cause feto-maternal haemorrhage? *The Lancet* **i**: 691.
Westgren M, Selbing A and Strangenberg M (1988) Fetal intracardiac transfusion in patients with severe rhesus isoimmunisation. *British Medical Journal* **296**: 885–886.
White CA, Goplerud CP, Kisker CT, Stehbens JA, Kitchell M and Taylor JC (1978) Intrauterine fetal transfusion, 1965–1976, with an assessment of the surviving children. *American Journal of Obstetrics and Gynecology* **130**: 933–940.
Whitfield CR (1970) A three year assessment of an Action Line method of timing intervention in rhesus isoimmunisation. *American Journal of Obstetrics and Gynecology* **108**: 1239–1244.

6

Normal and disordered coagulation

B.E.S. Gibson

Royal Hospital for Sick Children and Queen Mother's Maternity Hospital, Glasgow

INTRODUCTION

At birth the newborn's haemostatic mechanism is immature and does not develop fully until 6 months of age. Many of the procoagulants, anticoagulants and proteins involved in fibrinolysis are gestation-dependent. Although this does not appear to present a clinical problem in the healthy newborn, it may contribute to morbidity in the sick and pre-term infant. The development of neonatal haemostasis and the common problems associated with coagulation and platelet abnormalities in the newborn will be discussed.

THE DEVELOPMENT OF HAEMOSTASIS IN THE NEONATE

Platelets

Megakaryocytes are evident in the haemopoietic tissue of the liver and spleen by the 6th and 12th week of gestation, respectively. They are well-represented in the bone marrow during the last trimester, when this becomes the main site of haematopoiesis. Fetal magakaryocytes have recently been reported to be smaller in size and less mature than those of adults during the second trimester (Graeve and De Alarcon, 1989). Using immunohistochemical staining techniques, these workers compared the size and maturational stage of fetal magakaryocytes from 20 human fetuses of 12–21 weeks gestation with those from normal adults. They reported the mean diameter of fetal megakaryocytes to be 14.0 μm when stained with anti-glycoprotein IIb and 15.2 μm when stained with anti-factor VIII, compared with 18.4 and 20.6 μm, respectively, for adult megakaryocytes.

Platelets have been identified in the fetal circulation from an early stage of gestation onwards (see Chapter 1). The newborn's platelet count has been thoroughly studied, and current reports confirm that both healthy full-term

Table 6.1 Fetal platelet counts on blood obtained by fetoscopy.*

Gestational age (weeks)	Number of samples	Platelets ($\times 10^9$ per litre) Mean	SD
15	6	190	31
16	5	208	57
17	16	202	25
18	18	192	45
19	29	211	48
20	12	170	60
21	13	223	61

* Adapted from Millar DS *et al.* (1985).

and pre-term infants have values within the adult range (Sell and Corrigan, 1973; Millar *et al.*, 1985). Earlier work suggesting that the pre-term infant had a lower platelet count than the term infant arose from the inclusion of sick infants, who are commonly thrombocytopenic, in the studies. Millar reported platelet counts measured on pure, undiluted fetal blood obtained by fetoscopy performed for a variety of diagnostic indications. The gestational age of the 116 fetuses sampled ranged from 15–21 weeks and the results (Table 6.1) show no significant change over the period studied. On the basis of this information, it would appear that neonates should be considered thrombocytopenic if they have a platelet count below 150×10^9 per litre regardless of their gestational age. The platelet count tends to rise to 300×10^9 to 400×10^9 per litre during the first month of life in both full-term and pre-term infants.

Platelet function has not been particularly well studied in the infant because of the difficulty in obtaining platelet-rich plasma samples of adequate volume for the necessary tests. Pandolfi reported defective aggregation at 20 weeks' gestation in response to adrenaline, collagen and ADP in a small group of fetuses (Pandolfi *et al.*, 1972). The term infant similarly has impaired aggregation compared with adult controls. A number of studies have shown that platelet aggregation in the neonate can be improved by using a higher concentration of platelets or aggregating agents in the test system. For example, Bleyer reported maximum collagen-induced platelet aggregation with a platelet concentration of 700×10^9 per litre in the newborn; an equivalent response being achieved with a platelet concentration of 250×10^9 per litre in the infant's mother (Bleyer *et al.*, 1971). In contrast, ristocetin-induced platelet aggregation is increased, which may be attributed to the newborn's elevated level of von Willebrand factor (vWF).

The underlying abnormality responsible for defective platelet aggregation in the neonate remains unclear. A defect in the platelet release reaction is favoured, although some studies suggest a storage-pool type of abnormality. Adrenaline-induced platelet aggregation is particularly impaired and this may be related to a deficiency of α-adrenergic receptor sites on the neonatal platelet membrane. The neonate's platelets appear to have a normal ultrastructure and normal expression of the major platelet membrane glycoproteins (GPIb and GPIIB/IIIa) and antigens (Pl^{A1} and Bak^a). GPIIb/IIIa and GPIb appear as early as 16 weeks' gestation, when Pl^{A1} and Bak^a are also completely expressed. Reduced platelet factor 3 and serotonin content and release have been reported. Premature infants may have a more pronounced aggregation abnormality than term infants.

Although platelet aggregation in the newborn is defective, this does not appear to be clinically significant and it does not produce a bleeding tendency. However, the newborn is more susceptible to inhibition of platelet aggregation by maternally ingested aspirin. Acetyl salicyclic acid, an inhibitor of platelet cyclo-oxygenase, is known to cross the placenta. Similarly, antenatal ingestion of promethazine has been associated with a prolonged bleeding time in the newborn.

Despite impaired platelet function, the newborn has a bleeding time that is normal or shorter than that of the adult (Feusner, 1980; Andrew *et al.*, 1987). This may be due to either elevated levels of vWF (Andrew *et al.*, 1987) or reduced prostaglandin I_2-like regenerating activity (Stuart, 1981), both of which are present in the newborn.

Procoagulants

Coagulation factors do not appear to cross the placental barrier to any significant degree. A newborn male infant with an inherited deficiency of factor VIII has a very low level of that procoagulant in the cord blood, although his mother has normal values, confirming that clotting factors in the circulation of the newborn have been synthesized by the fetus. When dealing with coagulation problems in the newborn infant it is important to be aware of the normal physiological gestation-dependent ranges. The majority of studies on the development of the clotting factors have been carried out on cord-blood samples taken at the time of delivery of pre-term and term infants. Results may be compromised by several factors. Firstly, it is difficult to obtain clean samples of adequate size from very small premature babies. Secondly, only healthy neonates should be included in studies aimed at establishing normal values. Despite efforts to adhere to this rule, it is difficult to ensure that sick infants with risk factors for disseminated intravascular coagulation (DIC) are not unwittingly included. Thirdly, the birth process itself alters a number of the coagulation parameters. Johnson reported significantly higher levels of vWF:Ag in infants delivered vaginally compared to those delivered by caesarean section (Johnson *et al.*, 1981). The advent of fetal blood sampling by fetoscopy has provided data on a range of normal haematological values at varying gestations. However, this technique for determining normal ranges has its own intrinsic problems, and care with interpretation is as important as with data obtained from cord blood at birth.

The information available suggests that factors I, V, VIII:C and vWF are within the normal adult range from the beginning of the third trimester onwards. All other procoagulants are reduced at birth to variable levels and are dependent on gestational age. This is illustrated in Figure 6.1 and Table

Table 6.2 Values for the procoagulants in the fetus and newborn infant.*†

		Cofactors ($U\ ml^{-1}$)			Vitamin K dependent factors ($U\ ml^{-1}$)				Contact factors ($U\ ml^{-1}$)				
	$Ig l^{-1}$	V	VIII:C	vWF:Ag	II	VII	IX	X	XI	XII	PK	HMWK	XIII ($U\ ml^{-1}$)
Adult	3.40	1.00	1.00	1.00	1.00	1.00	1.00	1.00	1.00	1.00	1.00	1.00	1.00
Term newborn													
37–41 weeks	2.40	1.00	1.50	1.60	0.52	0.57	0.35	0.45	0.42	0.44	0.35	0.64	0.61
Pre-term newborn													
33–36 weeks	3.00	0.82	0.93	1.66	0.45	0.59	0.41	0.44	—	0.25	0.33	—	—
25–32 weeks	2.50	0.80	0.75	1.50	0.32	0.37	0.22	0.38	0.20	0.22	0.26	0.28	0.11–0.40
Fetus													
≃ 20 weeks	0.96	0.70	0.50	0.65	0.16	0.21	0.10	0.19	—	—	—	—	*c.* 0.30

* One unit is the amount of factor in 1 ml of normal plasma; means are given. All values are venous and for the first 24 h of life. All subjects received vitamin K at birth.

† Adapted from Hathway and Bonnar, 1987, *Hemostatic Disorders of the Pregnant Woman and Newborn Infant*, published with kind permission of Elsevier Science Publishing Company Inc.

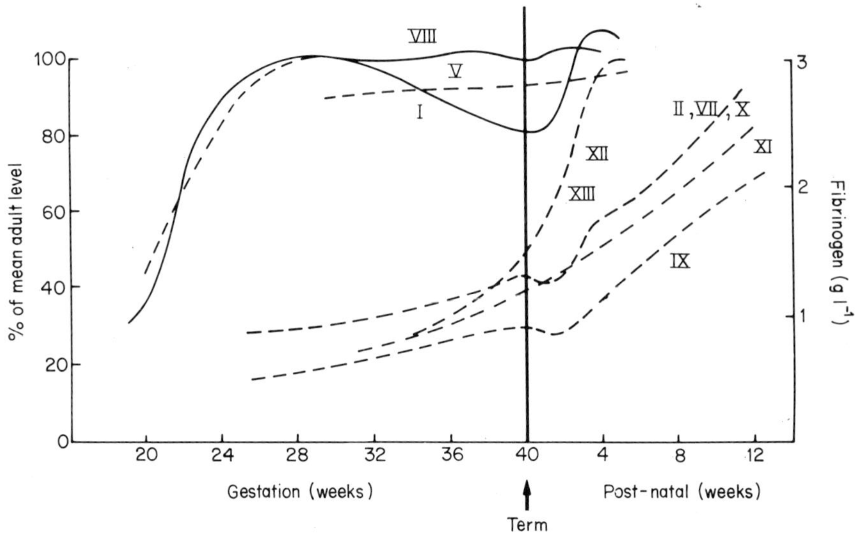

Figure 6.1 Approximate mean levels of clotting factors in pre-term and full-term infants related to gestation. (From Hardisty RM and Weatherall DJ, 1982, *Blood and Its Disorders*, 2nd edn, with permission of Blackwell Scientific.)

6.2. Tables 6.3 and 6.4 give data on fetuses of early gestation obtained by fetoscopic sampling. Differences between individual mean clotting values may reflect recognized intrinsic problems in sampling, and this emphasizes the need for control data in any laboratory using fetoscopy for prenatal diagnosis of coagulation disorders. Hopefully, as fetoscopy becomes a common tool, reliable information on normal coagulation values at all gestations in the fetus and neonate will become available.

Table 6.3 Fetal haemostatic values obtained by fetoscopy at 17–21 weeks' gestation.*

Factor	*n*	Mean	Range
Fibrinogen			
Coagulant assay (gl^{-1})	12	0.63	0.49–0.76
Antigen assay (gl^{-1})		0.96	0.70–1.22
Factor V (% *n*)	40	52	3 67
Factor II			
Coagulant assay (% *n*)	10	17	15–20
Antigen assay (% *n*)		17	15–20
Factor VII (% *n*)	10	19	16–23
Factor X (% *n*)	10	20	16–25
Antithrombin III			
Amidolytic assay (% *n*)	14	27	20–33
Antigen assay (% *n*)		28	20–39

* Adapted from Mibashan and Millar, 1983, *British Medical Bulletin 39* (4): 392–398, with kind permission of Churchill Livingstone.

Table 6.4 Coagulation factors (%) obtained by fetoscopy of 103 normal fetuses at various gestations (means ± SD).*

Age (week of gestation)	*n*	VIII:C	vWF:Ag	IX:C	V:C	II:C
19–21	51	40 ± 12	59 ± 12.5	9 ± 2.5	39 ± 11	13 ± 4
22–24	44	39 ± 13.5	64 ± 13	9 ± 3	40.5 ± 5	14 ± 2
25–27	44	42.5 ± 12	63 ± 13	12 ± 4	39 ± 9	14 ± 3.5

* Adapted from Forestier *et al.*, 1986, *Pediatric Research 20(4):* 342–346, with kind permission of International Pediatric Research Foundation Inc.

Fibrinogen

Fibrinogen synthesis has been demonstrated in cultures of fetal liver at 5.5 weeks' gestation. Holmberg reported mean levels of just under 1 g l^{-1} in fetuses between 14 and 24 weeks' gestation (Holmberg *et al.*, 1974). Infants from this gestation onwards have mean fibrinogen values within the adult range (Holmberg *et al.*, 1974; Hathaway and Bonnar, 1978). Current information suggests that a fibrinogen level of 1.5 g l^{-1} at birth should be regarded as the lower limit of normal in both the term and pre-term infant.

A number of observations point to the existence of a fetal fibrinogen structurally distinct from the 'adult' molecule. Firstly, thrombin and reptilase times are generally prolonged in the newborn. The thrombin clotting time measures the thrombin-mediated conversion of fibrinogen to fibrin and is prolonged in the presence of a low fibrinogen, an abnormal fibrinogen, or inhibitors such as heparin and fibrinogen degradation products (FDPs). It was at one time suggested that the prolongation of the newborn's thrombin clotting time might be due to increased levels of FDPs resulting from fibrinolysis *in vitro*. Although the concentration of plasminogen activator is high in the neonate, increased FDPs are not found in samples collected properly to prevent *in vitro* fibrinolysis. The newborn's thrombin clotting time is therefore prolonged in the presence of both normal fibrinogen and FDP levels, and can best be explained by a dysfibrinogenaemia. Secondly, fibrinogen levels based on heat precipitation or protein estimations are often higher than those obtained by clotting assays.

Fetal fibrinogen is relatively insensitive to thrombin-induced proteolysis (Mills and Karpatkin, 1972). Sodium dodecyl sulphate polyacrylamide gel electrophoresis (SDS–PAGE) studies and tryptic peptide maps are identical for fetal and adult fibrinogen (Teger-Nilsson and Ekelund, 1974), whilst their chromatographic patterns on diethylaminoethanol (DEAE)-cellulose are reported to be different. Adult and fetal fibrinogen have the same content of amino acids (Witt *et al.*, 1969) and of hexoses, but fetal fibrinogen has been shown to contain twice as much phosphorus (Witt and Müller, 1970). More importantly, fetal fibrinogen has an increased sialic acid content which correlates with the degree of prematurity and prolongation of the thrombin clotting time. Although the role of sialic acid in the conversion of fibrinogen to fibrin is controversial, its removal from the fibrinogen molecule enhances clot formation by thrombin. There is no firm evidence that fetal fibrinogen is structurally distinct from adult fibrinogen and, as such, comparable to fetal haemoglobin and coded for by a specific gene. Since similar abnormalities of fibrin formation are found in liver disease in adult patients, fetal fibrinogen may represent a post-synthetic modification of a basic fibrinogen protein which is hypersialated in the fetal liver.

Factor V

At birth, factor V levels are within the normal adult range in both term and pre-term infants and are only slightly lower during the second trimester (Sell and Corrigan, 1973; Holmberg *et al.*, 1974; Mibashan and Millar, 1983).

Factor VIII

At birth, the term infant has a factor VIII:C level above the normal adult value, whilst that of the pre-term infant is within the normal adult range. The factor VIII molecule does not cross the placenta and there is no correlation between maternal and infant factor VIII:C concentrations. At 20 weeks' gestation mean values in normal fetal samples obtained by fetoscopy have been reported as factor VIII:C 43.5 U dl^{-1}, factor VIII:CAg 22.3 U dl^{-1} and vWF:Ag 60.1 U dl^{-1} (Mibashan *et al.*, 1979, 1980). Sell reported mean factor VIII:C values of 90 U dl^{-1} at 27–30 weeks' gestation and 168 U dl^{-1} at term (Sell and Corrigan, 1973). Forestier found lower values at the beginning of the third trimester when fetoscopically obtained blood was assayed (Forestier *et al.*, 1986). Both term and premature infants have raised vWF:Ag values.

Neonatal and fetal plasma contains unusually large von Willebrand factor multimers (ULvWFM) not present in normal adult plasma, and similarly elevated proportions of high molecular weight multimers (Weinstein *et al.*, 1989). The testing of infants for von Willebrand's disease (vWD) subtypes may be more complicated than appreciated. A loss of the high molecular weight multimers (HMW) of the vWF has been noted in disseminated intravascular coagulation and ventricular septal defects (VSD), and these have returned to normal with resolution of the DIC or closure of the VSD (Gill *et al.*, 1984).

Vitamin K-dependent clotting factors

Levels of the vitamin K-dependent factors (II, VII, IX and X) are gestation-dependent and are approximately 50% of the normal adult value at term and about half of that value at 24 weeks' gestation. A further reduction is commonly observed in the first 3 days of life in infants who have not received vitamin K at birth, and results from defective γ-carboxylation of the glutamic acid residues. Breast-fed infants are particularly vulnerable.

Contact factors

All factors involved in the initial contact-activated phase of the intrinsic coagulation pathway (XI, XII, prekallikrein (PK) and high molecular weight kininogen — HMWK) are reduced in both the term and pre-term infant. The levels are dependent on gestational age with ranges of 20–30% and 30–50% reported in the pre-term and term infant, respectively (Barnard *et al.*, 1979; Gordon *et al.*, 1980). A deficiency of these factors usually results in a greater prolongation of the activated partial thromboblastin time (APTT) than a corresponding deficiency of FVIII:C or FIX:C.

Factor XIII

Levels of factor XIII in the term infant are about 50–60% of adult values. As only small quantities are required for clot stabilization, this minor decrease in activity has no clinical significance.

Anticoagulants

In the healthy adult, procoagulants are carefully balanced by their reciprocal anticoagulants, and an imbalance leads to pathology. However, an imbalance would appear to exist in the normal neonate, and to what extent this contributes to morbidity has not been clearly defined. Although levels of the inhibitors antithrombin III (ATIII), protein C and protein S are in the range at which thrombotic disorders occur in the heterozygously affected adult, healthy infants do not develop spontaneous thrombosis. A number of anticoagulants, which act as inhibitors in different areas of the coagulation cascade, have been identified to date. Antithrombin III, heparin cofactor II (HCII), protein C and protein S are all reduced at birth and are dependent on gestational age, α_2-macroglobulin is not (Table 6.5).

Antithrombin III

Antithrombin III (ATIII) levels in the term infant are in the range of 50–60% of adult values and further reduced in the pre-term infant. ATIII inhibits factors II and X. As concentrations parallel those vitamin K-dependent coagulation proteins, a balance of procoagulants and anticoagulants exists (Table 6.6). Many neonates have ATIII levels which would be associated with thrombotic episodes in adults, but even in congenital ATIII deficiency thrombosis in childhood is exceptional.

Table 6.5 Values (U ml^{-1})* for the anticoagulants in the fetus and newborn infant.†

	ATIII	α_2-Antiplasmin	C1-Esterase Inhibitor	a_2-Macroglobulin	Plasminogen	Protein C:Ag	Protein S:Ag
Adult	1.00	1.00	1.00	1.00	1.00	1.00	1.00
Term newborn							
37–41 weeks	0.56	0.78	1.00	1.80	0.49	0.50‡	0.24‡
Pre-term newborn							
33–36 weeks	0.40	—	—	1.29	0.38	0.38	
25–32 weeks)	0.35	—	—	1.58	0.35	0.29	
Fetus							
≃ 20 weeks	0.23	—	—	—	—	0.10	

* One unit is the amount of factor in 1 ml of normal plasma; means are given. All values (except ‡) are venous and for the first 24 h of life. All subjects received vitamin K at birth.

† Adapted from McDonald and Hathaway, 1983, *Seminars in Perinatology, 7 (3)*, with kind permission of Grune and Strattan Inc., and from Hathaway and Bonnar, 1987, *Hemastatic Disorder of the Pregnant Woman and Newborn Infant*, published with kind permission of Elsevier Science Publishing Company Inc.

‡ Cord blood.

Table 6.6 Procoagulant and anticoagulant levels (U ml^{-1}).*†

	Vitamin K-dependent				
	II	VII	IX	X	ATIII
Adult	1.00	1.00	1.00	1.00	1.00
Term newborn 37–41 weeks	0.52	0.57	0.35	0.45	0.56
Pre-term newborn 33–36 weeks	0.45	0.59	0.41	0.44	0.40
25–32 weeks	0.32	0.7	0.22	0.38	0.35

* One unit is the amount of factor in 1 ml of normal plasma; means stated. All values are venous and for the first 24 h of life. All subjects received vitamin K at birth.
† Adapted from Hathaway and Bonnar, 1987, *Haemostatic Disorders of the Pregnant Woman and Newborn Infant*: 58–59, published with kind permission of Elsevier Science Publishing Company Inc.

Proteins C and S

The anticoagulants protein C and protein S are vitamin K-dependent factors and reduced to levels similar to those of the other vitamin K-dependent proteins in the term and pre-term infant. Mean day-1 protein C values of 0.32, 0.39 and 0.35 U ml^{-1} have been reported (Polack *et al.*, 1984; Schettini *et al.*, 1985; Andrew *et al.*, 1987). Andrew *et al.* reported a mean day-1 protein S value in term infants of 0.36 U ml^{-1}. Protein S acts as a cofactor for protein C, which in its activated form inhibits activated factors V and VIII. Unlike proteins C and S, factors V and VIII are not reduced at birth, and consequently an imbalance in favour of thrombosis exists in the newborn (Table 6.7). This physiological imbalance does not appear to lead to clinical problems in the healthy infant. However, the very low level of protein C found in homozygous congenital deficiency has been associated with fatal thrombosis. In the normal adult plasma, protein S exists in a free active form (40%) and in an inactive form (60%) complexed to the regulating complement protein, C4b-binding protein (C4bBP).

Schwarz measured immunological and functional levels of protein S and C4bBP in the plasma of 20 newborn infants with a range of gestational ages from 29–34 weeks (Schwarz *et al.*, 1988). Total protein S antigen levels averaged 23% (range 14–27%), which was similar to the levels of the other vitamin K-dependent factors. However the protein S anticoagulant activity was 74% (range 46–94%) of that of adult normal plasma. The discrepancy between activity and antigen is due to low or undetectable levels of C4bBP in the newborn, which results in most, if not all, protein S existing in its free and active form. In 11 neonates, the C4bBP level was less than 8% of that found in adult normal pooled plasma. In the remaining nine infants, C4bBP levels averaged 20%.

A further study (Malm *et al.*, 1988) reported pre-term infants to have a mean free protein S concentration of 3.3 mg l^{-1}, which represented 82% of

Table 6.7 Procoagulant and anticoagulant levels (U ml^{-1}).*†

	Procoagulants		Anticoagulant
	V	VIII	protein C
Adult	1.00	1.00	1.00
Term newborn			
37–41 weeks	1.00	1.50	0.50‡
Pre-term newborn			
33–36 weeks	0.82	0.93	0.38
25–32 weeks	0.80	0.75	0.29

* One unit is the amount of factor in 1 ml of normal plasma; means are given. All values (except ‡) are various and for the first 24 h of life. All subjects received vitamin K at birth.
† Adapted from Hathaway and Bonnar, 1987, *Haemostatic Disorders of the Pregnant Woman and Newborn Infant*: 58–59, published with kind permission of Elsevier Science Publishing Company, Inc.
‡ Cord blood.

their total plasma protein S and corresponded to approximately 43% of the normal adult concentration. The mean concentration of free protein S in term infants was 4.6 mg l^{-1}, which represented 68% of their total plasma protein S and corresponded to approximately 60% of the adult concentration. The mean concentration of C4bBP was 6 and 18% of that of adult plasma for pre-term and term infants, respectively (Malm *et al.*, 1988). Sthoeger *et al.* (1989) reports the level of total protein S in the term infant to be in the adult range by 10 months of age. In contrast the mean level of free protein S was similar to adult values by 2–4 months of age.

α_2-Macroglobulin

Levels of α_2-macroglobulin are elevated above the adult range in both the term and pre-term infant. α_2-Macroglobulin complexes with serine proteases and relies upon reticuloendothelial clearance rather than inactivation (Harpel and Rosenberg, 1976). The elevated level of this inhibitor may play a protective role against thrombosis at a time when levels of the other major anticoagulants are low and in a range associated with thrombosis in the adult. Similarly, the relatively high level of active protein S in infants may enhance the potential of the protein C pathway and partially compensate for deficiencies of the other inhibitors.

Fibrinolysis

Fibrinolytic activity appears to be increased in the newborn (Ekelund *et al.*, 1970). Increased fibrinolytic activity, as reflected in a short euglobin lysis time, has been reported from as early as 16 weeks' gestation onwards.

Plasminogen activator activity is high from then until term, but falls to adult levels within 4 hours of birth. Plasminogen concentrations are gestation-dependent and are about 50% in the term infant, reaching adult levels at about 6 months of age (Table 6.5). Tissue plasminogen activator (tPA) and plasminogen activator inhibitor (PAI) are both high at term, whilst the major inhibitor of plasmin, α_2-antiplasmin (α_2 AP) is within the normal adult range (Barnard, 1984).

Although there are published reference values for both term and pre-term infants for most coagulation factors at birth, the data beyond birth are very scanty. Andrew addressed this problem in a study aimed at determining the postnatal development of the human coagulation system in a large number of consecutive healthy full-term infants (Andrew *et al.*, 1987). One hundred and eighteen infants were recruited and components of their coagulation, fibrinolytic and inhibitor systems measured on days 1, 5, 30, 90 and 180 of life. Between 40 and 79 full-term infants were studied on each day for each of the coagulation tests. The results are given in Figures 6.2 to 6.8. All of the neonates were healthy and had received 1 mg vitamin K intramuscularly at birth, at least 12 hours prior to the first blood sample being drawn.

The study confirmed the previously known facts:

(1) coagulation tests vary with postnatal age;
(2) different coagulation factors show different postnatal patterns of maturation;
(3) most coagulation factors achieve near adult values by 6 months of age.

Reference ranges have now similarly been published from 137 healthy premature infants evenly distributed in age between 30 and 36 weeks (Andrew *et al.*, 1988). The postnatal maturation towards adult levels is generally accelerated in premature infants and, like full-term infants, they achieve mean adult values for most components of the coagulation system by 6 months of age. The overall pattern of the coagulation system is similar in premature and full-term infants and the differences are minor compared with those between adults and premature infants. Thus, the period between 30 and 40 weeks of gestation does not appear to be a time of rapid change in the haemostatic parameters. As Andrews *et al.* (1988) point out, one of the more important purposes of reference ranges is to aid the correct diagnosis of specific congenital or acquired coagulopathies. Their studies establish several interesting facts:

(1) Mild, moderate and severe haemophilia A can be confidently diagnosed in both term and pre-term infants.

(2) Mean values for factor IX suggests that severe haemophilia B can be diagnosed with confidence in the newborn period in term and premature infants, but that mild or moderate haemophilia B cannot.

(3) Diagnosis of the more common forms of von Willebrand's disease are difficult in the first months of life because vWF behaves as an acute-phase reactant and is markedly elevated in the early postnatal period in term and pre-term infants.

(4) Accurate diagnosis of the heterozygote state for specific inhibitors (e.g. ATIII, protein C and protein S) is difficult, although homozygosity has

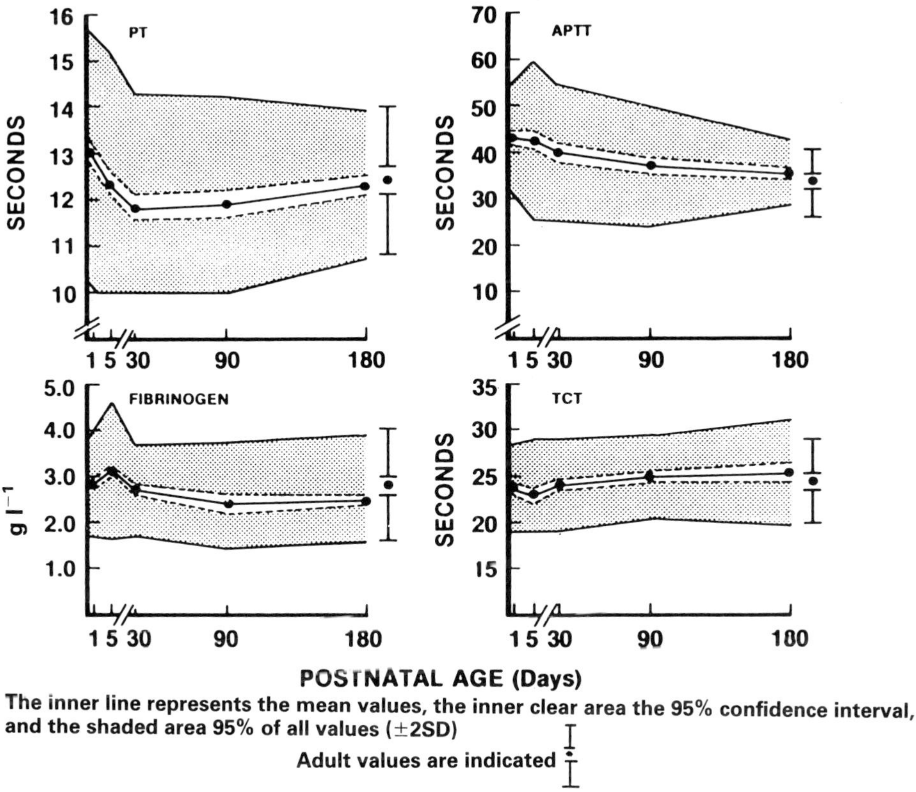

Figure 6.2 APTT, PT, Fibrinogen level and TCT in 118 healthy full-term infants throughout the first 6 months of life. From Andrew *et al.*, 1987, *Blood 70*: 167–170, with permission of Grune and Stratton.

been and should be diagnosed at birth.

(5) Acquired disorders, for example DIC and liver disease, should be easily diagnosed in view of the adult levels for fibrinogen and factors V and VIII in the term and premature newborn.

(6) Vitamin K deficiency is difficult to diagnose in the newborn, particularly in the premature infant, because of their very low levels of the four vitamin K-dependent factors. Assays that measure discrepancies between the amount of existing protein and its activity may be more helpful.

(7) Mean values for protein C are still low at 6 months of age. α_2-Macroglobulin is elevated at birth and C1 esterase inhibitor (C_1E-INH) and heparin cofactor II (HCII) become elevated during the first 6 months of life compared with adult values. The significance is unknown, but the authors speculate that a compensatory mechanism is in play.

(8) It must be remembered that only healthy pre-term and full-term infants were included in these studies. Some coagulation parameters have lower values in sick infants and rise more slowly. Antithrombin III is a particularly well-recognized example of this, and values are significantly lower in neonates with respiratory distress syndrome than in healthy term infants.

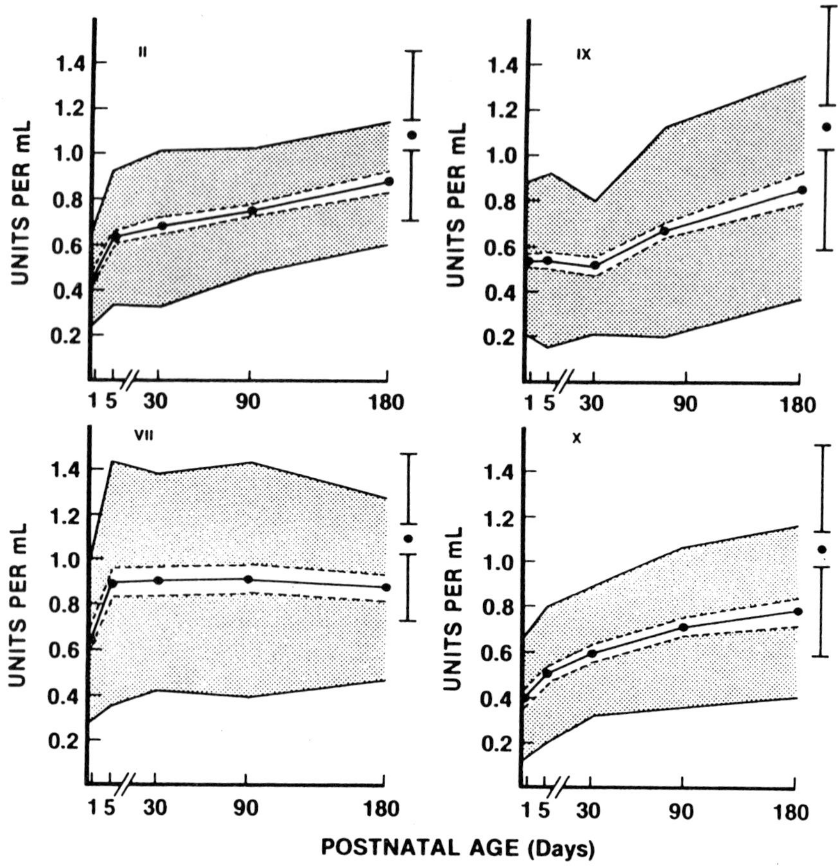

Figure 6.3 The vitamin K-dependent factors (II, VII, IX, X) in 118 healthy full-term infants throughout the first 6 months of life. (See Figure 6.2 for key.) From Andrew *et al.*, 1987, *Blood 70*: 167–170, with permission of Grune and Stratton.

NEONATAL THROMBOCYTOPENIA

Although healthy pre-term and term infants have a platelet count in the adult range, thrombocytopenia is a common occurrence in sick infants. A unique set of conditions surrounds the newborn, producing unusual susceptibility to thrombocytopenia, for example maternal antibodies, congenitally acquired infections and hypoxia. The incidence of thrombocytopenia has been variably reported, but few studies have attempted to define the natural history and identify the cause. Castle and her colleagues reported a one-year prospective study of 807 infants admitted consecutively to a regional neonatal intensive care unit (Castle *et al.*, 1986). Platelet counts for 174 infants (22%) were below 150×10^9 per litre and for 97 infants the values were below 100×10^9 per litre. In 75% of the thrombocytopenic infants, the nadir of the platelet count occurred on day 4 and the

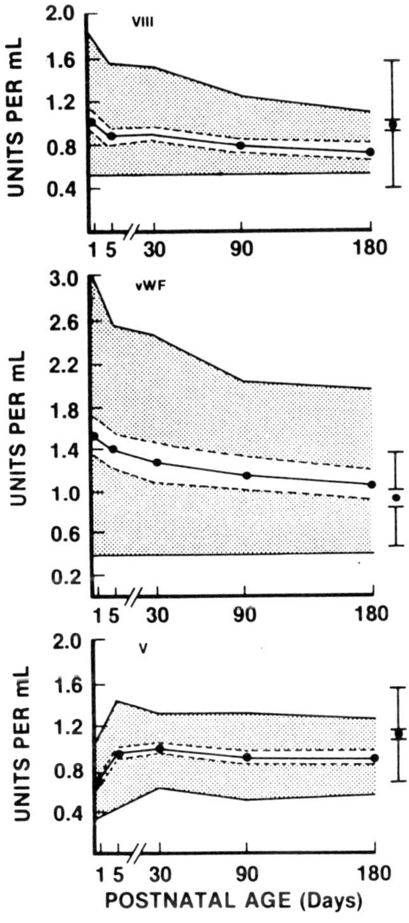

Figure 6.4 Factors V, VIII and vWF in 118 healthy full-term infants throughout the first 6 months of life. (See Figure 6.2 for key.) From Andrew *et al.*, 1987, *Blood 70*: 167–170, with permission of Grune and Stratton.

thrombocytopenia had resolved by day 10. Investigations supported increased platelet consumption as the underlying mechanism. Fifty-two per cent had elevated levels of platelet-associated IgG (PAIgG), 21% had evidence of DIC and 12% had received exchange transfusion. Of the many risk factors assessed, the authors considered birth asphyxia to be most strongly associated with the subsequent development of a low platelet count. It occurred in 70% of the thrombocytopenic infants compared with 30% of the controls. Only 7% of the thrombocytopenic infants had evidence of sepsis in the form of a positive blood culture. A minority of mothers had measurable amounts of IgG on their platelets or free in their serum, and the frequency was similar for mothers of thrombocytopenic and non-thrombocytopenic infants.

It is difficult to assess the clinical impact of thrombocytopenia on the

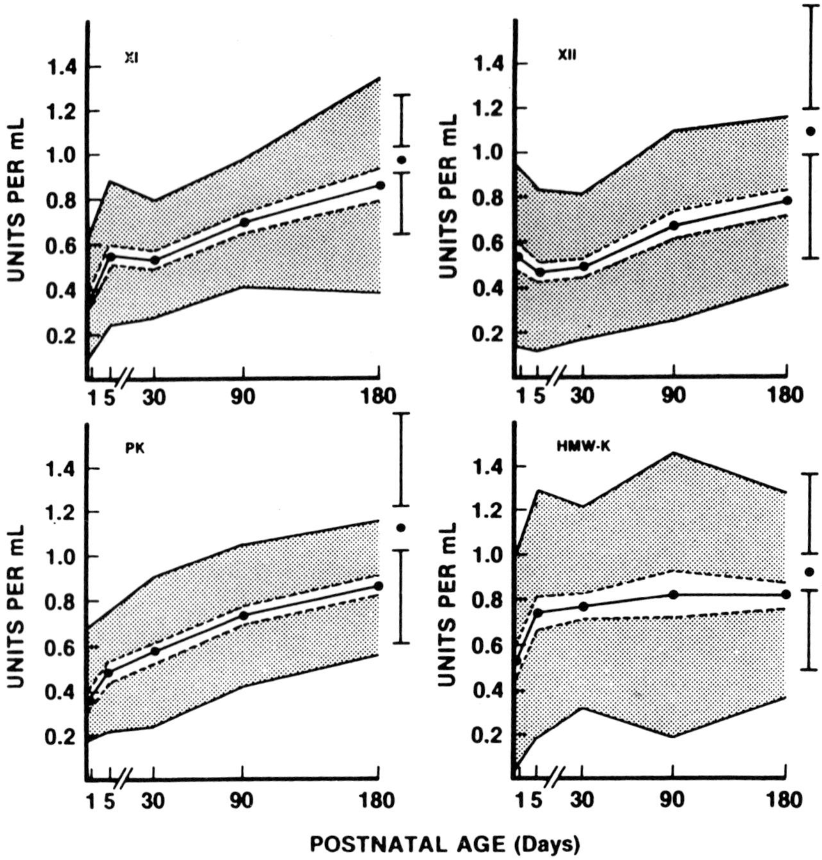

Figure 6.5 The contact factors (XII, XI, PK, HMWK) in 118 healthy full-term infants throughout the first 6 months of life. (See Figure 6.2 for key.) From Andrew *et al.*, 1987, *Blood 70*: 167–170, with permission of Grune and Stratton.

newborn, because thrombocytopenic infants are usually sick and/or premature and have a variety of medical complications that by themselves can contribute to morbidity and mortality. Andrew *et al.* (1987) reported the clinical outcome of thrombocytopenia in the same cohort of neonates previously described. The incidence of intraventricular haemorrhage (IVH) in 39 thrombocytopenic infants (platelet count $< 100 \times 10^9$ per litre) weighing less than 1500 g at birth was 78% compared with 50% for 26 non-thrombocytopenic control infants matched for age, weight and disease. The thrombocytopenic infants more frequently had severe grades of IVH. Forty-four per cent of thrombocytopenic infants had grade III or IV IVH compared with 16% of the control group. When infants with DIC were excluded from analysis, the results remained basically unchanged. Seventy-nine per cent of thrombocytopenic infants without DIC had ultrasonic evidence of IVH, and 53% had grade III or IV IVH. Overall, thrombocytopenic infants of less than 1500 g had three-and-a-half times the risk of IVH compared with non-

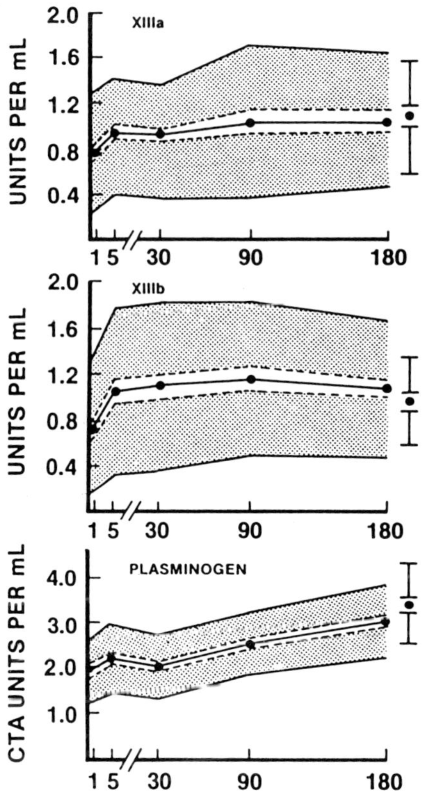

Figure 6.6 Factor XIIIa, XIIIb and plasminogen in 118 healthy full-term infants throughout the first 6 months of life. (See Figure 6.2 for key.) From Andrew *et al.*, 1987, *Blood 70*: 167–170, with permission of Grune and Stratton.

thrombocytopenic infants matched for age, weight and disease. Thirty-three per cent of thrombocytopenic and 17% of non-thrombocytopenic infants weighing less than 1500 g died. Forty-one per cent of thrombocytopenic and 7% of non-thrombocytopenic surviving infants developed serious neurological morbidity.

The causes of thrombocytopenia in the newborn are multiple (Table 6.8), with infections being the commonest in both term and pre-term infants. The infants general condition is helpful in identifying the underlying aetiology. For example, infection and DIC are likely in a sick pre-term infant, whilst immune-mediated thrombocytopenia should be considered in a full-term infant who appears otherwise to be well. It is important to take a careful perinatal history with particular reference to maternal immune thrombocytopenic purpura and infections, drugs and obstetrical disorders associated with thrombocytopenia. Appropriate laboratory investigations should include coagulation tests to identify DIC, bacterial and viral studies for infection, and a blood count and film to exclude an associated haematological disorder.

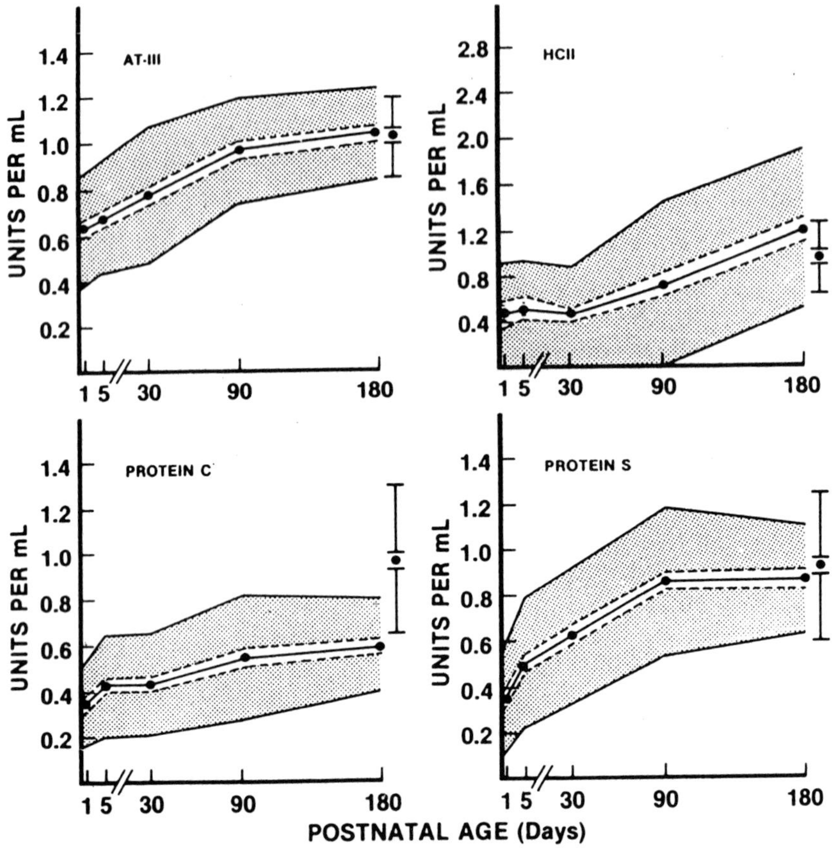

Figure 6.7 The inhibitors ATIII, HCII, protein C and protein S in 118 healthy full-term infants throughout the first 6 months of life. (See Figure 6.2 for key.) From Andrew *et al.*, 1987, *Blood 70*: 167–170, with permission of Grune and Stratton.

Immune-mediated thrombocytopenia

Neonatal alloimmune thrombocytopenia

Neonatal alloimmune thrombocytopenia (NAIT) is confined to the neonate and is the platelet counterpart of haemolytic disease of the newborn. The infant possesses a platelet antigen lacking in the mother. The infant's platelets enter the maternal circulation where they result in the production of IgG maternal antibodies, which cross the placenta to the fetal circulation and destroy the infant's platelets. Maternal antibodies can be directed against either platelet-specific or histocompatibility (HLA) antigens on fetal platelets. Because the antibody recognized an antigen lacking on the mother's platelets, her platelet count will be normal, which differentiates this disorder from immune thrombocytopenia secondary to maternal

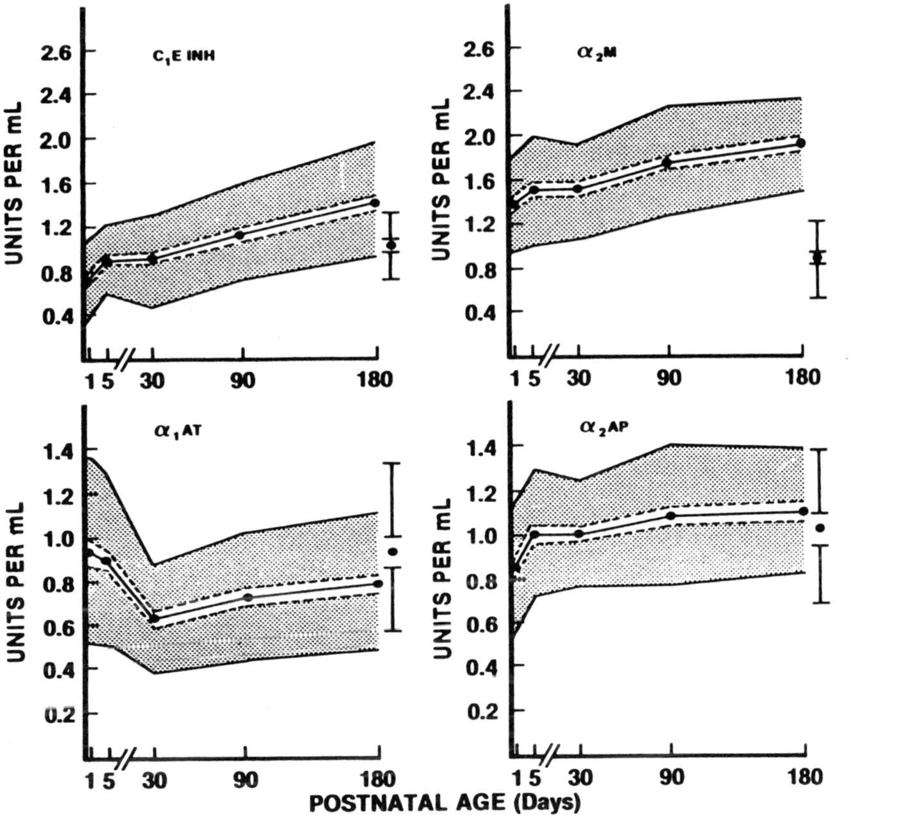

Figure 6.8 The inhibitors C_1E-INH, α_s-M, α_2-AP, and α_1-AT in 118 healthy full-term infants throughout the first 6 months of life. (See Figure 6.2 for key.) From Andrew *et al.*, 1987, *Blood 70*: 167–170, with permission of Grune and Stratton.

idiopathic thrombocytopenic purpura (ITP) or systemic lupus erythematosus (SLE). A number of platelet specific antigens have been incriminated, namely Pl^{A1}, Pl^{E2}, $DUZO^{a}$, Bak^{a}, as have two histocompatibility antigens $PlGrLy^{B1}$ and $PlGrLy^{C1}$.

Pl^{A1} is the most important antibody in terms of frequency and severity of symptoms. The majority of Pl^{A1}-negative mothers who become sensitized have the histocompatibility phenotype HLA-B8-DR3, which may be associated with the immune response.

Approximately 20% of cases are due to maternal-fetal incompatibility to antigens other than Pl^{A1}. The clinical significance of HLA antibodies is unclear. HLA antibodies may fail to enter the fetal circulation because of prior absorption onto placental tissue which expresses HLA antigens. Cases of alloimmune thrombocytopenia thought to be associated with HLA antibodies have generally been much milder than those due to platelet-specific antibodies. As antigens of the HLA system are not confined to the platelet membrane but have a broader specificity, the affected infant may also show transient leukopenia.

Table 6.8 Neonatal thrombocytopenia.

Immune-mediated
Neonatal alloimmune thrombocytopenia
Maternal ITP or SLE (autoantibody production)
Drug-induced

Infection
Viral: rubella, cytomegalovirus, herpes simplex, HIV
Bacterial
Congenital syphilis
Toxoplasmosis

Disorders of intravascular coagulation
DIC
Maternal pre-eclampsia
Hypothermia, hypoxia, shock, sepsis
Rhesus isoimmunization
Major vessel thrombosis (aortic, renal vein)
Necrotizing enterocolitis, congenital heart disease
Congenital heart disease

Congenital megakaryocytic hypoplasia
Thrombocytopenia with absent radii
Fanconi's anaemia
Trisomy syndromes — 13 and 18

Hereditary thrombocytopenia
Wiskott–Aldrich syndrome
Bernard–Soulier syndrome
May–Hegglin anomaly

Giant haemangioma

Bone marrow infiltration
Congenital leukaemia
Familial erythrophagocytic lymphohistiocytosis
Langerhans' cell histiocytosis
Neonatal neuroblastoma
Osteopetrosis

Miscellaneous
Type IIB von Willebrand's disease
Ventilation
Drugs administered to neonate
Metabolic disorders: hyperglycinaemia, methylmalonic acidaemia, isovaleric acidaemia
Post-exchange transfusion
Maternal drugs: tolbutamide, hydantoin
Perinatal pulmonary syndromes

Pearson reported an incidence of NAIT of 1:5000 births (Pearson *et al.*, 1964), but it is now appreciated that this estimate is too low and as many as 1 in 1000–2000 newborn babies may be affected (Mueller-Eckhard *et al.*, 1989). The incidence of platelet antigens in the general population, associated with NAIT are as follows: Pl^{A1} 98%, $PlGrLy^{B1}$ (HLA-A2) 46%, $PlGrLy^{C1}$ 30%, Pl^{E2} 5%, Bak^{a} 91%, $DUZO^{a}$ 22%. NAIT frequently occurs in the first pregnancy (about 50% without previous sensitization), and there is a *c.* 75% chance of recurrence in subsequent pregnancies. By comparison with the index case, subsequent affected siblings are usually similarly or more severely thrombocytopenic. One should therefore be alerted to this problem, if the mother has delivered a previously affected infant.

Bruising, if not present at birth, generally appears within the first 24 hours of life. Haemorrhagic manifestations after this time suggest an aetiology other than immune-mediated, for example infection. In immune-mediated thrombocytopenia the infant is otherwise healthy. Intracranial haemorrhage (ICH), which affects about 10–20% of infants with this disorder, constitutes the greatest risk. Minor changes in vital signs or parameters should be taken seriously. It should be remembered that intracranial haemorrhage can occur *in utero* (5–10%), with porencephaly and hydrocephaly as sequelae. Other symptomatology includes bleeding from the gastrointestinal tract, oozing from the umbilical cord, haematuria or prolonged bleeding from heel stabs or venepuncture sites. Bruising of the presenting parts may be seen, especially if the delivery was traumatic. The thrombocytopenia resolves as the maternal antibody disappears from the infant's circulation, which occurs well within the first few months of life.

Confirming the diagnosis is only within the capability of a small number of specialized laboratories, which have the facilities to adequately type platelets and detect specific IgG antibodies on the infant's platelets and in the maternal serum. NAIT occurs only when fetal platelets possess an antigen which is inherited from the father and is not present on maternal platelets. If the father is homozygous for the antigen, all subsequent children will be affected. If the father is heterozygous, 50% of the children may be affected. The tests required to firmly establish the cause are very complex. In many instances one will accept the diagnosis if the mother has a normal platelet count and is Pl^{A1}-negative. Ideally, for a 'cast-iron' diagnosis, an antigen absent on maternal platelets should be demonstrated to be on neonatal and paternal platelets, in addition to demonstration of the corresponding IgG antibody in maternal serum and on the infant's platelets.

Management

There is much controversy about the most appropriate management of alloimmune neonatal thrombocytopenia — aimed at reducing the incidence of ICH. In NAIT, intracranial haemorrhage can occur both *in utero* and after delivery. Platelet antibodies have been shown to cross the placenta by 14 weeks gestation, at which stage platelets can be identified circulating in the fetal blood. It is now appreciated that antenatal haemorrhage is not rare and management strategies are aimed at raising fetal platelet numbers and preventing this complication. Skill in fetal blood sampling by cordocentesis has made it possible to confirm the infant's Pl^{A} status and to assess the severity of the thrombocytopenia as early as 20 weeks' gestation. Additionally, the technique can be used to transfuse compatible platelets and reduce the risk of bleeding.

Repeated in-utero platelet transfusions have been given because of a previous severely brain-damaged baby (Nicolini *et al.*, 1988). Such an aggressive approach is questionable for a number of reasons. Although it is likely that the greatest risk of haemorrhage is in the last trimester, thrombocytopenia may already be present at 20 weeks' gestation, when the technique becomes possible. Additionally, platelet transfusion would be required every 4–5 days because of their short lifespan, and this is not only technically difficult but the risk of transfusion-transmitted infection must be considered. Despite increasing awareness of the risk of antenatal ICH, the highest morbidity is still probably associated with delivery. Previously caesarean section was advocated for all suspected cases of NAIT. However, even infants delivered by this method have suffered ICH. A single platelet transfusion immediately prior to delivery may allow a normal birth. This of course does not offer any protection against haemorrhage in the last trimester. Platelet concentrates should be gamma-irradiated, to prevent transfusion-induced graft-versus-host-disease in the fetus, and should be of the same type as the mother.

A non-invasive approach to prenatal treatment of NAIT is now being recommended by some authorities. Bussel advocates the use of high-dose immunoglobulin (Bussel *et al.*, 1988). He reports a successful outcome in seven cases of NAIT with weekly maternal administration of high-dose intravenous immunoglobulin (1 g kg^{-1}, once weekly) given for a period of 6–17 weeks before delivery. In all cases, fetal platelet counts (monitored by fetal blood sampling) increased and the infants suffered no haemorrhagic complications. Daffos reported the successful outcome in one case treated by prednisolone (10 mg daily) from 23 weeks' gestation (Daffos *et al.*, 1988). It is important that the benefits of immunoglobulin and steroid therapy given antenatally are properly assessed, because if they prove successful then repeated invasive procedures can be avoided.

Not all infants with NAIT will require treatment but, because of the severity of the problem, they should be carefully observed in the immediate perinatal period, until the extent of the problem is clear. Compatible platelets should be available for immediate transfusion if delivery of an affected infant is anticipated. Transfused platelets should be of the same type as the mother (e.g. Pl^{A1}-negative). If maternal platelets are given, they should be washed to remove alloantibodies in the plasma and resuspended in AB plasma. Alternatively, large centres may have access to a platelet donor pool whose platelet types are known. Severely affected infants with serious bleeding or with a platelet count less than 25×10^9 per litre should receive platelet concentrates. Recently, high-dose intravenous immunoglobulin (1 g kg^{-1} on two consecutive days) has been shown to be useful, but it will not raise the platelet count as rapidly as a platelet transfusion. Combined therapy may be the most appropriate approach. High-dose intravenous immunoglobulin may have a role in less severely affected infants who do not require transfusion. Steroids have been shown to be of no benefit.

Neonatal thrombocytopenic purpura due to maternal autoantibodies

Maternal chronic ITP and SLE frequently result in neonatal thrombocytopenia, because of placental transfer of maternal IgG antiplatelet autoantibodies. The mothers themselves will be thrombocytopenic, unlike the mothers of infants with NAIT. Thrombocytopenia caused by maternal autoantibodies accounts for 80% of all cases of immune-mediated neonatal thrombocytopenia, alloimmune thrombocytopenia being responsible for the remaining 20%.

There is no completely reliable non-invasive means of predicting which infants will be severely thrombocytopenic. Infants born to mothers with active disease or those with normal platelet counts but a previous history of

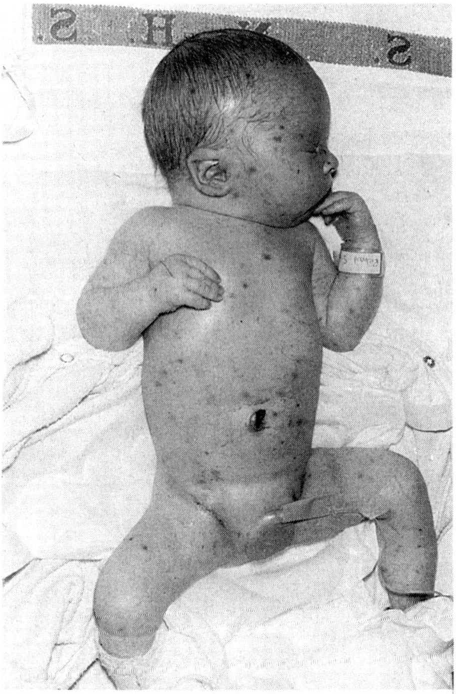

Figure 6.9 Purpura and petechiae in a neonate with immune-mediated thrombocytopenia; reproduced with permission of Salford Health Authority.

splenectomy, in whom circulating antiplatelet antibodies may persist, are said to be at particular risk of delivering an affected infant. However, recent studies have shown no consistent correlation between the infant platelet count and either the maternal platelet count or previous maternal splenectomy. Kelton found that only 50% of women at risk of delivering a thrombocytopenic infant did so (Kelton, 1983). The severity of the infant's thrombocytopenia may be proportional to the amount of antiplatelet antibody transferred across the placenta and is probably related to the characteristics of the antibody (quantity, subclass and ability to activate complement). Kelton reported a close correlation between maternal platelet-associated IgG and neonatal thrombocytopenia, although it was not predictive of severity (Kelton *et al.*, 1982). In contrast, Cines found a correlation between neonatal thrombocytopenia and the level of free antiplatelet antibodies in the maternal serum, but not with platelet-associated IgG (Cines *et al.*, 1982).

The clinical problems may be confined to bruising (Figure 6.9) or may be more serious. Intracranial haemorrhage is the commonest cause of death. However the disorder is self-limiting and the platelet count usually starts to rise by the third week, reaching normal values by the second or third postnatal month. The infant is generally otherwise healthy, although possibly anaemic from blood loss or icteric from absorption of haematoma.

Management. There are a number of controversial areas in the management of this disorder. Antenatally, autoimmune thrombocytopenia differs in two major aspects from neonatal alloimmune thrombocytopenia; the mother herself has a low platelet count and intracranial haemorrhage *in utero* is extremely rare.

The mother with ITP only requires treatment if her platelet count falls below 25×10^9 per litre. This level is adequate for haemostasis in pregnancy which does not require a higher platelet count than the non-pregnant state. If treatment is necessary, it should be with prednisolone 1 mg kg^{-1} per day and tapered quickly to the lowest dose that will maintain a safe platelet count. High-dose intravenous immunoglobulin (an infusion of 400 mg kg^{-1} on five days consecutively or 1 g kg^{-1} on two consecutive days) may be used for mothers who do not respond to steroids. The platelet count rises rapidly within a few days in responders. However, at delivery, the platelet count should be at least 50–100 $\times 10^9$ per litre, which is acceptable for delivery both vaginally and by caesarean section. Epidural anaesthesia should be avoided if the platelet count is less than 100×10^9 per litre. Splenectomy during pregnancy should not be undertaken lightly, because of the appreciable risk to both infant and mother.

Not all mothers with ITP or SLE will deliver a thrombocytopenic neonate and argument continues as to the best means of delivery. The period of greatest risk for an affected infant is at the time of delivery, which should be managed in a way designed to minimize trauma to the head. Although caesarean section is not without some risk in the presence of maternal thrombocytopenia, many obstetricians would elect to deliver all affected infants by this route. Unfortunately, there is no totally reliable non-invasive method of predicting whether an infant will be thrombocytopenic. Direct measurement of the platelet count is becoming common practice. This can be done by cordocentesis or fetal scalp capillary blood sampling early in labour (Scott *et al.*, 1982). The former carries a fetal mortality rate of less than 1% in experienced hands, but is not generally available. There are also problems associated with the latter technique. Platelet clumping leading to false low counts is common and the procedure is not without risk to the fetus, from haemorrhage, if the count is low. Any infant with a platelet count of less than 50×10^9 per litre (measured on fetal scalp capillary blood) should be delivered by caesarean section. Infants with counts above this level should be delivered according to obstetrical indications.

Both the need for and the efficacy of antenatal therapy designed to raise the fetal platelet count remain unclear. Two strategies have been employed. The antenatal administration of prednisolone (10–20 mg per day) for 12–14 days prior to delivery (as described by Karpatkin *et al.*, 1981) has not been found by other workers to be consistently successful. It has been suggested that the dose of prednisolone may be crucial and may have to be as high as 60 mg per day (Strother and Wagner, 1988). High-dose intravenous immunoglobulin (administered as previously described) has also been reported with variable success.

Once safely delivered, many infants, particularly those mildly affected, will require no further treatment. Postnatal therapeutic options include steroid therapy and high-dose intravenous immunoglobulin. Infants who have a platelet count of less than 50×10^9 per litre complicated by petechiae or purpura should receive a short course of prednisolone (2 mg kg^{-1} per day), tapered to maintain the platelet count above this level until the thrombocytopenia resolves. Intravenous immunoglobulin (1 g kg^{-1} per day on two consecutive days or 400 mg kg^{-1} per day for five days) will raise the platelet count more rapidly than steroids and should be reserved for severely thrombocytopenic infants and those with significant haemorrhage. In the event of significant haemorrhage, random donor platelets should be transfused but these will be rapidly destroyed unless exchange transfusion is concurrently performed to remove the causative platelet antibodies.

Neonatal thrombocytopenia due to maternal ingestion of drugs

An exceptionally rare cause of immune-mediated neonatal thrombocytopenia is maternal ingestion of certain drugs, for example quinine and quinidine. The maternal serum contains circulating IgG drug-induced antibodies, which pass into the fetal circulation. However, before these antibodies can result in neonatal thrombocytopenia, the drug must be present in the neonate's circulation.

Thrombocytopenia secondary to intra-uterine infection

Congenital rubella, toxoplasmosis, syphilis, cytomegalovirus and herpes simplex are all associated with thrombocytopenia. Herpes simplex is acquired from contact with vaginal or cervical secretions, whilst the others are acquired *in utero*. Although the incidences vary considerably between studies, approximately 50% of neonates with congenital rubella or cytomegalovirus will become thrombocytopenic. Infants with congenitally acquired toxoplasmosis and syphilis are much less commonly affected. Unlike infants with immune thrombocytopenia these babies are ill, have hepatosplenomegaly and may have characteristic congenital malformations. The platelet count usually resolves within the first few weeks of life and the problem is not as clinically severe as immune thrombocytopenia.

The underlying mechanism remains unclear. Impaired platelet production has been inferred from the presence of megakaryocytic hypoplasia, but this finding may merely reflect problematic sampling. Both defective platelet production and increased consumption may play a role, the latter resulting either from DIC or immune complexes on the platelets. HIV infection should now be considered in any neonate with persistent thrombocytopenia, in the absence of any other obvious cause. Bacterial infections are commonly associated with postnatal thrombocytopenia resulting from increased consumption.

Disseminated intravascular coagulation

Sepsis, hypoxia and shock are all recognized stimuli for DIC. Such critically ill infants require treatment of the underlying problem as well as management of the consumptive coagulopathy. Correction may require fresh frozen plasma (FFP), cryoprecipitate and platelets. In the newborn infant, exchange transfusion may be the best means of replacing these blood products and preventing circulatory overload. Infection and intravascular coagulation are the most common causes of thrombocytopenia in both term and pre-term infants.

Fanconi's anaemia

Fanconi's anaemia, with an autosomal recessive inheritance, rarely presents haematologically at birth although this has been described. Neonatal thrombocytopenia may be the first expression of progressive bone-marrow failure, although pancytopenia usually does not develop until 5–10 years of age. Variable congenital anomalies commonly affecting the musculoskeletal and genitourinary systems are characteristic. Abnormalities of the thumb are particularly common. Cytogenic abnormalities with multiple chromatid breaks are diagnostic (see Chapter 8).

Thrombocytopenia with absent radii

Thrombocytopenia with absent radii (TAR), with an autosomal recessive inheritance, is characterized by neonatal thrombocytopenia and bilateral absent radii. The thumbs are present, which may help to distinguish the problem from Fanconi's anaemia. In some cases the radii are extremely hypoplastic but not absent. Affected infants have been reported with failure to thrive, diarrhoea and symptoms of milk allergy. Thrombocytopenia is present at birth, with platelet counts in the region of 15×10^9 to 30×10^9 per litre. Symptoms range from petechiae and purpura to gastrointestinal or intracranial haemorrhage.

Examination of the bone marrow usually shows an absence of megakaryocytes or, occasionally, reduced numbers of small, immature megakaryocytes. Leukaemoid reactions are common in the first few months of life and the bone marrow then shows evidence of myeloid hyperplasia. Some cases have been reported with functional platelet defects and platelet aggregation abnormalities suggestive of storage pool disease.

The risk of bleeding is greatest in the first year of life, when the mortality rate is about 30 per cent. The platelet count begins to rise towards the end of the first year and the life expectancy approximates to normal. These infants should therefore be vigorously supported with platelets and blood transfusion when necessary. If they survive the first year of life their outlook is very good. However, the excessive use of platelets should be discouraged because of the risk of refractoriness. Corticosteroids and splenectomy have no proven role. Orthopaedic procedures should be postponed until after infancy, when the risk of haemorrhage may have resolved. The chance of further affected infants being born to the same parents is one in four, and absent radii can be detected antenatally by ultrasound.

Thrombocytopenia associated with trisomy

Hypoplastic thrombocytopenia is an uncommon finding in both trisomy 13 and trisomy 18 syndromes.

Wiskott–Aldrich syndrome

Wiskott–Aldrich syndrome is an X-linked recessive disorder characterized by chronic thrombocytopenia, eczema and a complex immunological defect predisposing the infant to recurrent infections. The immunological abnormality includes both cellular and humoral deficiencies. A forme fruste of the disorder is recognized in which thrombocytopenia is the predominant problem, although affected infants may develop immunodeficiency at a later date. Small platelets are infrequently seen on the blood film. The thrombocytopenia results from a combination of ineffective thrombopoiesis and decreased autologous platelet survival. The small defective platelets have a qualitative defect, failing to aggregate with adrenaline, ADP and collagen. A membrane-protein abnormality has been identified on both platelets and lymphocytes. Some affected individuals have an absence of a 115 000 Da glycoprotein on their lymphocytes and a reduction in GPIb on their platelets. Bruising is common, and bleeding responds normally to random donor platelets, which should be irradiated to prevent graft-versus-host-disease. Death may occur in infancy from haemorrhage or infection. Later progression to a lymphoproliferative state may occur, contributing to the mortality. Bone-marrow transplantation has been successful in a number of cases. Splenectomy has improved the thrombocytopenia but obviously increases the already high susceptibility to infection, and should not be carried out in the neonatal period; it may be of particular benefit in the forme fruste with thrombocytopenia as the main problem. Corticosteroids are of no value.

Bernard–Soulier syndrome

The thrombocytopenia in this disorder is mild to moderate and characterized by giant platelets on the peripheral smear. The bleeding time is prolonged and, although platelet aggregation with standard agents is normal, ristocetin-induced platelet aggregation is defective. Platelets from affected individuals have a deficiency of GPIb, which is the critical platelet membrane receptor site for vWF. Haemorrhage is most often from mucous membranes and may occur in the first few weeks of childhood. It can be terminated by platelet transfusions but these should be restricted because of the high risk of sensitization. The absent GPIb is a potent immunogen. Normal platelets carry this glycoprotein and can stimulate antiplatelet antibodies in Bernard–Soulier individuals.

Giant haemangioma (Kasabach–Merritt syndrome)

Thrombocytopenia results from the sequestration of large numbers of platelets in the vascular channels of these tumours (Figure 6.10). Localized consumption of both platelets and coagulation factors may occur and is generally low grade and chronic. A large-sized tumour is not a prerequisite for the development of thrombocytopenia. Lesions may enlarge during the first year of life and then regress. If the anatomical situation of the lesion compromises vital functions, surgical removal or radiotherapy-induced involution is indicated.

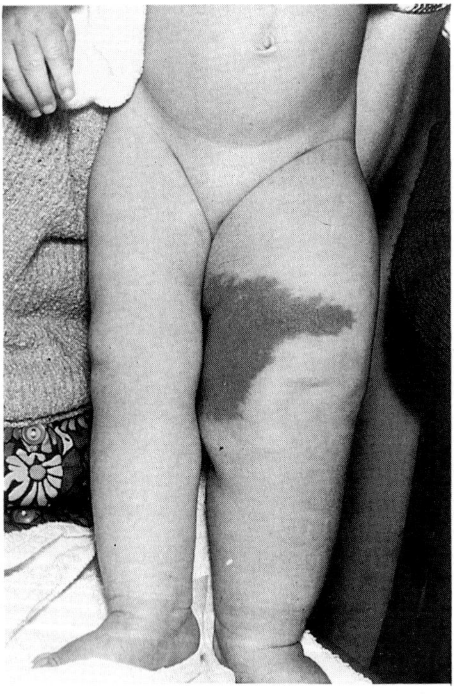

Figure 6.10 Kasabach–Merritt syndrome (giant haemangioma associated with thrombocytopenia) involving the left thigh; reproduced with permission of Salford Health Authority.

Congenital leukaemia and histiocytosis

A number of cases of congenital leukaemia, predominantly acute myelomonocytic leukaemia, have been reported. The white cell count is usually very high, with massive organ infiltration. Bluish nodules of leukaemic cell infiltrates are often seen on the skin and placenta. The response to treatment is poor (see Chapter 10). Similarly, a number of infants have been reported presenting with profound thrombocytopenia secondary to congenital Langerhans' cell histiocytosis and familial erythrophagocytic lymphohistiocytosis (FEL).

Thrombocytopenia and type IIB von Willebrand's disease

Three infants from two families have been reported who exhibited all the laboratory characteristics of type IIB vWD and severe thrombocytopenia (Donnér *et al.*, 1987). Type IIB vWD is generally believed to be inherited in an autosomal dominant manner, but in these families autosomal recessive inheritance was considered more likely. The thrombocytopenia in type IIB vWD is thought to result from increased vWF–platelet interaction leading to platelet aggregation *in vivo* and increased platelet consumption.

Mechanical ventilation

A causal relationship between mechanical ventilation and thrombocytopenia has been reported (Ballin *et al.*, 1987). This is independent of the underlying indication for ventilation. Ballin *et al.* reported decreased platelet counts during mechanical ventilation of newborn infants with respiratory distress syndrome (RDS), congenital diaphragmatic hernia and tracheoesophageal fistula. The thrombocytopenia is thought to result from increased utilization, but why this should occur is not clear.

Disorders of platelet function in the presence of a normal platelet count

Platelet function disorders can be inherited or acquired. Indomethacin, which may be given to the neonate to induce closure of a patent ductus arteriosus, is associated with impaired platelet function. Glanzmann's thrombasthenia is a well-recognized example of an inherited thrombocytopathy. This autosomal recessive disorder is characterized by a normal platelet count and a prolonged bleeding time. Clot retraction is absent or deficient and platelet aggregation impaired with ADP, adrenaline or collagen, but normal with ristocetin. The platelets lack platelet-membrane GPIIb/IIIa complex and have defective platelet–platelet interaction. The platelet-specific alloantigen PL^{A1} is carried on GPIIIa and Bak^a on GPIIb. The disorder may present in the neonatal period with minor or major haemorrhagic symptoms. Although bleeding can be terminated by platelet concentrates, unnecessary transfusion should be rigorously avoided because of the high risk of alloimmunization.

Management of a low platelet count in the neonate

With the exception of infants with immune-mediated thrombocytopenia, platelet transfusion is the only means of increasing the neonate's platelet count and terminating haemorrhage. The platelets should be ABO-compatible with the infant and suspended in as small a volume of plasma as possible. They should be HBsAg-, HIV- and CMV-negative. One unit of platelets should increase the platelet count of the newborn by at least 50×10^9 per litre, unless the thrombocytopenia is immune-mediated, when transfused platelets will be rapidly consumed. The survival of donor platelets should be documented by serial platelet counts in order to determine subsequent therapy. Platelet transfusion is warranted for serious bleeding or a platelet count less than 25×10^9 per litre. The special requirements of platelets for transfusion to infants affected by neonatal alloimmune thrombocytopenia have already been mentioned. Platelets transfused to infants of mothers with idiopathic thrombocytopenia will rapidly be consumed by maternal anti-platelet autoantibodies. However, it may be necessary to quickly raise the neonate's platelet count in the presence of serious haemorrhage, particularly intracranial haemorrhage. Such infants are best treated by exchange transfusion to remove antibody, followed by random donor platelet transfusion. Platelets for antenatal transfusion should be irradiated to prevent graft-versus-host-disease.

SPECIFIC INHERITED COAGULATION DEFECTS

Haemorrhage is common in the neonate and is usually due to an acquired coagulation problem. However, inherited coagulation defects also present at this time and although a family history is usually available, it is not always. The clinician should be alert to the possibility of a hereditary coagulation problem in an otherwise healthy infant with haemorrhage, especially if the neonate has been bottle-fed. Isolated haemorrhage is particularly suggestive of an inherited coagulation defect, and common presenting sites include bleeding following circumcision, umbilical and intracerebral haemorrhage. The latter can include both subdural and subarachnoid haematoma and may result in hydrocephalus. Haematomas, particularly cephalohaematomas, are common. Factor deficiences associated with neonatal haemorrhage include factors VIII:C, IX, vWF, afibrinogenaemia, XIII, VII and X. Generally, only severely affected infants present with problems in the newborn period. Haemophilia A and B and von Willebrand's disease account for more than 90% of inherited clotting factor deficiencies, and between 5 and 10% of affected infants will present in the neonatal period (Baehner and Strauss, 1966). The reader is referred to the excellent review, by Barnard (1984), of inherited bleeding disorders in the newborn infant.

Haemophilia A

This X-linked recessive disorder has an incidence of 1:10 000 newborn males. The clinical severity of the condition varies considerably and patients are classified into mild, moderate or severely affected according to their level of factor VIII:C. Severely affected males have a factor VIII:C level of less than 2% and will bleed spontaneously without trauma. Moderately affected males have a factor VIII:C level of 2–10% and bleed following minor trauma. Those individuals with factor VIII:C levels of 10% and above are considered mildly affected and bleed only after trauma or surgery. The relationship between activity level and clinical severity is not as straightforward as this classification implies. At least 50% of haemophiliacs have factor VIII:C levels of less than 2% and are severely affected. The severity of the deficiency is consistent within members of the same family.

Less than 10% of haemophiliac infants present with bleeding problems in the newborn period and they will be severely affected. Diagnosis can be made on the cord blood as the factor VIII:C level is within the normal adult range at birth. Haematoma following an intramuscular vitamin K injection or oozing after heel-prick screening for phenylketonuria (PKU) may highlight the underlying coagulopathy. Bleeding may occur from the cord or from a circumcision site, if it has been performed on an undiagnosed haemophiliac. Intracranial bleeding is rare, although cephalhaematoma is seen. Splenic and adrenal haemorrhage have also been described (Jannaccone and Pasquino, 1981; Schmidt and Zipursky, 1986). Caesarean section is only indicated for documented cephalopelvic disproportion or causes that would indicate caesarean section in a normal infant. Forceps delivery should be avoided. The majority of affected males will have no problems in the neonatal period and will not present until the second year of life, when they start walking and exploring their environment.

About 30% of cases have no family history and may go undetected in the neonatal period unless the infant has a clinical problem, the diagnosis is realized and the appropriate testing done. However, the majority of haemophiliacs will have a family history and many families now seek prenatal diagnosis. In the past, many women who knew themselves to be carriers of haemophilia A would not risk the birth of a haemophiliac son and elected to terminate all male pregnancies, half of which would in fact be unaffected. The advent of prenatal diagnosis offers a rational approach to family planning for obligate or possible carriers. Termination of affected pregnancies will not eradicate haemophilia because of the 30% of cases which arise from new mutations, and the many obligate carriers will not consider termination and decline prenatal diagnosis. Two basic methods are available and both have their own intrinsic limitations which the clinician must be aware of when interpreting the results. Prenatal diagnosis can be based on DNA analysis or immunological assays of factor VIII:CAg and vWF:Ag on fetal blood (see Chapter 9).

If treatment is necessary in the neonatal period, factor VIII:C replacement can be given with either factor VIII concentrate or cryoprecipitate. When it was realized that factor VIII concentrates were implicated in the spread of HIV infection, it became policy to treat all 'virgin' haemophiliacs up to the age of 4 years with cryoprecipitate. However, now that factor VIII concentrate is heat-treated it may in fact be a safer product than cryoprecipitate, particularly in terms of transmission of non-A, non-B hepatitis. One unit of factor VIII:C (the amount of factor VIII:C contained in 1 ml of plasma) per kilogram will raise the recipient's factor VIII:C level by 2%. The half-life of factor VIII:C is 8–12 h. Desmopressin acetate (DDAVP), which releases endogenous factor VIII–vWF complex from its stores, may be a useful agent in the mild or moderate haemophiliac. However, this is not an alternative therapeutic option for the severely affected haemophiliac, who is most likely to present in the newborn period.

Christmas disease (haemophilia B)

Haemophilia B is clinically indistinguishable from haemophilia A and has a similar inheritance pattern. It is less common with about 1:30 000 newborn males being affected. Patients are classified into severely (< 2%), moderately (2–10%) or mildy affected (> 10%), according to their level of functional factor IX. The characteristics of haemophilia B differs widely between families, some families making normal amounts of an inactive protein and others low levels or no active protein.

Diagnosis in the newborn period is complex. Factor IX is a vitamin K-dependent factor with gestationally dependent low values at birth. It may, therefore, be impossible to diagnose with confidence, mild or moderately affected individuals in the newborn period, although diagnosis should be possible for severely affected boys. Prenatal diagnosis may be possible by DNA analysis, but diagnosis based on fetal blood sampling is complicated by the heterogeneity of the disorder and the gestation-dependent low levels of factor IX. Factor IX can be provided by fresh frozen plasma or factor IX concentrate. The latter may produce a tendency to thrombosis in the newborn infant who has physiological deficits of ATIII and protein C. One unit of factor IX per kilogram of body weight will raise the factor IX level by 1%.

Von Willebrand's disease

Von Willebrand's disease is characterized by lack of vWF which causes platelet dysfunction and sometimes factor VIII deficiency. It is probably the most common of the inherited disorders of haemostasis (1–3% of the population), but the incidence is difficult to determine because mild cases often go undiagnosed. The factor VIII deficiency is characterized by a corresponding decrease in factor VIII:C and vWF:Ag. vWF normally facilitates platelet adhesion to sub-endothelium, and its absence is demonstrated in the laboratory by a prolonged bleeding time (BT), defective ristocetin-induced platelet aggregation and reduced vWF activity (measured by the ristocetin cofactor assay). The disorder is very heterogeneous and can be classified according to the multimeric structure of vWF.

Three types can be identified. Type I vWD (classical) and type II vWD (variant) are transmitted by an autosomal dominant gene whilst type III vWD has an autosomal recessive inheritance. Type I vWD has reduced levels of all components of the factor VIII–vWF complex, including factor VIII:C, vWF:Ag and ristocetin-cofactor activity. Although reduced, vWF multimers are normal in pattern. Type II can be differentiated from type I by a qualitative abnormality of vWF. Large and intermediate multimers are absent from both plasma and platelets in type IIA, whilst large multimers are absent from plasma but present in normal amounts in the platelets of individuals with type IIB. Such individuals have enhanced platelet aggregation with low concentrations of ristocetin, which distinguishes this subtype from type IIA. Subtypes IIC to IIH have been reported in a few individuals and are characterized by aberrant multimeric patterns. Type III vWD represents homozygous or doubly heterozygous vWD and all components of the factor VIII–vWF complex are present in minute amounts only. This severe form, although uncommon, is the most likely to present in infancy, usually with mucous membrane bleeding. The diagnosis of vWD may be difficult during the neonatal period. The physiological stress of delivery may increase factor VIII–vWF complex values to within normal limits in infants with mild to moderate von Willebrand's disease (type I vWD). However, severely affected individuals should be identifiable at birth because they are not able to respond to stress by increasing their factor VIII–vWF complex values. Type II vWD has a qualitative abnormality of vWF. Multimeric analysis of the von Willebrand protein may be diagnostic but care must be exercised in the interpretation, because infants, as well as adults with DIC, may have structurally altered vWF with loss of the large molecular weight multimers similar to that seen with type IIB vWD. Additionally, a recent report by Weinstein that normal fetal and neonatal blood contains unusually large von Willebrand factor multimers (ULvWFM), and similarly elevated proportions of HMWvWF multimers may further complicate diagnosis of subtypes (Weinstein *et al.*, 1989).

Factor VIII concentrate rich in HMW multimers is the preferred treatment for patients not responsive to DDAVP. Some patients with vWD respond to DDAVP, but severely affected individuals with type III vWD do not and this is the subtype likely to have problems in the neonatal period. Similarly, factor VIII concentrates are not always effective in correcting the bleeding time because many products do not contain enough of the HMW multimers of vWF. Cryoprecipitate contains the entire factor VIII–vWF complex and can be used if factor VIII concentrates do not achieve haemostasis: however, cryoprecipitate that is not heat-treated carries the risk of hepatitis and HIV infection. One bag of cryoprecipitate per 5 6 kg body weight is the recommended dose.

Table 6.9 gives recommendations for treatment. In general, the use of commercial concentrates prepared from large pools of donors have not been recommended in the neonatal period because of the risk of viral transmission especially HIV, hepatitis B and non-A, non-B hepatitis. However, the new heat-treated factor VIII and factor IX concentrates are considered safe from HIV transmission and concentrates are less likely to transmit non-A, non-B hepatitis than cryoprecipitate. Affected individuals should be vaccinated against hepatitis B. Cryoprecipitate may be used for severe vWD and afibrinogenaemia. It should be remembered that neonates

Table 6.9 Haemostatic therapy in the newborn.

Deficiency	Product	Dose and recommendations
Haemophilia A	FVIII concentrate (heat treated) Cryoprecipitate	1 U kg^{-1} will raise VIII:C level by 2% t½ of FVIII:C = 12 h One bag of cryoprecipitate = 100 units FVIII:C
Haemophilia B	FIX concentrate (heat treated) FFP	1 U kg^{-1} will raise FIX:C level by 1% t½ of FIX = 18–24 h
von Willebrand's disease	FVIII concentrate (heat treated) Cryoprecipitate	1 U kg^{-1} will raise FVIII:C level by 2% 1 bag/6 kg will raise vWF by 0.5 U ml^{-1}
	DDAVP	0.3 μg/kg^{-1} (dissolved in 20 ml saline and infused over 20 min)
Afibrinogenaemia	Cryoprecipitate	1 bag/6 kg will raise the fibrinogen by 100 mg dl^{-1} t½ of FI = 3–4 days
Factor XIII	Cryoprecipitate/FFP	5–10 ml kg^{-1} t½ of FXIII 4–6 days
Other factor deficiencies	FFP	10–15 ml kg^{-1} gives a rise of 20% in factors
ATIII	FFP	10 ml kg^{-1}
Protein C	FFP FIX concentrate (heat treated)	10 ml kg^{-1} q12h 50–75 U kg^{-1} on alternate days
Thrombocytopenia	Platelet concentrates	1 unit/5 kg will give a rise of $50 \times 10^9\ l^{-1}$
Thrombosis	Urokinase Heparin	4400 U $kg^{-1}\ h^{-1}$ Loading dose of 50 U kg^{-1} followed by continuous infusion of 20–25 U $kg^{-1}\ h^{-1}$
DIC	FFP	10–15 ml kg^{-1}
Vitamin K	Vitamin K	1 mg parenterally at birth repeated 3- to 4-weekly in severe malabsorption disorders

with inherited coagulation defects should not receive aspirin or intramuscular injections.

All congenital coagulation disorders other than haemophilia A and B and vWDs are rare. Some are associated with such mild bleeding problems that they are likely to go undetected in the newborn period unless a family history prompts investigation. Others are associated with a significant bleeding problem and may present symptomatically in the newborn period. The differential diagnosis includes a physiological depression of those factors reduced at birth, vitamin K deficiency or consumption associated with DIC. A definitive diagnosis is made by demonstrating an absence or disproportionate reduction of an isolated factor. However, it may not always be possible to confirm the diagnosis in the newborn period.

Congenital afibrinogenaemia

Congential disorders of fibrinogen synthesis include afibrinogenaemia, hypofibrinogenaemia and dysfibrinogenaemia. Congenital afibrinogenaemia is a rare, inherited bleeding disorder characterized by complete absence of fibrinogen in the plasma. Inheritance is by an autosomal recessive gene resulting in afibrinogenaemia in the homozygote and normal or reduced fibrinogen levels in the heterozygote. Neonatal presentation is common and symptoms range in severity from bruising to intracranial haemorrhage. Mucous membrane bleeding (presenting as melaena or haematemesis), haematomas secondary to trauma at delivery and bleeding from the umbilical cord are particularly common. Spontaneous haemarthosis can occur in childhood. Heterozygotes are asymptomatic. Patients with dysfibrinogenaemia may have a mild to moderate bleeding diathesis or a tendency to thrombosis, or they may be asymptomatic depending on the variant inherited. In the homozygote, fibrinogen is completely absent when measured by clotting techniques but immunological assays may detect trace amounts. The results of all screening tests based on fibrin formation, i.e. prothrombin time (PT), activated partial thromboplastin time (APTT) and thrombin clotting time (TCT) will be abnormal. Heterozygotes may have reduced levels of fibrinogen.

Bleeding episodes can be controlled by replacement of fibrinogen with FFP or cryoprecipitate. The half-life of fibrinogen is approximately 80 h, and therefore treatment need only be given every 4–5 days.

Congenital prothrombin deficiency

This exceedingly rare disorder appears to be inherited in an autosomal recessive manner. Both a true deficiency and synthesis of an abnormal molecular variant have been described. The deficiency is not complete and most homozygotes produce approximately 10% of the normal amount of functional prothrombin. The bleeding disorder is usually mild to moderate and characterized in the neonatal period by umbilical or post-circumcision bleeding. Haematemesis and intracranial bleeding have been reported. Patients with dysprothrombinaemia may be asymptomatic or have problems comparable to those of patients with hypoprothrombinaemia. The prothrombin time is moderately prolonged and the differential diagnosis is from vitamin K-deficiency. The diagnosis depends upon a discrepancy between the level of prothrombin and the other vitamin K-dependent factors. Synthesis of an abnormal prothrombin molecule can be demonstrated by an immunological assay. Accurate diagnosis of hypoprothrombinaemia or dysprothrombinaemia is difficult in the newborn. Treatment is rarely necessary, but if required FFP should be given. Treatment need only be given every 2–3 days, because of the long half-life of the protein. Vitamin K is of no value.

Congenital factor V deficiency

This autosomal recessive disorder is associated with a mild bleeding tendency usually from the mucous membranes. It is unlikely to manifest itself in the neonatal period but, if it does, it is generally by umbilical bleeding. The deficiency is due to failure of production of the protein with a complete absence in the homozygous state. Factor V levels correlate poorly with clinical severity. The PT and APTT are prolonged. Both the term and preterm infant have normal levels of factor V at birth and therefore diagnosis is not complicated and can be confirmed by a factor V assay. The half-life of the transfused protein is 36 hours and replacement is with FFP.

Congenital factor VII deficiency

This rare clotting disorder is thought to be inherited as a highly penetrant, incompletely recessive, autosomal trait. The severity of the bleeding problem depends on the degree of deficiency. The more mildly affected individuals rarely have bleeding problems, but the severely affected may experience serious mucous membrane bleeding, haemarthrosis and muscle haematomas. Neonates have been reported with fatal bleeding usually due to intracranial haemorrhage. Other neonatal presentations include oozing from the umbilical cord, bleeding post circumcision, cephalohaematoma, ecchymoses and haematemesis. Heterozygotes may have clinical problems. Two types of homozygotes have been identified, those who produce no protein and those who produce a (presumably) non-functional protein. The PT is abnormally prolonged for the infant's gestation, but the APTT is not affected. The addition of Russell's viper venom corrects the PT to a normal value for the infant.

Factor VII is a vitamin K-dependent factor and physiologically reduced at birth. A specific assay for factor VII should be disproportionately low compared to the other vitamin K-dependent factors. The half-life of the protein is 5 h, and treatment, if required, should be with FFP. Vitamin K is of no value.

Congenital factor X deficiency

This is an extremely rare coagulation disorder inherited as an incompletely recessive trait. Several forms of defect have been described including patients with a complete deficiency of the protein, patients with an abnormal, non-functional molecule and patients with a small amount of non-functional molecule. The bleeding manifestations are moderately severe or severe, and infants have been reported with intracranial haemorrhage and bleeding from the umbilical cord and gastrointestinal tract. Heterozygotes may bleed. The definitive diagnosis is dependent on demonstrating absent or disproportionately low levels of factor X in the presence of normal values for the other vitamin K-dependent factors. Factor replacement, if required, should be given with FFP. Vitamin K is of no value.

Congenital factor XI deficiency

Congential factor XI deficiency is a mild bleeding disorder. Most reported cases have been in Jewish patients and the inheritance is as an autosomal, incompletely recessive trait. Even in the most severely affected, the bleeding problem is usually mild but does not necessarily correlate with the factor XI coagulant activity. Diagnosis in the neonatal period is difficult, because of the physiological depression of this contact factor. The PT is normal, but the APTT is prolonged. A specific factor XI assay will be disproportionately low for gestation. Diagnosis may not be possible until the physiological depression has resolved. FFP is the best source of factor XI available.

Congential factor XII deficiency

This disorder is not associated with haemorrhagic manifestations and therefore diagnosis is by chance rather than by investigation of a clinical problem. The APTT is markedly prolonged and a specific factor XII assay is required for definitive diagnosis.

Other contact factors

Congenital deficiencies of prekallikrein (Fletcher factor) and high molecular weight kininogen (Fitzgerald factor) have also been reported. However, although these result in a prolongation of the APTT, there are no associated haemorrhagic problems.

Congenital factor XIII deficiency

This disorder is inherited as an autosomal recessive trait and is characterized by poor wound healing and late wound bleeding. In the absence of factor XIII an unstable friable clot is formed. The molecule is composed of two subunits, subunit A and subunit B (or S). Only subunit A has fibrin-stabilizing activity. Two types of factor XIII deficiency exist. In the first type, both subunits A and S are immunologically decreased, whilst in the second form only subunit A is defective, subunit S being normal or near normal. Infants with congenital deficiency commonly bleed from the umbilicus. Intracranial bleeding has also been reported. Wounds heal slowly and although clotting takes place at the time of surgery, secondary bleeding occurs 24–36 hours later. In the absence of factor XIII, cross-linkage of the fibrin polymer does not take place, resulting in an unstable clot that is more susceptible to digestion by plasmin. The PT, APTT and TCT are normal. The diagnosis is confirmed by the rapid solubility of the fibrin clot in 5 M urea or in 1% solution of monochloracetic acid. This screening test does not detect heterozygotes. The factor XIII activity can be measured using a chromogenic assay and the subtypes differentiated by immunological techniques.

Although the normal neonate has a reduced level of factor XIII, this does not cause problems because only tiny quantities are required for fibrin stabilization. Replacement, if required, should be given with FFP. Factor XIII has a half-life of 6 days.

INVESTIGATION OF THE NEONATE WITH A BLEEDING PROBLEM

The investigation of the neonate with a bleeding problem starts with a coagulation screen, i.e. PT, APTT and TCT and a platelet count. A bleeding time need only be done if a defect of platelet function is suspected. There are inherent problems related to the interpretation of these results in the newborn infant. Firstly, *in vitro* artefacts are common due to problems in obtaining adequate blood samples and, secondly, the values obtained have to be interpreted in the light of the normal physiological immaturity of the newborn's haemostatic mechanism.

Blood sampling

Small volumes

Standard coagulation screening and, more particularly, platelet aggregation studies require volumes of blood which cannot safely be taken from neonates. Laboratories providing a service to neonatal units should establish microtechniques for routine coagulation screening. These methods must be well standardized and reproducible with respect to reagents, techniques and volumes employed. One to two millilitres of blood are sufficient to perform a coagulation screen and full range of factor assays (Andrews *et al.*, 1987). As little as 20 μl of plasma suffice for each of the screening tests (PT, APTT and TCT). Factor assays employing dilutions of 1 in 10 (10 μl plasma diluted in 90 μl buffer), rising to 1 in 100, require very small quantities of plasma. Once a dilution has been prepared this can theoretically be used for more than one factor assay. Although coagulation tests are generally performed in duplicate, this may not be possible in the neonate. It is important that all clinical information is available to the haematologist, so that the most appropriate tests are carried out first and precious plasma not wasted.

In vitro *artefacts*

It is important to obtain a venous sample that is not contaminated by intravenous solutions, has flowed freely and has neither activated nor clotted in the process of sampling. Activation of the specimen characteristically shortens the APTT. Specimens should always be checked for fibrin strands or clots as such artefacts are particularly common in samples taken from very small babies. The development of immunological assays has helped to overcome some of the problems of contaminated or partially activated specimens, as they measure total and not just functional protein. However, at the present time we rely heavily on functional assays, particularly for screening tests which can only be measured this way. It is therefore important that any abnormal result not in keeping with the clinical picture is repeated in the first instance. However, the problems of repeatedly taking blood from the neonate may make this difficult or impossible.

Heparin contamination of specimens

Heparin contamination of specimens obtained from arterial or venous catheters, through which heparin is being infused to prevent thrombosis, is a common problem. At least 4 ml of blood must be withdrawn prior to sampling to prevent contamination. A blood sample that potentially might be contaminated with heparin should always be checked for the presence of a circulating anticoagulant.

Table 6.10 Volume of anticoagulant for nine volumes of whole blood (used in newborns to correct volume of anticoagulant for high haematocrit).

Haematocrit (%)	Anticoagulant volume (ml)
45	1.0
50	0.9
51	0.9
53	0.85
55	0.8
57	0.8
59	0.75
60	0.7
63	0.65
65	0.65
67	0.6
69	0.55
70	0.55
71	0.5
73	0.5
75	0.45
77	0.4
79	0.4
80	0.35
81	0.35
83	0.3
85	0.3
87	0.25
89	0.2
90	0.2

From Corrigan Jr, (1989). *Perinatal Haematology* **21**: 167, with permission of Churchill Livingstone.

Anticoagulant

The anticoagulant ratio should be based on the plasma volume and not on the total volume of whole blood. The volume of anticoagulant should be reduced proportionately to the increased haematocrit value (Table 6.10). This is particularly important for infants with very high haematocrits.

Coagulation tests

A clinical interpretation should be put on a coagulation screen (PT, APTT and TCT) only after the haematologist has satisfied him or herself that there is no artefactual or technical error influencing the result. The next step is to decide if the results are normal for a baby of that gestation. This demands that any laboratory handling a large number of samples from neonates has established gestation-dependent normal ranges. If the result is considered abnormal for that infant, a more definitive diagnosis can be arrived at by specific factor assays. As already stated, these require very small amounts of plasma. It is usually not helpful to measure the level of one factor only. For example a low factor IX can occur congenitally, in DIC, in vitamin K deficiency and in liver disease. In this situation a number of factor assays are necessary to identify the underlying problem. Congenital deficiencies of both factors IX and XI may be difficult to diagnose with confidence in the newborn period and confirmation may have to be deferred until 3–6 months of age.

Both the term and pre-term infant have a bleeding time within the normal adult range. A modified template bleeding time should be used to assess platelet function, as unacceptably large volumes of plasma are required for formal platelet aggregation studies. Newer aggregometers have been modified for small volumes, but many still require about 150 μl of platelet rich plasma per aggregating agent. Monoclonal antibodies are now available for the detection of GPIb and GPIIb/IIIa on the platelet surface, making the diagnosis of Bernard–Soulier syndrome and Glanzmann's thrombasthenia possible using small volumes of whole blood. Andrew reported a shortened bleeding time in neonates, compared with adults, using a modified template bleeding time developed for infants. The mean bleeding time of 61 non-thrombocytopenic infants was 142 ± 37 s (mean ± SD) (Andrew *et al.*, 1987a). Other workers have also reported the newborn's bleeding time to be shorter than that of the adult, despite its impaired platelet function (Feusner, 1980). Andrew postulated that the short bleeding time may be related to the high haematocrit or elevated vWF in the infant. Stuart gives an alternative suggestion for a normal bleeding time in the presence of impairment of platelet aggregation (Stuart, 1981). She reported the neonate to have a markedly reduced ability to regenerate prostaglandin I_2 (PGI_2) compared with the adult. The PGI_2-like regenerating activity normalizes by 3–5 months of age, at a time when platelet function is no longer impaired. She suggests that the physiological impairment in platelet function provides a safety mechanism to counteract the prothrombotic state induced by a deficiency of PGI_2. The impaired ability of neonatal blood to regenerate

Table 6.11 Reference values (means + SD) for screening tests in the healthy full-term infant during the first six months of life *

Tests	Day 1	Day 5	Day 30	Day 90	Day 180	Adult
PT (s)	13.0 ± 1.43	12.4 ± 1.46	11.8 ± 1.25	11.9 ± 1.15	12.3 ± 0.79	12.4 ± 0.78
APTT (s)	42.9 ± 5.80	42.6 ± 8.62	40.4 ± 7.42	37.1 ± 6.52	35.5 ± 3.71	33.5 ± 3.44
TCT (s)	23.5 ± 2.38	23.1 ± 3.07	24.3 ± 2.44	25.1 ± 2.32	25.5 ± 2.86	25.0 ± 2.66

* Adapted from Andrew *et al.*, 1987, *Blood 70(1)*, with kind permission of Grune and Stratton Inc.

Table 6.12 Reference values for screening tests in healthy premature infants (30–36 weeks' gestation) during first six months of life.*

	Day 1		Day 5		Day 30		Day 90		Day 180		Adult	
Tests	M	B	M	B	M	B	M	B	M	B	M	B
PT (s)	13.0	(10.6–16.2)	12.5	(10.0–15.3)	11.8	(10.0–13.6)	12.3	(10.0–14.6)	12.5	(10.0–15.0)	12.4	(10.8–13.9)
APTT (s)	53.6	(27.5–79.4)	50.5	(26.9–74.1)	44.7	(26.9–62.5)	39.5	(28.3–50.7)	37.5	(21.7–53.3)	33.5	(26.6–40.3)
TCT (s)	24.8	(19.2–30.4)	24.1	(18.8–29.4)	24.4	(18.8–29.9)	25.1	(19.4–30.8)	25.2	(18.9–31.5)	25.0	(19.7–30.3)

* M = mean, B = lower and upper boundary encompassing 95% of the population. (Adapted from Andrew *et al.*, 1988, *Blood, 72(5)*: 1653, with kind permission of Grune and Stratton Inc.)

PGI_2-like activity may be related to its markedly decreased antioxidant potential, as correction follows the addition of vitamin E *in vitro*.

The PT measures the clotting activities of factors I, II, V, VII and X. The APTT measures the coagulant activity of factors I, II, V, VIII, IX, X, XI, XII, prekallikrein and HMWK. The value is dependant on the activating agent used, and much of the prolongation reflects low levels of the contact factors. The TCT in the term and pre-term infant is slightly prolonged due to the relative thrombin insensitivity of fetal fibrinogen. The addition of calcium to the buffering system brings the TCT into the adult range.

The values in Table 6.11 and Figures 6.2–6.8 are based on a large number of healthy full-term infants studied longitudinally over a 6-month period (Andrew *et al.*, 1987a), and Table 6.12 gives those for healthy pre-term infants (Andrew *et al.*, 1988). Venous samples only were tested and all infants had received 1 mg of vitamin K at birth. This comprehensive study showed that although the variability of the PT was greater in the pre-term and term newborn infant, the mean values were not significantly different from the adult. The PT shortened during the first month of life. It has already been stated that low levels of the contact factors in infants may greatly prolong the APTT such that the test becomes of little diagnostic value. Andrew *et al.* used a reagent containing ellagic acid rather than kaolin as an activating agent and, by doing so, narrowed the normal range, increasing the usefulness of the APTT as a screening test. They reported the APTT to be prolonged at birth, and to reach adult values by 3 months of age in the full-term infant. The APTT was further prolonged in the pre-term infant at birth and remained statistically significantly longer than the adult value, until 6 months of age. The TCT performed with calcium present in the buffering system was in the adult range at birth and a narrow normal range delineated.

THROMBOSIS

The peak incidence of thrombosis in the paediatric age group falls in the neonatal period (Table 6.13). Thrombosis in the newborn is most frequently iatrogenic and associated with indwelling catheters, although not exclusively so. The reviews referenced in Table 6.13 illustrate the increased incidence of spontaneous thrombosis in the first month of life. Most vessels have been affected, including renal, adrenal, portal and hepatic veins, peripheral, cerebral, pulmonary, coronary, renal and mesenteric arteries, and the aorta and inferior vena cava.

The triad of factors attributed to Virchow to predispose to thrombosis are (Virchow 1956): (1) abnormalities of the vessel wall, (2) disturbances of blood flow, and (3) changes in blood coagulability. These factors will be considered in the pathogenesis of neonatal thrombosis.

Abnormalities of the vessel wall

All intra-arterial and intravenous catheters carry a risk of thrombosis. Indwelling catheters induce thrombosis for a number of reasons. Most

Table 6.13 Thrombotic disease in paediatric age groups: peak incidence (%) in the newborn period and early infancy.*

		Age at diagnosis			
Entity	Study design	< 1 month	> 1 month to < 1 year	> 1 year	Reference
Renal venous thrombosis	Literature review of case reports ($n = 95$);	63	21	16	Kaufman (1958)
	Clinicopathological survey ($n = 115$)	73	20	7	Arneil (1973)
Pulmonary embolism (no intravascular catheters)	Pathological survey ($n = 25$)	20	52	28	Emery (1962)
Severe arterial thrombosis and embolism in the systemic circulation (no intravascular catheters)	Literature review of case reports ($n = 47$)	96	2	2	Gross (1945)

* From Schmidt B and Zipursky A, 1984, *Clinics in Perinatology 11(2)*: 462, with permission of WB Saunders Co.

importantly, the foreign surface has thrombogenic properties and is a nidus for thrombus formation. Furthermore, the catheter damages the endothelium of the vessel wall, predisposing to thrombus formation. Additional contributing factors include mechanical occlusion, vasospasm and alterations in blood flow. Catheter-associated thromboembolism has been reported in association with radial, pulmonary, temporal and femoral arterial lines, as well as with central venous catheters inserted into the jugular and femoral veins. However, in this age-group, it is because of their popularity that umbilical catheters are associated with the majority of catheter-related thrombosis.

The incidence of catheter-related thrombosis varies widely between studies, due particularly to the different criteria employed for diagnosis. In 1976 Tyson *et al.* reported a 59% incidence of umbilical artery catheter-associated thrombosis at autopsy. The incidence has been reported to vary between 20 and 95% in studies detecting thrombotic lesions by aortography. These data suggest that clinically evident thrombotic complications grossly underestimate the extent of the problem, as many events are clearly silent. Catheterization of the umbilical vein is also associated with thrombotic lesions, but the incidence is unclear. Two factors strongly correlate with the risk of thrombosis at this site. Firstly, the incorrect placement of the catheter tip in the portal or hepatic vein and, secondly, the infusion of hyperosmolar solutions. Correct placement of the catheter tip in the inferior vena cava significantly reduces the risk of portal vein thrombosis. Infants of low birth weight and early gestation, and sick infants, appear to be particularly susceptible to catheter-related thrombotic episodes. However, as these are the newborns most likely to be catheterized, this observation may be biased.

The sequelae of catheter-related arterial thrombosis include renal hypertension, necrotizing enterocolitis, paraplegia, peripheral gangrene, organ infarction and death. Follow-up studies of clinically silent, radiologically diagnosed thrombosis have been limited but have not revealed significant sequelae. Catheter-related thrombus may provide a focus for bacterial colonization, contributing to the higher rate of infection seen in patients with catheters.

Worthy of special mention is the high incidence of renal vessel thrombosis in the neonatal period. About 70% of cases of neonatal renal vein thrombosis have been reported in infants of less than 1 month of age and it can even be an antenatal event. The small calibre of the renal vessels and the low renal blood flow in the perinatal period are thought to be contributing factors. Haematuria or enlarged kidneys should always alert the physician to the possibility of renal vein thrombosis. Over 90% of cases of hypertension in the neonate are associated with renal vascular disease.

The use of low-dose heparin has been advocated to prolong patency and reduce the incidence of catheter-related thrombosis. In 1987 Horgan *et al.* reported the effect of low-dose heparin on the incidence of large-vessel thrombosis and serious thrombotic complications in 111 consecutive infants requiring umbilical artery catheterization. Fifty-nine infants were randomized to receive prophylactic heparin and 52 infants served as controls. The mean dose of heparin was 0.9 $U\ kg^{-1}\ h^{-1}$ (range 0.46–3.4 $U\ kg^{-1}\ h^{-1}$). The numbers of thrombotic episodes in the two groups were not significantly different: 16 in the heparin group and 18 in the control group. Aortic thrombosis was documented by ultrasonography in 30 infants, by autopsy in two infants and by clinical criteria in two infants. Of the 30 infants diagnosed radiologically, 24 had sleeve clots and six had bulky intraluminal and mural thrombi. Only nine infants (26.4%) with thrombosis were symptomatic, which suggests a high incidence of occult thrombus formation. There was no correlation between the length of time that the umbilical arterial cather (UAC) was *in situ* and the development of large vessel thrombus. Although low-dose heparin did not appear to reduce the incidence of catheter-related thrombus formation, the number of clotted and non-functional UACs was reduced (10 of 52 in the control group versus two of 59 in the heparin group). However, the addition of low-doses of heparin to UACs did appear to have an effect on thrombotic complications as the incidence of hypertension, a serious UAC-associated thrombotic complication, was lower in the heparin group (none out of 16 versus nine out of 18 infants with aortic thrombi).

From the available data it would appear that continuous infusions of low-dose heparin or heparin 'flushes' do little to prevent catheter-related thrombosis, although these measures do prolong catheter patency. Recently, the use of low doses of heparin has been implicated as a risk factor for intraventricular haemorrhage in the infant of low birth weight. However, these babies are not only the infants most likely to be catheterized but also those with the highest incidence of intraventricular haemorrhage. It is clearly important to clarify the situation, which is complicated by our poor understanding of the role of abnormal haemostasis in the pathogenesis of intraventricular haemorrhage and by the many other risk factors in infants of low birth weight.

Two other vessel-wall anomalies may occasionally play a role in neonatal thrombosis. Firstly, although thrombosis does not occur during normal closure of the ductus arteriosus, if this does not undergo normal involution, thrombi may form within the vessel, providing a source of emboli to both the systemic and pulmonary circulation. Secondly, thrombi can be found in fetal–placental veins in a number of maternal disorders, particularly pre-eclampsia, and are a potential source of embolus.

Disturbances of blood flow

Alterations of blood flow have been documented in infants with abnormally high haematocrits. In newborns, as in adults, there is a strong correlation between blood viscosity and haematocrit. Submaximal limb blood flow as measured by strain-gauge plethysmography decreases in polycythaemic newborns with increasing haematocrit (Bergquist and Zetterström, 1975). There appears to be a consistent relationship between viscosity and haematocrit within the normal range, but at the relatively high haematocrit values found in the newborn infant, a small rise (above or around 70%) in packed cell volume (PCV) produces a considerable rise in blood viscosity. True polycythaemia and dehydration both result in an elevated haematocrit. Additionally, the red cell diameter is important for platelet adherence and the larger diameter of neonatal red blood cells is associated with significantly increased platelet adherence (Piet *et al.*, 1983).

Changes in blood coagulation

Any imbalance between the activators and inhibitors of either the coagulation or fibrinolytic mechanisms may predispose towards thrombosis. Hereditary protein C, protein S, ATIII, HCII and plasminogen deficiences are associated with venous thrombosis in the adult but very rarely with arterial thrombosis. Likewise, dysfibrinogenaemias and excess fibrinolytic inhibitors have been incriminated in the pathogenesis of venous thrombosis in adults. Neonates with homozygous protein C deficiency have been reported with fatal fulminant thrombosis. A small number of infants born to mothers with congenital ATIII deficiency have died in the newborn period of aortic thrombosis (Bjorke *et al.*, 1974). Congenital ATIII deficiency was suspected in these babies, but was not verified by assay. Despite this, there is no real evidence that the physiological reduction of natural anticoagulants in the neonate contributes to thrombosis. The physiological depression of ATIII in the neonate is balanced by an equal reduction of the procoagulants, factors II, VII, IX and X. However, the reduction in protein C is not balanced by a depression of factors V and VIII, which are within the normal adult range at birth. This imbalance is in favour of a thrombotic tendency. Other physiological changes compensate. Fibrinolysis is increased in the neonate and neonatal platelet function is impaired.

Specific thrombotic disorders

In the absence of an obvious identifiable cause for thrombosis the infant should be investigated for a congenital deficiency of one of the natural anticoagulants, particularly protein C. Purpura fulminans, multiple thrombotic lesions and evidence of intra-uterine thrombosis are particularly suggestive.

Homozygous protein C deficiency

As already stated, protein C is a vitamin K-dependent factor and is reduced in the newborn infant. To function as an anticoagulant, protein C is first activated by limited proteolysis. Thrombomodulin, a thrombin receptor present on the surface of endothelial cells, functions as a cofactor in the activation of protein C. Thrombomodulin has a high affinity for thrombin and binds with it to form a 1:1 M complex, which activates protein C at least 1000 times faster than free thrombin (Figure 6.11). Thrombomodulin, by binding thrombin, has an important role in regulating haemostasis. When thrombin is complexed to thrombomodulin it is no longer able to activate factor V or convert fibrinogen to fibrin. Activated protein C destroys activated factors V and VIII:C and enhances fibrinolysis. The rate of inactivation of factor Va by activated protein C is enhanced by protein S, which acts as a cofactor in this reaction. The role of activated protein C in the regulation of haemostasis is illustrated in Figure 6.11.

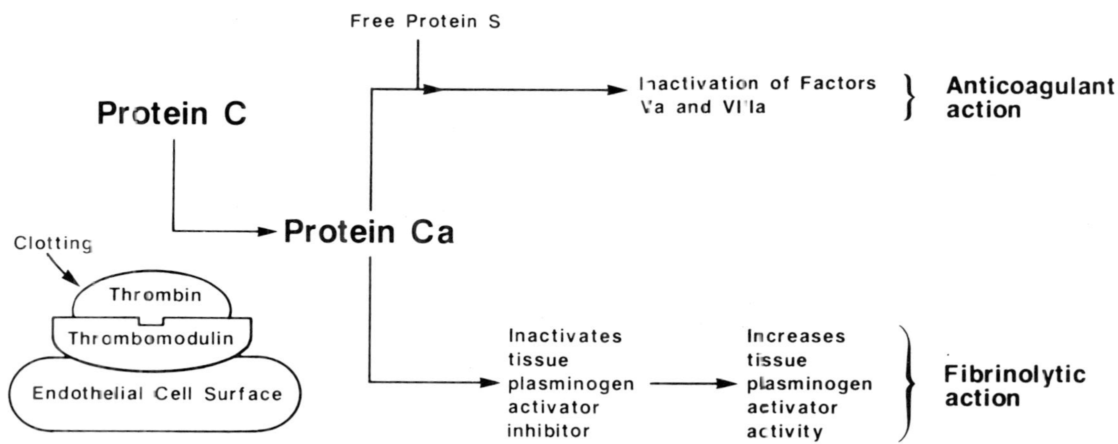

Figure 6.11 Thrombin–thrombomodulin model of the anticoagulant and fibrinolytic action of protein C. From Clouse and Comp, 1986. The regulation of hemostasis: the protein C system. Reprinted by permission of *The New England Journal of Medicine*, 314(20): 1298–1304.

Protein C in inherited as an autosomal dominant trait. The anticoagulant can be measured by both immunological and functional assays. This identifies two distinct patterns. In the commonest type both protein C antigen and protein C functional activity are reduced. Rare cases of a non-functional protein have been reported, characterized by a normal protein C antigen but reduced protein C activity. A 50% reduction of protein C appears to be sufficient to predispose the adult to venous thrombosis, although symptoms do not occur until young adulthood or later.

A small number of neonates have been reported with homozygosity for protein C deficiency, characterized by virtual absence of the anticoagulant (Estellés *et al.*, 1984; Seligsohn *et al.*, 1984; Marciniak *et al.*, 1985). These infants have presented with fulminant thrombosis and purpura fulminans. Untreated homozygous protein C deficiency is probably incompatible with life. Seligsohn *et al.* (1984) reported a family in which two infants had died of massive venous thrombosis shortly after birth. Protein C antigen was undetectable by immunologic assays of plasma available from one infant. The parents were first cousins and had plasma protein C levels on electroimmunoassay of 47 and 60%, respectively, and on radioimmunoassay of 44 and 40%, respectively (Seligsohn *et al.*, 1984). Marciniak *et al.* (1985) have reported two unrelated infants who presented in the neonatal period with purpura fulminans. The first had computer tomography scan evidence of superior sagittal sinus and cortical vein thrombosis and died at 32 days of age. Protein C antigen was undetectable in the infant's plasma. Both parents were defined as heterozygotes; the maternal protein C level was 47% and the paternal 37%. The second infant died at 25 days of age with evidence of widespread thrombosis at autopsy. Protein C was not measured in this infant, but again the parents were shown to be heterozygotes: the maternal protein C level was 50% and the paternal 36% (Marciniak *et al.*, 1985). Branson *et al.* reported the combination of purpura fulminans and disseminated intravascular coagulation presenting at 11 hours of age in a heterozygote for protein C deficiency (Branson *et al.*, 1983). The infant had repeated thrombotic and haemorrhagic episodes. He was latterly treated with coumarin and died 3 months later of a fatal subarachnoid and intracerebral haemorrhage. His protein C level on coumarin was less than 6%. The mother and siblings had protein C levels in the heterozygote range and the father was unaffected. The very low value found in this infant can best be explained by a combination of heterozygous protein C deficiency, coumarin therapy and DIC.

A small number of cases have now been reported where diagnosis was suspected early and treatment instigated. Anticoagulation with heparin alone has not been helpful. Initial treatment should always be with FFP (10 ml kg^{-1}, twice daily). However, the half-life of protein C is about 7 h and treatment has to be given at such regular intervals to maintain adequate levels that this is not a practical long-term solution. Hopefully, protein C concentrates or recombinant protein C will become available in the near future and make it possible for those individuals to receive specific therapy. At present, two therapeutic approaches are available for long-term management.

Firstly, the successful use of factor IX concentrate as a vehicle for administering protein C has been reported (Sills *et al.*, 1984). It appears that every-other-day infusions of 50–75 U kg^{-1} of protein C are sufficient to stop thrombotic episodes, although levels approach zero by the end of 48 h. The factor IX concentrate should be selected with care to minimize its thrombotic risk, and levels of protein C, and factors II, IX and X monitored carefully to prevent excessive rises (Montgomery *et al.*, 1985). Heat-treated concentrates should be used and the risk of transmission of hepatitis not underestimated.

Alternatively, warfarin has also been used with some success and is now recommended by the International Committee on Thrombosis and Haemastasis (see below): it is suggested that affected neonates are initially treated with infusions of fresh frozen plasma (10 ml kg^{-1} every 12 hours) until the infant is 2–3 months old, all symptoms have resolved and the other vitamin K-dependent factors have approached adult levels. Warfarin is then started at a daily dose of 0.15–0.40 mg kg^{-1} until a minimum maintenance dose is established to keep the child symptom-free. The prothrombin time will range from 1.0–1.5 to 2.5 times the control value and the International Normalized Ratio (INR) will be between 2.5 and 4.4. FFP should be administered for the first 5–7 days of oral anticoagulant therapy as protection against recurring purpuric lesions. It should be reinstituted if purpura fulminans recurs on oral anticoagulation (Marlar, *et al.*, 1989; report on the Working Party on Homozygous Protein C Deficiency of the Subcommittee on Protein C and Protein S, International Committee on Thrombosis and Haemostasis). The dose of oral anticoagulant and the monitoring range should be individualized on the basis of a number of factors: (1) minimum dose to remain symptom-free, (2) age, (3) weight, (4) drugs the infant may be receiving. It is difficult to achieve a stable therapeutic dose in neonates, and this therapy does nothing to raise the level of protein C or to correct the imbalance between protein C and its procoagulants. Bone growth and development (followed by densitometry) should be monitored every 6–12 months, because the long-term effects of vitamin K antagonist use in childhood are not fully understood.

Protein S deficiency

Protein S is a cofactor for protein C, and is also a vitamin K-dependent plasma protein. Protein S and activated protein C form a lipid-bound complex that inactivates factor Va more rapidly than does activated protein C alone. Adults deficient in protein S are predisposed to recurrent venous thrombotic disease. There have as yet been no cases reported of thrombosis in the neonatal period associated with protein S deficiency.

Antithrombin III deficiency

Homozygous ATIII deficiency is probably incompatible with life. Half of the infants born to heterozygous ATIII-deficient mothers will be ATIII-deficient themselves. This, combined with the gestational-dependent reduction in ATIII levels, may predispose the neonate to thrombosis. A small number of infants born to mothers with congenital ATIII deficiency have died in the newborn period with thrombotic complications (Bjarke *et al.*, 1974). Because of this, infants born to mothers with ATIII deficiency should have their level measured at birth. An ATIII-deficient infant would be expected to have a cord-blood ATIII level of 20–30%. It has been recommended that affected infants should receive prophylactic ATIII concentrate or FFP to maintain values appropriate for the newborn (60%) until the infant's own level has risen to around 50% at 3 months of age (Hambley *et al.*, 1983). However, these infants have a relatively small risk of thrombosis and such an aggressive therapeutic approach may produce greater morbidity from transfusion-related viral infections despite the availability of heat-treated ATIII concentrates. On balance, a more conservative approach seems appropriate, although the neonate's ATIII level may be useful in finally determining the need for prophylaxis.

Pregnancy in women with congenital ATIII deficiency is associated with an extremely high risk of thrombosis, in the order of 70%. About 75% of thrombotic events will occur in early pregnancy and the remainder in the puerperium. These women require full therapeutic heparinization throughout pregnancy. Warfarin should be discontinued and heparin introduced before conception because of the teratogenicity attributed to warfarin therapy. Sodium heparin should be started subcutaneously at a dose of 12 500 units every 12 hours, and adjusted to prolong the APTT by at least 10 s. At delivery, heparin is discontinued or reduced to 5000 units twice daily s.c. and ATIII concentrate given at a dose of 50–70 units kg^{-1} initially, followed by daily infusions of 20–30 units kg^{-1} to maintain plasma ATIII levels at 80% of normal (Winter *et al.*, 1982). Warfarin therapy is re-established at 7–10 days post-delivery. The use of subcutaneous heparin at such high doses throughout pregnancy is not without some risk, particularly of osteoporosis and heparin-induced thrombocytopenia.

Treatment of thrombosis in the neonate

Thrombosis, when suspected, can be confirmed by appropriate investigation. If a catheter is *in situ* it should be removed, but first it may provide a route for radiological confirmation. Anticoagulant therapy, thrombolytic drugs and surgery have all been employed therapeutically.

Heparin

Heparin is a prophylactic drug and is used in the primary prevention of thrombosis and thrombus extension. It is the drug of choice in mild to moderate vessel occlusion, but surgery or thrombolytic agents should be used when there is arterial impairment of blood flow. The neonate may require a greater amount of heparin than an adult in order to achieve a therapeutic effect because of the low level of ATIII in the newborn. The initial loading dose required is 50 U kg^{-1}. Continuous infusion is the optimal route of administration, beginning with a dose of 20 U kg^{-1} h^{-1} for small pre-term infants and 25 U kg^{-1} h^{-1} for infants weighing more than

1500 g (McDonald and Hathaway, 1982). The partial thromboplastin micro time (PTT) is already prolonged in the neonatal period, particularly in the premature infant, and therefore is not as helpful in the monitoring of heparin therapy. McDonald and Hathaway (1982) recommend the use of the Laidlaw micro whole blood clotting time. A modified PTT incorporating contact product has been suggested as an alternative approach (Andrew and Karpatkin, 1982). Low levels of the contact factors are largely responsible for the prolongation of the PTT. Contact product contains factor XIa and, when substituted in the PTT for kaolin, bypasses the contact factors and shortens the newborn PTT to within 3–9 s of the control. More simply, modified APTT reagents have replaced the need for such an approach by narrowing the normal range and increasing the usefulness of the APTT as a test (Andrew *et al*, 1988).

Urokinase

Urokinase may have a role to play in the treatment of major thromboses which are not amenable to surgery. Urokinase is a plasminogen activator that does not need to form a complex with plasminogen to exert its effect. It is preferable to streptokinase for use in the newborn as it has a linear dose–effect curve (Montgomery *et al.*, 1985). Because it will lyse all clots, not just those causing vascular occlusion, it cannot be used within 10 days of surgery or if the infant has a pre-existing bleeding problem. A loading dose of 4400 U kg^{-1} is given intravenously followed by a continuous infusion of 4400 U kg^{-1} h^{-1} (Montgomery *et al.*, 1985). This will produce a fall in fibrinogen and significant levels of fibrin degradation products. Successful results are more often achieved with young, small clots, where blood flow in the affected vessels is reasonable and the plasminogen content high. Thrombolytic agents are not given without risk and require careful monitoring. Suggested assays for monitoring include the fibrinogen level, fibrinogen degradation products and euglobulin lysis time.

Warfarin

Oral anticoagulants have little place in the treatment of neonatal thrombotic disease, perhaps with the exception of homozygous protein C deficiency. The thrombotic episodes for which warfarin is most frequently prescribed in adults do not occur in neonates. In adults, coumarins are not indicated in the immediate treatment of an acute thrombotic episode, but later in treatment to prevent recurrence. There is no evidence that thrombotic episodes in the neonatal period have a high risk of recurrence. Dosage recommendations are given above.

Surgery

Surgical intervention is indicated for the management of major arterial thrombosis when occlusion is total. In the adult, surgery is usually the chosen mode of treatment of occlusive vascular disease. This is because the clot has generally formed on an atheromatous section of vessel wall and has a high chance of recurrence without endarterectomy. This situation is not seen in the neonatal period, and the small calibre of the neonate's vessels reduces the chance of success by surgery. The role of surgery is therefore limited in this age group, and so thrombolytic agents may have a greater role to play than in the adult.

MISCELLANEOUS HAEMORRHAGIC DISORDERS

A number of haemorrhagic problems are peculiar to the neonate because of its physiological immaturity.

Haemorrhagic disease of the newborn

Several investigators have played important roles in the understanding of the aetiology of this disorder. In 1894 Townsend first used the term 'haemorrhagic disease of the newborn' (HDN) when he reported a series of infants who presented with self-limiting bleeding, usually from the gastrointestinal tract, on the second or third day of life. Vitamin K was discovered in 1929 by Dam. In 1939, vitamin K was shown to shorten the prolonged prothrombin time seen in the neonatal period and its role in the prevention and cure of HDN reported (Nygaard, 1939; Wadell and Guerry, 1939). In 1961 the Committee on Nutrition of the American Academy of Pediatrics recommended that prophylactic vitamin K be administered parenterally to all newborn infants at a dose of 0.5–1.0 mg.

Haemorrhagic disease of the newborn results from a deficiency of the procoagulant factors II, VII, IX and X. Vitamin K is required for the post-translational carboxylation of glutamic acid residues on the vitamin K-dependent coagulation factors. The conversion of glutamic acid to γ-carboxyglutamic acid is essential for formation of effective calcium-binding sites which are necessary for activation of the clotting factors. In the non-carboxylated state these proteins are unable to bind calcium and are functionally defective. Vitamin K-dependent carboxylation is shown in Figure 6.12 and takes place in the rough endoplasmic reticulum of the hepatocyte. Immaturity of the biosynthetic hepatic enzyme system is responsible for the reduction of the vitamin K-dependent coagulation factors at birth. However, a further fall is commonly observed in the first 3 days of life, which can be prevented by the prophylactic administration of vitamin K at birth and is therefore at least in part due to deficiency of this vitamin (Lane and Hathaway, 1985).

When faced with the clinical problem of a bleeding neonate, it is

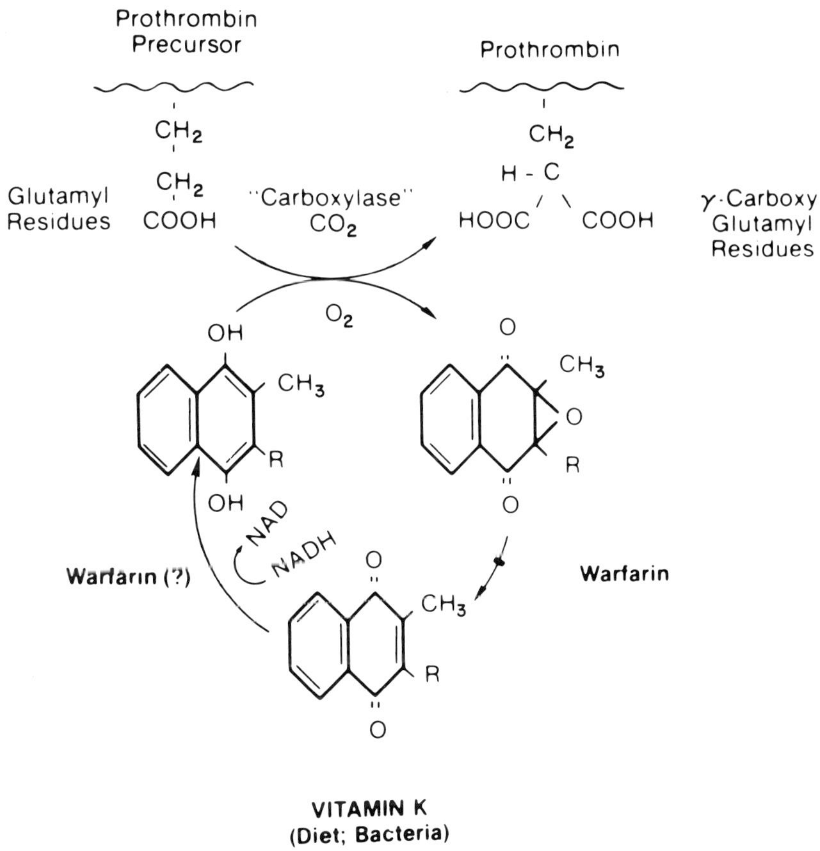

Figure 6.12 Vitamin K cycle and the carboxylation reaction. From Corrigan, 1985, *Hemorrhagic and Thrombotic Diseases in Childhood and Adolescence* 11, with permission of Churchill Livingstone.

necessary to differentiate between vitamin K deficiency and an acquired or congenital coagulation problem. It can be particularly difficult to differentiate vitamin K deficiency from hepatic dysfunction. A range of laboratory tests are available to help clarify the situation. A common presentation is that of generalized haemorrhage in an otherwise healthy term infant with a normal platelet count and fibrinogen level, but a prolonged PT and APTT.

Screening tests for vitamin K deficiency

The prothrombin time (PT), activated partial thromboplastin time (APTT) and thrombotest are prolonged in vitamin K deficiency. A shortening of these coagulation parameters following vitamin K administration is usually interpreted as indicating a previous vitamin deficiency.

Functional factor assays (II, VII, IX, X)

These will be depressed physiologically in the newborn and in vitamin K deficiency. Levels are usually lower in the latter when gestational age is balanced but, as the normal range is wide, overlap occurs. A rise in factor levels following the administration of vitamin K suggests a previous deficiency.

Immunological assays for vitamin K deficiency

In the absence of vitamin K a non-carboxylated, functionally abnormal but immunologically intact clotting protein is formed. This fact has been exploited in several assay systems described below to demonstrate the presence of vitamin K deficiency. However, the report by Blanchard *et al.* of small amounts of abnormal prothrombin in the plasma of patients with acquired liver disease has challenged the specificity of such assays (Blanchard *et al.*, 1981).

Prothrombin coagulant/antigen ratio. Prothrombin is measured by both a functional and immunological assay. Factor II antigen levels in plasma should be normal and a low coagulant/antigen ratio suggests vitamin K deficiency.

PIVKA-II (protein induced in vitamin K's absence: prothrombin). Normal carboxylated prothrombin is absorbed from plasma using barium carbonate. Any non-carboxylated prothrombin formed in the absence of vitamin K is left behind and is assayed immunologically.

Crossed electrophoresis. Abnormal, non-carboxylated prothrombin will migrate further than carboxylated prothrombin in the first dimension in a medium containing calcium, because of decreased calcium binding. If prothrombin antibody is added, the prothrombins will precipitate in the second dimension and a double peak indicates the presence of two species of prothrombin with different calcium binding; one carboxylated and one non-carboxylated.

Echis assay

This assay utilizes the fact that both carboxylated and noncarboxylated prothrombin can be activated to form thrombin by non-physiological activators, in this case venom from the snake *Echis carinatus*. As in immunological assays, the Echis assay measures total prothrombin, both caryboxylated and non-carboxylated. A high level, in the presence of a low level of prothrombin, measured by a functional clotting assay, suggests vitamin K deficiency.

Sources of vitamin K

The prevalence of vitamin K deficiency (measured as non-carboxy prothrombin = PIVAK-II) at birth is not agreed. Whilst some investigators have found no PIVKA-II in cord plasma, others have reported levels in healthy term infants of as high as 50%. Part, but not all, of the discrepancy may be explained by differences in the assay methods and in the infants studied. After birth the diet provides vitamin K_1. Vitamin K_1 is absorbed in the small intestine and requires the presence of bile acids. Breast milk is particularly deficient in vitamin K_1, with levels as low as 2 compared with 5 $\mu g\ l^{-1}$ for cow's milk and values greater than 50 $\mu g\ l^{-1}$ for many commercial formulae (Haroon *et al.*, 1982). In addition to vitamin K_1 provided by the diet, vitamin K_2 or fat-soluble menaquinone is produced endogenously by the intestinal flora. Antibiotic therapy inhibits absorption of vitamin K_1 from dietary sources and can lead to deficiency, especially in breast-fed infants.

Syndromes associated with vitamin K deficiency

Haemorrhagic disease of the newborn has three recognized patterns depending on the time of presentation; early HDN (within the first 24 hours of life), classic HDN (at 2–5 days of age) and late HDN (after the first postnatal month).

Haemorrhagic disease of the newborn presenting within the first 24 h of life may be associated with severe and sometimes fatal haemorrhage. Symptoms vary from bruising to internal bleeding. Intracranial, intrathoracic, intra-abdominal and gastrointestinal haemorrhages are all seen. Early haemorrhagic disease is typical of infants whose mothers have been prescribed drugs that affect vitamin K metabolism. Anticonvulsant drugs taken by epileptic mothers can cross the placenta and increase the catabolism of vitamin K by induction of the fetal hepatic enzyme system. The risk of HDN in infants of mothers on anticonvulsants remains undefined. In one survey of 111 such pregnancies, 20 infants had significantly prolonged prothrombin times and eight infants were symptomatic. Three of these haemorrhagic babies died and one developed neurological sequelae (Deblay *et al.*, 1982). The authors recommended that mothers taking anticonvulsant therapy should receive vitamin K prenatally. However, this opinion has been challenged recently by a study of the infants of 23 mothers on chronic anticonvulsant therapy, which showed that 1 mg of vitamin K given intramuscularly immediately after delivery was protective in 22 of the 23 infants (Hulac *et al.*, 1986). The antituberculous drugs rifampicin and isoniazid have also been reported to be associated with early HDN. Warfarin is the classic drug that can cross the placenta and result in serious bleeding problems and, although it is rarely prescribed to pregnant women because of its teratogenicity, it is still indicated for anticoagulation in mothers with artificial heart valves. It is not excreted in breast milk in significant amounts.

Classic HDN presents at 2–5 days of age and is generally manifest by bruising or bleeding from the gastrointestinal tract or following circumcision. Intracranial haemorrhage is less common. Classic HDN can be prevented by the administration of vitamin K_1 at birth.

Although one commonly associates vitamin K deficiency with the immediate newborn period, presentation may be delayed until after the first month of life. Typically this happens when an infant (usually breast-fed) has not received vitamin K prophylaxis or when an infant has an underlying condition predisposing to impaired vitamin K absorption. The former generally presents at between 1 and 3 months of age, whereas the latter may present at any time during the first year of life. Intracranial haemorrhage is the commonest problem and, if not fatal, may result in severe neurological damage. Vitamin K deficiency can develop in infants with chronic diarrhoea, malabsorption or oral antibiotic therapy, and HDN has been the initial manifestation of cystic fibrosis, biliary atresia, α_1-antitrypsin deficiency and abeta-lipoproteinaemia. An underlying cause should be sought in all cases of late onset HDN.

Prevention

Argument still continues as to whether all infants should receive vitamin K prophylaxis and, if so, whether this should be given parenterally or orally. Using specific assays for non-carboxylated vitamin K, some investigators have found evidence of vitamin K deficiency at birth and others have not. The true incidence has not been universally accepted. Shapiro *et al.* (1986) reported the prevalance of vitamin K deficiency in a prospective study of 934 infants. Of 934 cord blood samples assayed, 2.9% were positive for PIVKA-II indicating vitamin K deficiency. All infants received prophylactic vitamin K_1. No infant with PIVKA-II in the cord sample subsequently had clinical bleeding. Sixty-three per cent of infants with neonatal vitamin K deficiency were otherwise normal newborns.

It has been suggested that only infants at high risk of developing vitamin K deficiency, i.e. breast-fed babies or recipients of antibiotics, etc., need receive prophylaxis. However, vitamin K is a safe drug and virtually no infant in receipt of it develops classic haemorrhagic disease of the newborn. McNinch *et al.* (1983) reported a local recurrence of haemorrhagic disease of the newborn in an area in which prophylactic vitamin K was not routinely given. In a 17-month period he encountered six cases of HDN, i.e. 1:1200 live births. All infants were breast-fed and had not received vitamin K at birth; three of the six infants died. Although one infant was born to an epileptic mother receiving phenytoin, bleeding did not occur until day 10 of life and, as with the other infants, would undoubtedly have been prevented by prophylactic vitamin K_1. This experience has prompted McNinch *et al.* to reintroduce the administration of vitamin K_1 to all neonates in their hospital. Their example should be followed, as their experience highlights the risk of not adhering to a policy of vitamin K prophylaxis for all newborns, especially in a society where breast-feeding is increasingly popular.

Concern about administering vitamin K_1 orally relates to doubts about optimal absorption and possible regurgitation. There is little available information on the intestinal absorption of vitamin K_1 in neonates. In adults, 70–80% of an orally administered dose is absorbed. Plasma concentrations reach a peak at 2–4 hours and fall to 10–20% of the peak value by 24 hours. McNinch *et al.* (1985) compared the oral and parenteral administration of 1 mg vitamin K_1. The neonates who received oral vitamin K_1 achieved peak median plasma concentrations of 73 ng ml^{-1} at 4 hours compared to 1781 ng ml^{-1} at 12 hours for parenteral administration. Although the concentration following oral administration is considerably lower than with parenteral administration, it is still some 300 times the adult medium value and represents approximately 8.5 μg of vitamin K_1 in the plasma. No infant in the study developed haemorrhagic disease of the newborn although in two infants no vitamin K was detected. Oral administration appears an attractive alternative to parenteral administration, but further work is required to determine the percentage absorbed from an oral dose and, consequently, the optimal dosage. The study by McNinch *et al.* suggests an average absorption of 24%, but the range was wide. It is clear that vitamin K prophylaxis should be given to all newborns. An important question to address is whether infants who are exclusively breast-fed should receive further vitamin K supplementation after the immediate newborn period. A number of breast-fed infants have been reported who developed late haemorrhagic disease of the newborn despite receiving vitamin K at birth, although this appears to be a rare finding. Breast fed infants who develop diarrhoea and infants who receive antibiotic therapy are at particular risk of vitamin K deficiency. The American Academy of Paediatrics (Barness, 1979) state:

> Breast-fed infants who develop diarrhoea of longer than several days duration should be given one intramuscular injection of vitamin K (1.0 mg). Infants at continued risk of vitamin K deficiency (e.g. malabsorption, biliary atresia) should be given supplements of vitamin K at regular intervals.

Treatment

The bleeding manifestations of vitamin K deficiency can be both prevented and treated by the administration of parenteral vitamin K

(1) In the face of life-threatening haemorrhage, vitamin K-dependent factors can be immediately raised by giving FFP 10–15 ml kg^{-1}. Otherwise, 1 mg of vitamin K_1 will correct any degree of vitamin K deficiency in the neonate. After parenteral administration, correction will occur within a few hours. Vitamin K_1 is a safe drug without side effects. Only vitamin K_3 (Synkavit) given parenterally has been associated with haemolytic anaemia and kernicterus.

(2) All neonates should receive vitamin K prophylaxis as soon after birth as possible. Oral vitamin K appears to prevent classic HDN, but its efficacy in the prevention of late HDN is less well-established. In contrast, late HDN is extremely rare in infants who have received parenteral vitamin K at birth. At present, the best proven prophylaxis is vitamin K, 1 mg parenterally, although this may change with increasing knowledge of optimal oral therapy. The parenteral route should always be used for prophylaxis for the following categories of infants:

(i) infants of mothers on anticonvulsant therapy,
(ii) premature infants,
(iii) infants admitted to a special care baby unit,
(iv) babies born by traumatic delivery.

The optimal oral dose of vitamin K has not been clearly established. Dosages recommended range from 1 mg of vitamin K (Tripp and McNinch, 1987) to 5 mg (Hathaway and Bonnar, 1987).

(3) The guidelines of the American Academy of Paediatrics should be followed (Barness, 1979) for breast-fed infants who develop prolonged diarrhoea and for infants at continued risk because of underlying pathology. In the latter group, the interval of optimal supplementation will depend on the route of administration chosen.

Neonatal intraventricular haemorrhage

Intraventricular haemorrhage (IVH) is common in premature infants of low birth weight and, despite the recent improvement in their survival, it remains a major cause of morbidity and mortality. The incidence has been variably reported to be between 30 and 40% (Volpe, 1981; Tarby and Volpe, 1982; Beverley *et al.*, 1984; McDonald *et al.*, 1984). Several predisposing factors are well established, others are unproven.

Intracranial haemorrhage is the commonest manifestation of the coagulopathy associated with late-onset vitamin K deficiency. These infants are almost invariably breast-fed and will not have received vitamin K prophylaxis. Chaou *et al.* (1984) reported late-onset intracranial haemorrhage related to vitamin K deficiency in 32 breast-fed infants, 31 of whom had not received prophylactic vitamin K at birth. The one infant who had been given prophylaxis had Hirschsprung's disease and presented with intracranial haemorrhage at 5 months of age. In each case the intracranial haemorrhage was proven by computer tomography scanning. Most infants had subarachnoid haemorrhage (90.6%), either alone or in combination with subdural haemorrhage (37.5%), parenchymal haemorrhage (31.3%), or intraventricular haemorrhage (12.5%). In three infants (9.4%) the infratentorial region was involved. The mortality in the series was 9.4%. This form of late haemorrhagic disease of the newborn characteristically occurs at 1–2 months of age.

Lesko *et al.* (1986) noted an association between germinal matrix intraventricular haemorrhage and the use of low-dose heparin to maintain the patency of vascular catheters in low birth-weight infants. The association did not extend to the severity of the haemorrhage, dose of heparin or method of administration. The authors reported a four-fold increase in the risk of germinal matrix intraventricular haemorrhage in infants receiving heparin, but conceded that other factors may have contributed, and recommended a controlled trial to evaluate the true risk. Other investigators have similarly reported an association between intraventricular haemorrhage and the use of low-dose heparin to prolong catheter patency. It must be appreciated that it is the low birth-weight infant at the highest risk of intraventricular haemorrhage who is most likely to require an indwelling catheter for venous access and monitoring.

Intraventricular haemorrhage predominantly affects premature infants of low birth weight. Attempts have been made to evaluate the aetiological role of abnormal haemostasis by correcting coagulation parameters in the hope of preventing intraventricular haemorrhage. Beverley *et al.* (1985) reported on 73 premature infants of less than 32 weeks' gestation, or less than 1500 g, recruited to a prospective controlled trial. The newborns were randomized to receive FFP (10 ml kg^{-1}) on admission and at 24 h of age, or to act as controls and receive no treatment. All infants were given vitamin K_1 prophylaxis at birth. There was no difference in coagulation parameters [PT, APTT, fibrinogen, fibrin degradation products (FDPs), platelet count] on admission, and at 48 h of age, between the treatment and control groups. The diagnosis of IVH was made by ultrasound. Fifteen of 37 (41%) control infants sustained an IVH compared with five of 36 (14%) infants who received FFP. It appeared that FFP reduced the incidence of IVH but there was no noticeable effect on mortality and no association with a lasting improvement in the coagulation parameters. Although there was a consistent trend for more abnormal coagulation in the infants who developed IVH, the trend was not significant. The association between unstable blood pressure leading to variable cerebral blood flow and IVH is well recognized.

Beverley *et al.* questioned whether fresh frozen plasma may exert its effect by stabilizing the blood pressure rather than by improving coagulation. However, in this study, the number of babies with an unstable intra-arterial blood pressure tracing was the same in both groups. Turner *et al.* (1981) made similar observations. They looked at the effect of correcting coagulation parameters on the incidence of IVH in infants of less than 1500 g and 34 weeks gestation, premature infants with respiratory distress syndrome, and mature infants with asphyxia. Replacement therapy was given to completely correct any coagulation abnormality and maintain correction. Those allocated to the treatment group received prothrombin complex concentrate, cryoprecipitate or platelet concentrate as appropriate. Prothrombin complex concentrate was given to infants with a prolonged PT (PT $>$ 28 s), cryoprecipitate to infants with a low fibrinogen (fibrinogen < 1 g l^{-1}) and platelet concentrate to infants with a low platelet count (platelets $< 100 \times 10^9$ per litre). All infants received vitamin K_1. They did not observe IVH in infants who maintained normal haemostasis (i.e. did not have abnormal coagulation parameters by the investigators criteria). Replacement therapy did reduce the incidence of IVH to some extent, but this was not statistically signficant and did not result in any change in mortality or morbidity.

Vitamin E supplementation, which protects endothelial cell membranes from oxidative damage, has been reported to have a protective effect against IVH (Spear *et al.*, 1984; Sinha *et al.*, 1987). Other studies have shown conflicting results (Phelps, 1984). Sinha reported on infants of less than 32 weeks' gestation enrolled into a randomized, controlled trial to assess the efficacy of vitamin E in the prevention of periventricular haemorrhage. Two hundred and ten supplemented babies without haemorrhage on entry to the trial had a lower frequency of IVH than controls (8.8% versus 34.3%) and a lower frequency of combined intraventricular and parenchymal haemorrhage (10.8% versus 40.7%), determined ultrasonically. Vitamin E did not affect mortality, but surviving supplemented babies had a lower frequency of intraventricular or periventricular haemorrhage and, hopefully, reduced neurodevelopmental handicap. Haemorrhage originates in the subepenchymal region, where it may be confined or rupture into the ventricles or brain parenchyma. Vitamin E did not prevent subepenchymal haemorrhage but appeared to limit its extent. The authors suggested that vitamin E works by scavenging free radicals generated during ischaemic injury of the subepenchymal region and thereby limits tissue damage and the extent of periventricular haemorrhage on reperfusion. Similar results have been reported for ethamsylate (Benson *et al.*, 1986).

In 330 infants without evidence of periventricular haemorrhage on entry into the trial, there was little difference between ethamsylate and placebo groups with respect to subepenchymal haemorrhage, but intraventricular and parenchymal haemorrhages developed in 30 out of 162 infants (18.5%) in the treated group, compared with 50 out of 168 (29.8%) in the control group. The incidence of intraventricular and parenchymal haemorrhage in survivors was 20 out of 137 (14.6%) in the ethamsylate group and 37 out of 146 (25.3%) in the controls. Ethamsylate treatment appeared to limit parenchymal extension but had no effect on mortality. Ethamsylate reduces capillary bleeding probably by modifying prostaglandin synthesis, though its exact mode of action is unclear. The end-result may not be too dissimilar from the antioxidant action of vitamin E, which reduces the perodixation of lipids that are precursors of the prostanoids. The precise role of the neonate's hypocoagulable state in the pathogenesis of IVH has not been properly defined and, although coagulation factor replacement appears to reduce the incidence, the means by which this is achieved is unclear, as a measurable improvement in coagulation parameters has not been a consistent finding. However, replacement therapy may act by preventing haemorrhagic extension of an initial ischaemic lesion, a role not dissimilar from that of vitamin E or ethamsylate. It is therefore appropriate to correct any coagulation abnormalities that are defined as soon as possible. Further controlled studies are required to assess the different therapies available.

Disseminated intravascular coagulation

Sepsis, acidosis, hypoxia and shock are potent provokers of disseminated intravascular coagulation and are common in neonates. Factors V and VIII:C are regulating steps in the coagulation system and in the neonate are not balanced by their natural inhibitor, protein C. This relative inhibitor deficiency predisposes the neonate to a hypercoagulable condition. Although it seems sensible to replace consumed factors, the most important measure in the treatment of DIC is correction of the underlying cause. Gross *et al.* (1982) reported on 33 neonates with DIC and noted no benefit from specific therapy aimed at correction of the coagulation abnormalities, but did note that survival was related to successful treatment of the underlying cause. Consumed procoagulants and anticoagulants can be replaced by a combination of FFP, cryoprecipitate and platelets. However, adequate replacement is often restricted by volume, and in this situation exchange transfusion provides the best means of giving platelets, procoagulants and the physiological inhibitors, antithrombin III and protein C. These may be as important as clotting factors in correcting the coagulation abnormality. The newborn is at the added disadvantage of being unable to compensate for factor consumption because of its immature liver.

CONCLUSION

Neonates are at particular risk of both thrombotic and haemorrhagic problems. The difficulty in obtaining adequate volumes of blood for investigation often means that 'blunderbuss' therapy is given. The development and refinement of micro-methods and a better understanding of the careful interpretation of results should aid the investigation of these infants and allow more appropriate replacement.

REFERENCES

Andrew M and Karpatkin M (1982) A simple screening test for evaluating prolonged partial thromboplastin times in newborn infants. *Journal of Pediatrics* **101**: 610–612.

Andrew M, Castle V, Saigal S *et al.* (1987a). Clinical impact of neonatal thrombocytopenia. *Journal of Pediatrics* **110**: 457–464.

Andrew M, Paes B, Milner R *et al.* (1987b). Development of the human coagulation system in the full-term infant. *Blood* **70**: 165–172.

Andrew M, Paes B, Milner R *et al.* (1988) Development of the human coagulation system in the healthy premature infant. *Blood* **72**: 1651–1657.

Arneil GC, MacDonald AM, Murphy AV *et al.* (1973) Renal venous thrombosis. *Clincal Nephrology* **1**: 119–131.

Baehner RL and Strauss HS (1966) Haemophilia in the first year of life. *New England Journal of Medicine* **275**: 524–528.

Ballin A, Koren G, Kohelet D *et al.* (1987) Reduction of platelet counts induced by mechanical ventilation in newborn infants. *Journal of Pediatrics* **111**: 445–449.

Barnard DR (1984) Inherited bleeding disorders in the newborn infant. *Clinics in Perinatology* **11**: 309–337.

Barnard DR, Simmons MA and Hathaway WE (1979) Coagulation studies in extremely premature infants. *Pediatrics* **13**: 1330–1335.

Barness LA (1979) Vitamins. In *Pediatric Nutrition Handbook*. Evanston, Ill: American Academy of Pediatrics.

Benson JW, Drayton MR, Hayward C *et al.* (1986) Multicentre trial of ethamsylate for prevention of periventricular haemorrhage in very low birthweight infants. *The Lancet* **2**: 1297–1300.

Bergqvist G and Zetterström R (1975) Submaximal blood flow and blood viscosity in newborn infants. *Acta Paediatrica Scandinavia* **64**: 254–256.

Beverley DW, Chance GW and Coates CF (1984) Intraventricular haemorrhage — timing of occurrence and relationship to perinatal events: *British Journal of Obstetrics and Gynaecology* **91**: 1007–1013.

Beverley DW, Pitts-Tucker TJ, Congdon PJ *et al.* (1985) Prevention of intraventricular haemorrhage by fresh frozen plasma. *Archives of Disease in Childhood* **60**: 710–713.

Bjarke B, Herin P, Blomback M (1974) Neonatal aortic thrombosis: A possible clinical manifestation of congenital antithrombin III deficiency. *Acta Paediatrica Scandinavica* **63**: 297–301.

Blanchard RA, Furie BC, Jorgenson M *et al.* (1981) Acquired vitamin K-dependent carboxylation deficiency in liver disease. *New England Journal of Medicine* **305**: 242–248.

Bleyer WA, Hakami N and Shepard TH (1971) The development of haemostasis in the human fetus and newborn infant. *Journal of Pediatrics* **79**: 838–853.

Branson HE, Katz J, Marble R and Griffin JH (1983) Inherited protein C deficiency and coumarin-responsive chronic relapsing purpura fulminans in a newborn infant. *The Lancet* **2**: 1165–1168.

Bussel JB, Berkowitz RL, McFarland JG *et al.* (1988) Antenatal treatment of neonatal alloimmune thrombocytopenia. *New England Journal of Medicine* **319**: 1374–1378.

Castle V, Andrew M, Kelton J *et al.* (1986) Frequency and mechanism of neonatal thrombocytopenia. *Journal of Pediatrics* **108**: 749–755.

Chaou WT, Chou ML and Eitzman DV (1984) Intracranial hemorrhage and vitamin K deficiency in early infancy. *Journal of Pediatrics* **105**: 880–884.

Cines DB, Dusak B, Tomaski A *et al.* (1982) Immune thrombocytopenic purpura and pregnancy. *New England Journal of Medicine* **306**: 826–831.

Clouse LH and Comp PC (1986) The regulation of hemostasis: the protein C system. *New England Journal of Medicine* **314**: 1298–1304.

Committee on Nutrition, American Academy of Pediatrics (1961) Vitamin K compounds and the water soluble analogues: use in therapy and prophylaxis in pediatrics. *Pediatrics* **28**: 501–507.

Corrigan JJ (1985) *Hemorrhagic and Thrombotic Diseases in Childhood and Adolescence,* p 11. Churchill Livingstone Inc.

Corrigan JJ (1989) Neonatal coagulation disorders. *Perinatal Hematology* **21**: 167.

Daffos F, Forestier F and Kaplan C (1988) Prenatal treatment of fetal alloimmune thrombocytopenia. *The Lancet* **2**: 910.

Dam H (1929) Cholesterinstoffwechsel in Hühnereiern und Hühnchen. *Biochem. Zeitschr.* **215**: 475.

Deblay MF, Vert P, Andre M and Marchal F (1982) Transplacental vitamin K prevents haemorrhagic disease of infant of epileptic mother (letter). *The Lancet* **1**: 1247.

Donnér M, Holmberg L and Nilsson IM (1987) Type IIB von Willebrand's disease with probable autosomal recessive inheritance and presenting as thrombocytopenia in infancy. *British Journal of Haematology* **66**: 349–354.

Ekelund H, Hedner U and Nilsson IM (1970) Fibrinolysis in newborns. *Acta Paediatrica Scandinavica* **59**: 33–43.

Emery JL (1962) Pulmonary embolism in children. *Archives of Disease in Childhood* **37**: 591–595.

Estellés A, Garcia-Plaza I, Dasi A *et al.* (1984) Severe inherited 'homozygous' protein C deficiency in a newborn infant. *Thrombosis and Haemostasis* **52**: 53–56.

Feusner JH (1980) Normal and abnormal bleeding times in neonates and young children utilizing a fully standardized template technic. *American Journal of Clinical Pathology* **74**: 73–77.

Forestier F, Daffos F, Galacteros F *et al.* (1986) Hematological values of 163 normal fetuses between 18 and 30 weeks of gestation. *Pediatric Research* **20**: 342–346.

Gill JC, Wilson A, Marlar RA *et al.* (1984) Loss of the large von Willebrand factor (vWf) multimers from the plasma of patients with ventricular septal defect (VSD). *Clinical Research* **32**: 308A.

Gordon EM, Ratnoff OD, Saito H *et al.* (1980) Studies on some coagulation factors (Hageman factor, plasma prekallikrein, and high molecular weight kininogen) in the normal newborn. *American Journal of Pediatric Hematology/Oncology* **2**: 213–216.

Graeve JLA and De Alarcon PA (1989) Megakaryocytopoeisis in the human fetus. *Archives of Disease in Childhood* **64**: 481–484.

Gross RE (1945) Arterial embolism and thrombosis in infancy. *American Journal of Disease in Childhood* **70**: 61–73.

Gross SJ, Filston HC and Anderson JC (1982) Controlled study of treatment for disseminated intravascular coagulation in the neonate. *Journal of Pediatrics* **100**: 445–448.

Hambley H, Yates R, McNaughton MC *et al.* (1983) Congenital antithrombin III deficiency: extended use of a pasteurised antithrombin III concentrate in late pregnancy and puerperium. In *Proceedings of the British BTS,* 11.

Hardisty RM and Weatherall DJ (1982) Approximate mean levels of clotting factors in preterm and full-term infants related to gestation. In *Blood and its Disorders,* 2nd edn, p 90.

Haroon Y, Shearer MJ, Rahim S *et al.* (1982) The content of phylloquinone (vitamin K_1) in human milk, cow's milk and infant formula foods determined by high-performance liquid chromatography. *Journal of Nutrition* **112**: 1105–1117.

Harpel PC and Rosenberg RD (1976) Alpha 2-macroglobulin and antithrombin-heparin cofactor: modulators of hemostatic and inflammatory reactions. Alpha 2-macroglobulin. *Progress in Hemostasis and Thrombosis* **3**: 145–189.

Hathaway WE, Bonnar J (1978) Perinatal coagulation. In *Monographs in Neonatology,* pp 55–59. New York: Grune & Stratton.

Hathaway WE and Bonnar J (1987) *Hemostatic Disorders of the Pregnant Woman and Newborn Infant.* Elsevier Science Publishing Inc, New York.

Holmberg L, Henriksson P, Ekelund H *et al.* (1974) Coagulation in the human fetus: Comparison with term newborn infants. *Journal of Pediatrics* **85**: 860–864.

Horgan MJ, Bartoletti A, Polansky S *et al.* (1987) Effect of heparin infusates in umbilical arterial catheters on frequency of thrombotic complications. *Journal of Pediatrics* **111**: 774–778.

Hulac P, Shapiro A, Manco-Johnson M *et al.* (1986) Maternal anticovulsants and neonatal vitamin K deficiency. *Pediatric Research* **20**: 390A.

Johnson SS, Montgomery RR and Hathaway WE (1981) Newborn factor VIII complex: elevated activities in term infants and alterations in electrophoretic mobility related to illness and activated coagulation. *British Journal of Haematology* **47**: 597–606.

Jannaccone G and Pasquino AM (1981) Calcifying splenic haematoma in a haemophiliac newborn. *Pediatric Radiology* **10**: 183–185.

Kaufmann HJ (1958) Renal vein thrombosis. *American Journal of Disease in Childhood* **95**: 377–384.

Karpatkin M, Porges RF and Karpatkin S (1981) Platelet counts in infants of women with autoimmune thrombocytopenia: effects of steroid administration to the mother. *New England Journal of Medicine* **305**: 936–939.

Kelton JC, Inwood MJ, Barr RM *et al.* (1982) The prenatal prediction of thrombocytopenia in infants of mothers with clinically diagnosed immune thrombocytopenia. *American Journal of Obstetrics and Gynecology* **144**: 449–454.

Kelton JG (1983) Management of the pregnant patient with idiopathic thrombocytopenic purpura. *Annals of Internal Medicine* **99**: 796–800.

Lane PA and Hathaway WE (1985) Vitamin K in infancy. *Journal of Pediatrics* **106**: 351–359.

Lesko SM, Mitchell AA, Epstein MF *et al.* (1986) Heparin use as a risk factor for intraventricular hemorrhage in low-birth-weight infants. *New England Journal of Medicine* **314**: 1156–1160.

McDonald MM and Hathaway WE (1982) Anticoagulant therapy by continuous heparinisation in newborn and older infants. *Journal of Paediatrics* **101**: 451–457.

McDonald MM and Hathaway WE (1983) Perinatal hematology/oncology. *Seminars in Perinatology* **7**: 213.

McDonald MM, Koops BL, Johnson ML *et al.* (1984) Timing and antecedents of intracranial haemorrhage in the newborn. *Pediatrics* **74**: 32–36.

McNinch AW, Orme RL and Tripp JH (1983) Haemorrhagic disease of the newborn returns. *The Lancet* **1**: 1089–1090.

McNinch AW, Upton C, Samuels M *et al.* (1985) Plasma concentrations after oral or intramuscular vitamin K1 in neonates. *Archives of Disease in Childhood* **60**: 814–818.

Malm J, Bennhagen R, Holmberg L and Dahlback B (1988) Plasma concentrations of

C4b-binding protein and vitamin K-dependent protein S in term and preterm infants: low levels of protein S-C4b-binding protein complexes. *British Journal of Haematology* **68**: 445–449.
Marciniak E, Wilson HD and Marlar RA (1985) Neonatal purpura fulminans: a genetic disorder related to the absence of protein C in blood. *Blood* **65**: 15–20.
Marlar RA, Montgomery RR, and Broekmans AW (1989) Diagnosis and treatment of homozygous protein C deficiency. Report of the Working Party on Homozygous Protein C Deficiency of the Subcommittee on Protein C and Protein S. International Committee on Thrombosis and Haemostastis. *Journal of Pediatrics* **114**: 528–534.
Mibashan RS and Millar DS (1983) Fetal haemostatic values at 17–21 weeks gestation. *British Medical Bulletin* **39**: 392–398.
Mibashan RS, Rodeck CH, Thumpston JK *et al.* (1979) Plasma assay of fetal factors VIIIC and IX for prenatal diagnosis of haemphilia. *The Lancet* **1**: 1309–1311.
Mibashan RS, Peake IR, Rodeck CH *et al.* (1980) Dual diagnosis of prenatal haemophilia A by measurement of fetal factor VIIIC and VIIIC antigen (VIIIC Ag). *The Lancet* **2**: 994–997.
Millar DS, Davis LR, Rodeck CH *et al.* (1985) Normal blood cell values in the early mid-trimester fetus. *Prenatal Diagnosis* **5**: 367–373.
Mills DA and Karpatkin S (1972) Heterogeneity of human adult and fetal fibrinogen: detection of derivatives indicative of thrombin proteolysis. *Biochemica et Biophysica Acta* **285**: 398–403.
Montgomery RR, Marlar RA and Gill JC (1985) Newborn Haemostasis. *Clin Haematol* **14**: 443–460.
Mueller-Eckhardt C, Kiefel V, Grubert A *et al.* (1989) 348 cases of suspected neonatal alloimmune thrombocytopenia. *The Lancet* **1**: 363–366.
Nicolini U, Rodeck CH, Kochenour NK *et al.* (1988) In-utero platelet transfusion for alloimmune thrombocytopenia (letter). *The Lancet* **2**: 506.
Nygaard KK (1939) Prophylactic and curative effect of vitamin K in haemorrhagic disease of the newborn. *Acta Obstetrica et Gynecologica Scandinavica* **19**: 361.
Pandolfi M, Astedt B, Cronberg L and Nilsson IM (1972) Failure of fetal platelets to aggregate in response to adrenaline and collagen. Proceedings of the Society for Experimental Biology and Medicine **141**: 1081–1083.
Pearson HA, Shulman NR, Mardcer VJ and Cone TJ (1964) Isoimmune neonatal thrombocytopenic purpura: clinical and therapeutic considerations. *Blood* **23**: 154–177.
Phelps DL (1984) Vitamin E and CNS haemorrhage (Editorial) *Pediatrics* **74**: 1113–1114.
Piet AAMM, Piet BA, Kjell SS *et al.* (1983) Red blood cell size is important for adherence of blood platelets to artery subendothelium. *Blood* **62**: 214–217.
Polack B, Pouzol P, Amiral J and Kolodie L (1984) Protein C level at birth. *Thrombosis and Haemostasis* **52**: 188–191.
Schettini F, De Mattia D, Altomare M *et al.* (1985) Post-natal development of protein C in full-term newborns. *Acta Paediatrica Scandinavica* **74**: 226–229.
Schmidt B and Zipursky A (1984) Thrombotic disease in newborn infants. *Clinics in Perinatology* **11**: 462.
Schmidt B and Zipursky A (1986) Disseminated intravascular coagulation masking neonatal haemophilia. *Journal of Paediatrics* **109**: 886–888.
Schwartz HP, Muntean W, Watzke H *et al.* (1988) Low total protein S antigen but high protein S activity due to decreased C4b-binding protein in neonates. *Blood* **71**: 562–565.
Scott JR, Rote NS and Cruikshank DP (1982) Antiplatelet antibodies and platelet counts in pregnancies complicated by autoimmune thrombocytopenic purpura. *American Journal of Obstetrics and Gynecology* **145**: 932–939.
Seligsohn U, Berger A, Abend M *et al.* (1984) Homozygous protein C deficiency

manifested by massive venous thrombosis in the newborn. *New England Journal of Medicine* **310**: 559–562.

Sell EJ and Corrigan JJ Jr. (1973) Platelet counts, fibrinogen concentrations, and factor V and factor VIII levels in healthy infants according to gestational age. *Journal of Pediatrics* **82**: 1029–1032.

Shapiro AD, Jacobson LJ, Armon ME *et al.* (1986) Vitamin K-deficiency in the newborn infant: prevalence and perinatal risk factors. *Journal of Pediatrics* **109**: 675–680.

Sills RH, Marlar RA, Montgomery RR *et al.* (1984) Severe homozygous protein C deficiency. *Journal of Pediatrics* **105**: 409–413.

Sinha S, Davies J, Toner N *et al.* (1987) Vitamin E supplementation reduces frequency of periventricular haemorrhage in very preterm babies. *The Lancet* **1**: 466–471.

Spear ME, Blifeld C, Rudloph AJ *et al.* (1984) Intraventricular haemorrhage and vitamin E in the very low birth weight infant: evidence for efficacy of early intramuscular vitamin E administration. *Pediatrics* **74**: 1107–1112.

Sthoeger D, Nardi M and Karpatkin M (1989) Protein S in the first year of life. *British Journal of Haematology* **72**: 424–428.

Strother SV and Wagner AM (1988) Prednisone in pregnant women with idiopathic thrombocytopenic purpura. *New England Journal of Medicine* **319**: 178.

Stuart MJ (1981) Deficiency of plasma PGI_2-like regenerating activity in neonatal plasma. Reversal by vitamin E in vitro. *Pediatric Research* **15(6)**: 971–973.

Tarby TJ and Volpe JJ (1982) Intraventricular haemorrhage in the premature infant. *Pediatric Clinics of North America* **29**: 1077–1104.

Teger-Nilsson AC and Ekelund H (1974) Fibrinogen to fibrin transformation in umbilical cord blood and purified neonatal fibrinogen. *Thrombosis Research* **5**: 601–612.

Tripp JH and McNinch AW (1987) Haemorrhagic disease and vitamin K. *Archives of Disease in Childhood* **62**: 436–437.

Townsend CW (1894) The haemorrhagic disease of the newborn. *Arch Pediatr* **11**: 559–565.

Turner T, Prowse CV, Prescott RJ and Cash JD (1981) A clinical trial on the early detection and correction of haemostatic defects in selected high-risk neonates. *British Journal of Haematology* **47**: 65–75.

Tyson JE, deSa DJ and Moore S (1976) Thromboatheromatous complications of umbilical arterial catheterisation in the newborn period. Clinicopathological study. *Archives of Disease in Childhood* **51**: 744–754.

Virchow R (1856) Phlegose und Thrombose im Gefässystem. In Virchow. R, ed. Gesammelte Abhandlungen zür Wissenschaftlichen Medizin. Meidinger Sohn, 1856 pp. 458.

Volpe JJ (1981) Neonatal intraventricular haemorrhage. *New England Journal of Medicine* **304**: 886–891.

Waddel WW and Guerry D (1939) The role of vitamin K in the etiology, prevention and treatment of haemorrhage in the newborn infant. *Journal of Pediatrics* **15**: 802.

Weinstein MJ, Blanchard R, Moake JL *et al.* (1989) Fetal and neonatal von Willebrand factor (vWF) is unusually large and similar to the vWF in patients with thrombotic thrombocytopenic purpura. *British Journal of Haematology* **72**: 68–72.

Winter JH, Fenech A, Ridley W *et al.* (1982) Familial antithrombin III deficiency. *Quarterly Journal of Medicine* **51**: 373–395.

Witt I and Müller H (1970) Phosphorus and hexose content of human fetal fibrinogen. *Biochimica Biophysica Acta* **221**: 402–404.

Witt I, Müller H, Kunzer W (1969) Evidence for the existence of foetal fibrinogen. *Thromb Diath Haemorrh* **22**: 101–109.

7

Transfusion in the fetus and newborn

B.E.S Gibson

Royal Hospital for Sick Children and Queen Mother's Maternity Hospital, Glasgow

INTRODUCTION

The pattern of transfusion in the newborn has recently undergone considerable change. Following the widespread availability of anti-Rh immunoglobulin, the decrease in the incidence of haemolytic disease of the newborn has made intra-uterine transfusion a rare event and even exchange transfusions are much less commonly performed. Despite this, haemolytic disease of the newborn (HDN) is still with us and remains the main reason for which exchange transfusion is carried out (see Chapter 5).

Clarke *et al.* (1987) reported the perinatal mortality figures for haemolytic disease of the newborn in England and Wales for the period 1977–1985. The mortality rate fell from 18.3 in 100 000 in 1977 to 5.2 in 100 000 in 1983. The figure for 1985 was similar to that for 1983 suggesting that from now onwards the rate may remain static unless new therapeutic approaches are adopted. The data suggests that many women become immunised because they are not given anti-Rh immunoglobulin after an abortion. It is not always remembered that there are potentially sensitizing episodes other than delivery that are indications for intrapartum anti-Rh immunoglobulin, including spontaneous and therapeutic abortion, antepartum haemorrhage, amniocentesis and external version. Of even greater significance is the observation that of the mothers whose infants died in 1984 and 1985, about half could only have been protected by an antenatal anti-Rh immunoglobulin prophylaxis programme. The D antigen is well developed by 30–45 days of gestation. Fetal transplacental haemorrhage (TPH) is known to occur antenatally and complicates an increasing number of pregnancies as gestation advances. Women who are immunized after a relatively small TPH that occurred spontaneously, or following an abortion, are 'good responders' and their fetuses in subsequent pregnancies may be severely affected.

Outstanding improvements in neonatology have led to the survival of very small premature infants, who make special demands on the hospital blood bank. The resources of the blood bank, which were once directed at providing blood for exchange transfusions, are now being geared to the provision of blood and blood component therapy for repeated small volume transfusion.

SEROLOGICAL TESTING OF THE NEONATE

Haemolytic disease of the newborn is still with us despite the widespread availability of anti-Rh immunoglobulin. Neonates may require transfusion for immune-mediated haemolysis in this and a number of other situations. There is no way of preventing a pregnant or transfused woman from becoming immunized to red cell antigens other than the rhesus D antigen; over 30 blood group antigens have been incriminated in the pathogenesis of HDN. The increased use of blood and blood component therapy has resulted in an increase in the number of mothers immunized by transfusion, since transfused blood is only ABO and D compatible. Approximately 1–2% of people develop blood group antibodies after blood transfusion. Although the majority of such antibodies cause little or no haemolytic disease, antibodies to c, Kell and, less commonly, E, C, Fy^a and a few other antigens, may do so. It must also be remembered that autoimmune haemolysis in the mother may result in haemolytic disease of the newborn. In any of the above situations, the laboratory may be asked to provide, for the infant, blood which is lacking the antigen corresponding to the maternal antibody. Blood may be required for surgery or for top-up transfusion and, in addition, the laboratory has a duty to screen all neonates who are symptomatic or at risk of haemolytic disease. Such neonates include the following:

(1) All infants of rhesus negative mothers.

(2) All infants of mothers known to have red cell antibodies capable of causing haemolytic disease of the newborn. Some investigators might include all infants of group O mothers as their infants, if group A and B, are theoretically at risk of haemolysis. However, the workload would be considerable and screening is probably only justified for symptomatic infants of group O mothers.

(3) All symptomatic infants, i.e. infants who are anaemic or jaundiced.

Investigations required

The investigations required differ for different cases, and are outlined below.

(1) ABO and rhesus D typing of the mother and infant.

(2) Direct anti-human globulin (AHG) test on the cord or infant's red cells. A positive direct AHG test indicates the presence of maternal antibody attached to the corresponding antigen on the neonate's red cells. The strength of the direct AHG test does not correlate with the severity of the haemolysis. It may be negative or weakly positive in haemolysis due to ABO incompatibility but, with this one exception, a negative direct AHG test virtually excludes haemolytic disease of the newborn.

(3) If the direct AHG test is positive the antibody should be identified using maternal, cord or infant sera. The antibody is generally stronger in the mother's serum and a more generous sample can be obtained.

(4) Ideally an eluate should be prepared from cord or infant red cells and,

after elution, the antibody identified to confirm the maternal findings. Eluates are particularly useful if maternal serum is not available and may also be helpful in another situation; when the mother's serum contains several antibodies, the preparation and examination of an eluate will identify those responsible for the haemolysis.

(5) An acid elution demonstration of Hb F (Kleihauer) should be carried out on maternal blood to estimate the size of any fetomaternal haemorrhage. This test is based on the fact that fetal haemoglobin is resistant to acid and alkali denaturation, whilst adult haemoglobin is not.

(6) It must be emphasized that once blood has been selected, it should be cross-matched against maternal serum.

(7) In our laboratory we screen samples from infants who have necrotizing enterocolitis or sepsis with peanut lectins to detect T activation, which can result in a haemolytic transfusion reaction. Circulating neuraminidase, a product of several different bacteria, removes *N*-acetyl neuraminic acid from red blood cell (RBC) surface membranes and exposes the Thomsen–Friedenreich antigen. Most adults possess IgM anti-T as a naturally occurring antibody. When this antibody is inadvertently transfused in blood to infants with exposed T antigens, polyagglutination occurs and haemolysis results. A variety of bacteria have been incriminated and there have now been several reports of T activation occurring in infants with necrotizing enterocolitis (Placzek and Gorst, 1987). The use of washed cells overcomes this complication.

Problems related to the testing of neonatal samples

No problems should be encountered in ABO and rhesus grouping the mother. However, occasionally problems arise in typing the neonate. Wharton's jelly may produce false results, especially if the cells have not been washed adequately before testing. Additionally, interpretation of the group may be difficult if the infant has received an intra-uterine transfusion of group O rhesus-negative blood and is of a different ABO and rhesus type. Mixed-field agglutination may then result and careful interpretation is necessary.

ABO typing of the infant's red cells

Expression of the ABO antigens on cord cells are not fully developed and reactions may be weak. Only the red cells need be tested; testing the infant's serum is not helpful. The infant does not synthesize demonstrable amounts of anti-A and anti-B until 5–6 months of age. The majority of anti-A and anti-B present in cord or infant serum is IgG and is passively acquired from the mother.

Rhesus D typing of the infant's red cells

There is usually little difficulty in accurately establishing the infant's rhesus type, but problems may be encountered if the cord or infant cells are heavily sensitized with maternal antibody. A false-negative rhesus type may result from total blockage of the D antigens on the red cells by maternal antibody. Alternatively, a false-positive may occur when the typing serum has a high albumin content. A saline reagent should be used for rhesus-typing cord and infant cells and correct controls must be included. In the rare case when, despite the use of a saline typing reagent, the rhesus type of the infant is still not clear, examination of an eluate may be helpful. If the maternal serum contains anti-D and anti-D is eluted from the infant's cells, the infant must be rhesus-positive. After elution of the antibody the cord or infant cells can be correctly typed.

HAEMOLYTIC DISEASE OF THE NEWBORN ASSOCIATED WITH A POSITIVE DIRECT AHG TEST

In all cases where blood has to be provided for an infant having a positive direct AHG test, the responsible antibody must be correctly identified. An antibody screen should be performed on either the maternal or infant's serum or an eluate prepared from the neonate's red cells. The responsible antibody is then identified by further testing serum or eluate against a panel of reagent red cells. Blood negative for the corresponding antigen can then be issued for transfusion. A direct AHG test on maternal red cells should be included for identification of a maternal autoimmune process.

Positive antibody screen: maternal direct AHG test negative

Patterns obtained with a reagent red cell panel include the following:

Specific pattern of positivity. Testing against a panel of reagent cells may identify a specific antibody or a number of antibodies, e.g. anti-Kell, anti-Duffy (Fy).

All panel cells positive. All the cells in the reagent panel may give a positive reaction. This can occur in two situations:

(a) A mixture of antibodies may be present, which can usually be identified by the pattern of strength of reactions against specific cells in the reagent panel.

(b) A single antibody against a high-frequency antigen may be present. Such a 'public' antibody can be identified by testing against a panel of rare reagent cells.

Positive antibody screen: maternal direct AHG test positive

This pattern of positivity suggests a warm autoantibody in maternal serum associated with an autoimmune haemolytic anaemia (AIHA). This may occur with disorders such as systemic lupus erythematosus (SLE) and in these cases the haemolysis often improves with pregnancy. However, AIHA may present for the first time during pregnancy and resolve after delivery. This type of AIHA is unusual in two respects; the disorder is often severe and the direct AHG test surprisingly, frequently negative (Chaplin *et al.*, 1973; Yam *et al.*, 1980; Eldor *et al.*, 1975).

Negative antibody screen

Two situations result in a positive direct AHG test on cord cells in the presence of a negative antibody screen.

(1) The antibody may be directed against a low-frequency or 'private' antigen not present on the screening red cells. This can be demonstrated by testing the infant's serum or eluate against both maternal and paternal red cells. The mother's cells will be negative because they lack the antigen, but the father's cells will possess the antigen and be positive. The presence of a 'private' antigen can be further confirmed by testing the infant's serum or eluate against rare cells. This is, however, an unusual cause of haemolytic disease of the newborn, because most private antibodies are IgM and do not cross the placenta.

(2) The presence of an antibody directed against a drug in the serum has been reported as a rare cause of a positive direct AHG test in the neonate, and penicillins and cephalosporins have been most frequently incriminated. Testing the infant's eluate or serum or the maternal serum against pencillin-treated red cells gives a positive result, demonstrating the presence of an immune antipenicillin antibody.

Selection of blood

A number of factors are involved in the selection of blood for transfusion.

(1) If a single antibody or a mixture of antibodies are identified, blood negative for the corresponding antigens can be selected.

(2) It may be difficult to find compatible blood if a high frequency alloantibody is present. The mother's relatives should be screened or a rare donor panel may be available. The mother's blood will be compatible provided that her obstetrician is willing for her to donate. In the emergency situation, ABO-compatible blood, which is incompatible with the private antibody, may have to be given. These red cells will have a decreased survival, but will provide temporary oxygen-carrying capacity and will absorb some of the antibodies, until compatible blood is found.

(3) If an autoantibody is present incompatible blood may have to be transfused. Units which give reactions of similar or less strength than the

patient's own serum are usually preferred.

(4) There should be no difficulty finding blood lacking low frequency antigens and most donor blood will be compatible.

(5) If the problem is due to a drug-related antibody, there should be no problem finding blood, since the maternal serum will only react with red cells sensitized to the drug.

The donor blood should be cross-matched whenever possible against the maternal serum. If this is unavailable, an eluate prepared from cord cells or the infant's serum will have to be used. Both have disadvantages. The infant's serum will contain all the maternal antibodies in the infant's circulation with the possible exception of the antibody causing the haemolysis, which may go undetected due to absorption onto the infant's red cells. The eluate will contain the antibody responsible for the haemolysis but will lack any other haemolytic maternal antibodies in the infant's serum directed against antigens not present on the infant's red cells. These same antibodies could react with transfused red cells, if incompatible.

INTRA-UTERINE TRANSFUSION (IUT)

The prophylactic use of anti-Rh immunoglobulin at delivery has been widely employed since 1970 and has been extremely successful in preventing alloimmunization. However, in the United Kingdom 0.7–0.9% of rhesus-negative women at risk, without prior evidence of sensitization, become sensitized intrapartum (Gabra *et al.*, 1983; Tovey *et al.*, 1983). The combined antenatal and postpartum administration of anti-Rh immunoglobulin has further reduced the incidence of sensitisation to approximately 0.1% (Bowman *et al.*, 1978; Tovey *et al.*, 1983). Despite these measures, some women are still found to be sensitized with anti-D in their serum at their first antenatal visit (see chapter 5).

Specific considerations for blood used for IUT

For IUT, eight special considerations must be borne in mind.

(1) The blood must lack the red cell antigen corresponding to the antibody in the maternal serum. The Rh blood group antigen D is the most important cause of maternal alloimmunization and haemolytic disease of the newborn. Intra-uterine transfusion is nearly always carried out for rhesus incompatibility and group O rhesus-negative blood, cross-matched against maternal serum, should be transfused. Women who have become sensitized to produce anti-D are more likely to develop antibodies to other blood group antigens, such as Kell, Duffy and Kidd. Consideration should be given of the extent to which the blood used should be typed to ensure that it is negative for those antigens that the mother's red cells lack. The blood transfused should certainly be Kell-negative if the mother is Kell-negative, because the acquisition of anti-Kell will cause the next most severe haemolysis after anti-D. A maternal sample must be stored at the time of

each transfusion for subsequent testing should additional antibodies develop.

(2) The blood must be as fresh as possible, i.e. not more than 72 hours old, to ensure maximal viability of the red cells transfused. However, adequate time must be allowed for screening for hepatitis B surface antigen (HBsAg), cytomegalovirus (CMV) and human immunodeficiency virus (HIV) antibodies.

(3) The blood can be safely collected into a citrate phosphate dextrose (CPD) double pack. Citrate, K^+, Na^+ and H^+ are rapidly transported across the placenta and therefore do not constitute a risk to the fetus.

(4) The volume that can be infused into the fetal peritoneal cavity or fetal circulation is small and therefore the haematocrit should be high. The ideal haematocrit is the highest that will go through the fine catheters used for the procedure, approximately 70–75%. The cells should be packed tightly and the plasma removed. This also serves to remove from the plasma anti-A and anti-B, which might produce a transient drop in haemoglobin, if the infant belongs to group A or B. This potential problem can alternatively be overcome by washing the cells in saline and resuspending them in group AB plasma. However, this approach increases the risk of infection and is not necessary if sufficient plasma is discarded.

(5) The volume of blood transfused depends on the estimated age of gestation, which obviously reflects the capacity of the peritoneal cavity or blood volume. Several rules of thumb exist, but one commonly used formula is:

$$\text{volume (ml)} = \left(\begin{matrix}\text{estimated gestational}\\ \text{age (weeks)}\end{matrix} - 20\right) \times 10$$

i.e. 40 ml of blood at 24 weeks. Once a programme of intra-uterine transfusions has been started, these usually require to be repeated at 2-weekly intervals until the fetus is sufficiently mature to survive.

(6) Severe cases of graft-versus-host-disease (GVHD) have been reported following intra-uterine transfusion (Naiman *et al.*, 1969; Parkman *et al.*, 1974). The fetus is immunologically incompetent, and it may engraft viable and immunologically competent leucocytes transfused. Several methods of preparing the blood can minimize the number of leucocytes infused, but irradiation is the most effective and the simplest. In our laboratory we irradiate (1500 rad) all blood products transfused to the fetus *in utero*.

(7) It should be remembered at delivery that the infant has been transfused group O rhesus-negative blood and may type falsely as rhesus-negative. The direct AHG test may be negative or only weakly positive. Group O cells will have been given irrespective of the infant's own group, and he or she either may falsely type as group O or may show a mixed field pattern of agglutination. If exchange transfusion is necessary after delivery, group O rhesus-negative blood should be used, irrespective of the infant's own blood group.

(8) Following IUT the infant's blood will have the O_2 unloading characteristics of adult blood. The exact physiological significance of manipulation of the oxygen affinity of the infant *in utero* remains speculative.

EXCHANGE TRANSFUSION

The main aim of exchange transfusion is to prevent kernicterus by removing unconjugated bilirubin. Further production of bilirubin from red cell destruction is minimized by removing maternally derived antibody and by replacing incompatible red cells with red cells that lack the antigen corresponding to the maternal antibody.

Exchange transfusion is indicated for neonatal hyperbilirubinaemia of any aetiology, if the baby's unconjugated bilirubin would otherwise rise to a dangerous level. A haemoglobin concentration below 12–13 g dl^{-1} at birth and/or a bilirubin rising by 12 μmol l^{-1} h^{-1} or more are accepted criteria for exchange transfusion in our nursery, in addition to the guidelines given in Figure 7.1, although other neonatal units may employ different criteria. Rhesus incompatibility remains the most severe form of haemolytic disease of the newborn, despite the dramatic fall in its incidence since the availability of anti-Rh immunoglobulin. Although ABO incompatibility can be associated with haemolysis, it is rarely severe enough to require exchange transfusion. Other blood group incompatibilities are occasionally responsible, i.e. c, E, Kell. Hereditary red cell defects can result in haemolysis sufficiently severe in the newborn period to require intervention.

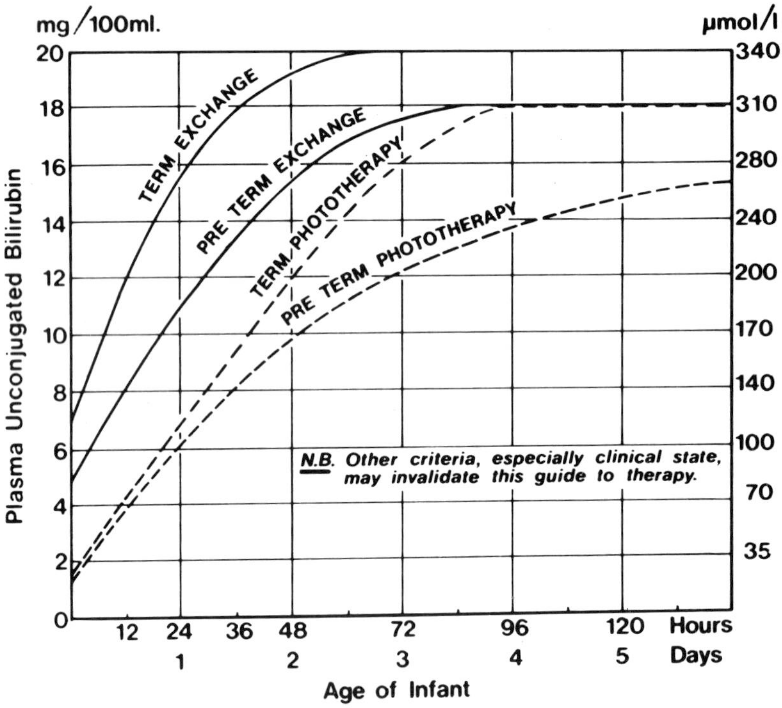

Figure 7.1 Guidelines for exchange transfusion and phototherapy in the term and pre-term infant. In addition, a haemoglobin concentration below 12–13 g dl^{-1} at birth and/or a bilirubin rising by 12 μmol l^{-1} h^{-1} or more are accepted criteria for exchange transfusion in the author's nursery.

The age of the infant, when the bilirubin starts to rise may suggest the cause. In rhesus incompatibility the bilirubin rises early, i.e. within the first few hours of life. In ABO incompatibility the rise is slower but often starts within the first 24 hours of life, reaching a maximum on the 3rd or 4th day. The degree of haemolysis is mild compared with that of rhesus incompatibility. Irrespective of the cause of hyperbilirubinaemia the haemolysis may be intensified by prematurity, acidosis, asphyxia and infection. It is now well recognized that kernicterus can develop at much lower levels of bilirubin than previously thought, particularly in pre-term infants. The initial exchange transfusion removes sensitized red cells destined for destruction, which would ultimately yield large amounts of bilirubin. Approximately 85% of cells can be removed in this way. Bilirubin and antibody removal, which are the main objectives of subsequent exchange transfusions, are less efficient. Irrespective of the cause of haemolytic disease of the newborn, it is the responsibility of the hospital blood bank to provide compatible blood, which meets the needs of the neonate, for exchange transfusion.

Specific considerations for blood used for exchange transfusion

ABO group and rhesus type

The blood must be ABO- and rhesus-compatible with both mother and infant. In the usual situation, where the haemolysis is due to rhesus incompatibility, rhesus-negative blood must be used. In the rare event of exchange transfusion being necessary for ABO-incompatibility, group O blood of the infant's rhesus type should be transfused. Group O cells can be safely employed for all exchange transfusions, but ABO-specific blood may be given where the baby and mother are of the same blood group. If group O blood is used there is a theoretical risk of destruction of the infant's red cells by A and B isoagglutinins. However, very little plasma is transfused with packed cells. When fresh frozen plasma is added to packed cells to adjust the haematocrit, this should be ABO compatible.

Compatibility

The transfused blood must lack the antigen corresponding to the maternal antibody. The offending antibody will be strongest in the maternal serum, which should be used for the initial cross-match. The infant's serum may be used if a maternal specimen is not available, although examination of an eluate prepared from the neonate's red cells is more likely to be rewarding.

Anticoagulant

CPD is now the anticoagulant of choice for routine blood collections. Although CPD blood may not be physiologically ideal for exchange transfusion, it can be used safely and is readily available. Acid citrate dextrose (ACD) blood should never be used for neonatal transfusion whether it be exchange or simple. Reasonably fresh CPD blood will have acceptable levels of K^+ and excellent levels of 2,3-diphosphoglycerate (2,3DPG). The advantages of CPD blood are many: it is readily available; it does not interfere with the infant's coagulation, and, because of the high glucose load, it does not produce hypoglycaemia during exchange. However, a rebound hypoglycaemia can occur due to insulin secretion in response to the glucose load and the infant's blood glucose requires to be carefully monitored. The citrate component binds calcium, which may result in hypocalcaemia. This is rarely symptomatic and calcium need only be given if symptoms develop. The elevated serum sodium of CPD stored blood may be a potential problem.

The main disadvantage of CPD blood is disturbance of the infant's acid–base balance. Although the pH of blood falls with storage, the acid load of CPD blood is insufficient to significantly lower the pH of a full-term infant (Bursaux *et al.*, 1973), but problems may arise with very small acidotic premature newborns. This problem can be overcome by washing the packed cells and resuspending them in ABO compatible fresh frozen plasma (FFP). This manoeuvre removes any undesirable electrolytes, but it should be remembered that many of the problems related to the transfusion of citrated blood to the neonate were evaluated when ACD was the routine anticoagulant for donor blood. Now that CPD has replaced ACD as the universally accepted anticoagulant, the problems, especially those of acid–base disturbance, are less. Despite this, some clinicians prefer to use heparinized blood for exchange transfusion. Heparinized blood has a shelf-life of only 12 h and 2,3DPG is not preserved in heparin. The anticoagulant effect is an additional disadvantage. Many infants requiring exchange transfusion already have abnormal coagulation and may well have risk factors for disseminated intravascular coagulation (DIC). The use of heparinized blood further deranges their already precarious clotting ability. Although most infants will metabolize heparin within 6–8 h, protamine may have to be given to reverse its effects. Hypoglycaemia may occur during the exchange. The advantage of heparinized blood lies in its more physiological pH and the lack of citrate- and calcium-related problems.

Packed cell volume

The PCV of the blood used for exchange transfusion should be in the region of 50–55% and the haematocrit of packed cells can be adjusted by the addition of fresh frozen plasma to achieve this. A very high PCV may present technical problems with the procedure or precipitate symptoms of hyperviscosity. For example, necrotizing enterocolitis has been attributed by some to local thrombosis of the mesenteric vessels, secondary to hyperviscosity following transfusion of blood with a very high haematocrit.

Age of blood for transfusion

CPD blood should be as fresh as possible to minimize the metabolic changes related to storage. It should preferably be less than 3 days old and definitely not more than 5 days of age. The use of CPD blood of this age should guarantee optimum red cell survival, acceptable K^+ levels and good levels of 2,3DPG.

Risks of exchange transfusion

The risks of exchange transfusion are many. Some depend on the anticoagulant of the blood and others do not.

Risks independent of the anticoagulant

(1) Hypothermia: the blood should be warmed as hypothermia can result in cardiac arrhythmia. Care should also be taken to keep the neonate warm.
(2) Thrombosis of the portal vein may occur as a result of cannulation and can progress to portal hypertension.
(3) Perforation of the umbilical vein.
(4) Air embolism.
(5) Septic thrombophlebitis.
(6) Hyperkalaemia: this should be insignificant if reasonably fresh blood is transfused.

Risks dependent on the anticoagulant

(1) Hypoglycaemia may occur during exchange with heparinized blood. It does not usually occur when CPD blood is used because of its high dextrose content. However, following exchange transfusion, a rebound hypoglycaemia may be seen secondary to insulin secretion in response to the high dextrose load.
(2) Acid–base balance disturbances are not seen with heparinized blood and they should not be significant with CPD blood in the full-term neonate. However, an already acidotic, small, premature infant may have problems handling the acid load of CPD blood.
(3) Hypocalcaemia: the citrate in citrated blood chelates calcium and may result in hypocalcaemia. This is rarely symptomatic.
(4) Hypocoagulability: the use of heparinized blood will accentuate any existing coagulation abnormality.
(5) An elevated level of free fatty acids is associated with the transfusion of heparinised blood and causes a reduction of albumin bilirubin binding.

Complications and mortality

The overall mortality related to exchange transfusion depends on the premorbid condition of the infant and has been variably reported but generally it is less than 1% (Boggs and Westphal, 1960; Cochran, 1978). Thrombocytopenia is a well-recognized complication of severe Rh erythroblastosis fetalis and usually corrects itself after 4–6 days. If the platelet count falls below $25 \times 10^9\ l^{-1}$, platelets should be transfused. In some instances, the thrombocytopenia appears to be the result of repeated exchange transfusions using platelet-poor blood. However, thrombocytopenia may precede the exchange transfusion and, more recently, accompanying neutropenia has been described by Koenig and Christensen (1989) who postulated that the marked increase in erythropoiesis in fetuses with Rh haemolytic disease can be accompanied by a down-modulation of neutrophil and platelet production. Regardless of the mechanism by which the neutropenia and thrombocytopenia is produced, these cytopenias are made worse by repeated exchange transfusions using neutrophil-poor and platelet-poor blood.

The procedure of exchange transfusion

Before starting the exchange transfusion every effort should be made to correct acidosis and hypoxia, if time permits. The infant's temperature, respiratory and cardiac status should be monitored throughout. The umbilical vein is cannulated and the positioning of the catheter tip in the inferior vena cava (IVC) confirmed radiologically.

The volume and rate of exchange are important, when hyperbilirubinaemia is the reason for exchange. A double exchange is generally performed initially:

$$\begin{aligned}\text{total volume exchanged} &= \text{baby's blood volume} \times 2\\ &= (85\text{–}100\ \text{ml kg}^{-1}) \times 2.\end{aligned}$$

A single-volume exchange is approximately 60–65% and a double-volume exchange 80–85% efficient in removing sensitized red cells. Aliquots of 5—10 ml of packed cells are exchanged at a time. A single-volume exchange can be completed in roughly 1 h and a double-volume exchange in 2 h. Bilirubin is in the extravascular as well as the intravascular fluid compartment and only about 25% of it is removed by a double-volume exchange transfusion.

TOP-UP TRANSFUSION

The success of Rh prophylaxis has greatly reduced the need for intra-uterine and exchange transfusion. Outstanding advances in neonatology have increased the numbers of premature and sick neonates surviving. These infants are repeatedly venesected for a range of laboratory tests and the resultant iatrogenically produced anaemia now constitutes the main reason for transfusion in the newborn intensive care unit.

Neonatologists continue to debate the optimal level at which an infant's haemoglobin should be maintained to facilitate adequate oxygenation of the tissues. Pre-term infants are particularly likely to require small volume transfusions to replace blood losses and for correction of refractory anaemia. The haemoglobin concentration or haematocrit is usually used to assess the severity of the anaemia and to calculate the volume of red cells to be transfused. In premature infants particularly, the haemoglobin and haematocrit values correlate poorly with the red cell mass. In addition to the red cell deficit, the plasma volume is contracted. This results in a falsely high haematocrit and underestimates the true degree of the anaemia. There are those who feel that red cell replacement should be based on the red cell mass and not the haemoglobin or haematocrit. If sufficient red cell replacement is given initially, the frequency of transfusion may be reduced. Such a purist approach is not practical in the everyday running of a busy laboratory. However, for those readers interested in this view, a rapid method for estimating the pre-transfusion red cell mass in neonates was recently reported (Phillips *et al.*, 1986). This method is based on the degree of dilution of autologous fetal haemoglobin (HbF) by donor adult haemoglobin after red cell transfusion, the percentages of HbF being estimated by an alkali denaturation method. The measured percentage of HbF in the infant's blood before (pre T) and after (post-T) transfusion of a small volume of red cells, together with the volume of red cells transfused (vol), allows calculation of the pre-transfusion red cell mass (RCM), which is expressed in millilitres per kilogram of body weight:

$$\text{RCM} = \frac{\text{vol} \times \text{post-T HbF}}{\text{pre-T HbF} - \text{post-T HbF}}$$

Neonatal top-up transfusions differ in two respects from most transfusions given to older children or adults. Firstly, these transfusions are of small volume, in the order of 15–30 ml. However, because the premature infant has a blood volume in the range of 100–200 ml and the full-term baby 200–340 ml, the transfused blood may constitute a significant proportion of the infant's total blood volume. Secondly, an increasing number of infants receive multiple, small-volume transfusions during their stay in the newborn intensive care unit. The blood used for these transfusions must be relatively fresh, fully compatible, HBsAG and HIV antibody-negative and, preferably, CMV screened. Each hospital blood bank must decide on the most convenient means of providing such blood for small volume transfusions.

Source of blood for top-up transfusions

There are basically two ways of obtaining small volume donations. The first is blood which has been collected by the Regional Blood Transfusion Service as a standard donation and then subdivided to provide a number of small volume units. Secondly, a 'walking donor' programme can be operated, where only a small volume of blood is taken from the donor at any one time.

Blood provided by the Regional Blood Transfusion Service

Using a small volume of blood from a standard donation and discarding the remainder appears very wasteful of a valuable resource. A number of alternative approaches exist to overcome this problem. However, demands vary and it may not be considered either cost-effective or worthwhile setting up a special collection system for neonates. Alternative approaches include division of donations and use of small aliquots of red cells.

Single donation of blood collected into a CPD quadruple blood pack. Packed cells are prepared by centrifugation and the plasma decanted into one of the four packs. The red cells are then divided aseptically into small aliquots for transfusion at the time of collection or transferred into the satellite bags when requested by the nursery (Figure 7.2). Commercial 'Pedi-Packs' are now available, allowing a greater number

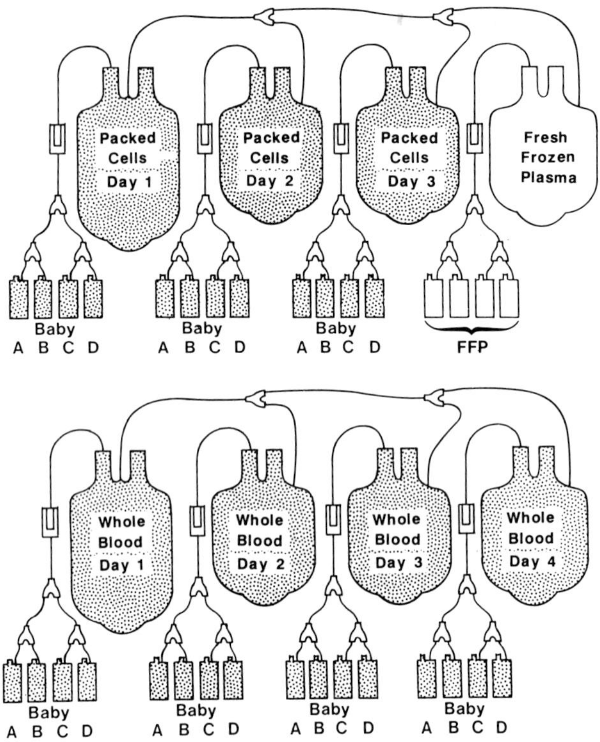

Figure 7.2 A single donation of blood is collected into a CPD quadruple blood pack. Packed cells are prepared by centrifugation and the plasma decanted into one of the four packs. The red cells are then divided aseptically into small aliquots for transfusion at the time of collection or transferred into the satellite bags when requested by the nursery. Commercial 'Pedi-Paks' are now available allowing a greater number of subdivisions of the original unit of blood. Whole blood (lower) and packed cells and fresh frozen plasma (upper) can be subdivided in this manner.

of subdivisions of the original unit of blood. This system is really only suitable if a policy of transfusing all neonates with group O blood has been accepted locally by the neonatologists. The blood can then be used for two or three neonates, irrespective of their blood group, utilizing the product most efficiently.

Reduced donation (225 ml) collected into a CPD triple blood pack containing an adjusted volume of anticoagulant. The plasma is removed and the remaining red cells can be divided aseptically to provide two units of packed cells of approximately 50 ml each. The advantage of having taken only half of a standard donation is that the donor can be recalled to provide a similar sized donation within a few days for the same neonate. This method provides reasonably fresh blood for a neonate who is receiving repeated blood transfusions several days apart and limits the exposure to a single donor, if this is considered important. However, this system does require a dedicated donor.

Single donation is collected into a CPD triple pack. The plasma is removed by centrifugation and a unit of packed cells remain. A small volume of red cells are transferred to a satellite bag leaving behind a volume which is still adequate for an adult transfusion. This method provides a single small-volume donation without wastage.

Blood provided by a 'walking donor' programme

'Walking donor' programmes for newborn intensive care units have operated successfully in many hospitals in the past as a means of providing small volumes of fresh blood for infants. A list of willing donors is kept by the hospital blood bank. The panel of donors is generally made up of hospital personnel (the staff of renal dialysis units are usually excluded because of their increased risk of hepatitis). The donors are ABO and rhesus typed and when blood is required for a neonate, a 'walking donor' of the appropriate blood group is called upon. Blood is withdrawn straight into a syringe containing a desired amount of heparin and then transfused to the neonate. The donor should meet the standard requirements of a donor to the Regional Blood Transfusion Service. His or her blood should be screened for the presence of red cell antibodies and for syphilis, hepatitis and HIV antibodies. In many institutions potential donors are regularly tested for antibodies to CMV, HIV and HBsAg, and any donor excluded who has had a blood transfusion or been unwell since he or she was last tested. Other centres operating a 'walking donor' system only for routine 'top-up' transfusions, which can generally be predicted, are able to screen blood for hepatitis, CMV and HIV the day before donation.

There are many advocates of this system and the advantages are threefold:

(1) It is a simple way of ensuring that the blood is fresh.

(2) A single donor can be asked to provide a small volume of blood on repeated occasions to meet the transfusion requirements of an individual

neonate throughout the neonate's time in the intensive care unit, thereby minimizing exposure to a single donor, if this is considered important.

(3) Small volumes of blood are taken from the donor, sufficient only to meet the neonate's transfusion requirements.

There are however many disadvantages to this type of programme, namely screening, organization and availability of donors.

(1) The most important problem lies with the difficulty in screening the blood for hepatitis, CMV and HIV antibodies after withdrawal and before transfusion, which would be the normal practice with blood supplied by the Regional Blood Transfusion Service. Screening blood donors at regular and frequent intervals does not guarantee that their antibody status has not changed. In addition to the risk to the neonate, there is also the problem of organizing the screening of the donors and acting on the results. Meticulous screening for hepatitis is important in a hospital-based donor population, which has a higher exposure rate. Particularly difficult is the sensitive issue of HIV testing. Some donors may refuse to be tested, because of the implications of a positive result: there is not just the concern of developing AIDS but also the threat to job security and the inability to obtain life insurance or mortgage facilities. Blood Transfusion Services are organized to deal with counselling such donors, whilst busy hospital blood banks and newborn intensive care units are not. Blood that has not been screened for HIV antibodies and found to be negative should never be transfused.

(2) The organization is time-consuming and a variable amount of the control of blood transfusion is unavoidably removed from the transfusion service. Donor and recipient records are less likely to be properly kept; this is very important in the event of an adverse reaction.

(3) Even the best motivated of donors are not always available when needed, especially at weekends or during the night.

Those who advocate the 'walking donor' approach generally list the freshness of the blood and the benefits of heparin over CPD as an anticoagulant in maintaining normal acid–base and electrolyte values. The Blood Transfusion Service should have little difficulty in supplying blood which is reasonably fresh. It is perfectly satisfactory to transfuse blood of this age to the neonate as the K^+ load is not excessive. Blood drawn into CPD will maintain reasonable 2,3DPG levels for the first week to 10 days of storage. The pH of CPD blood is lower than that of heparinized blood but the small volumes transfused will not alter the pH of the infant. Using packed cells, which have had much of the plasma removed, further minimizes the adverse effects of electrolyte and acid–base balance. There are also disadvantages to the use of heparinized blood. Blood drawn straight into a heparinized syringe is of a lower PCV than that of the healthy neonate, but it can be allowed to 'pack' in the syringe before transfusion. This blood is often being given to sick babies who have abnormal coagulation and heparinization compounds the problem. The risk of transmission of CMV is thought to be higher with fresh blood than with stored blood, which is an additional problem with a 'walking donor', if CMV screening is not possible.

In conclusion, CPD blood can be safely used for neonatal transfusion. Ideally the blood should be less than 5 days of age, if available, as its electrolyte content is little deranged. However, the age of blood is much less important for top-up transfusion than for exchange transfusion, and many neonatologists will happily use blood up to 14 days old for the former. The sensitive issue of HIV testing hospital personnel is now a major obstacle in the operation of a 'walking donor' programme. However, such a scheme may have a role to play if the Regional Blood Transfusion Service cannot provide blood suitable for administration to the newborn infant, for example small aliquots of CMV-screened, reasonably fresh packed cells.

Blood grouping and cross-matching for top-up transfusions

The donor cells must be ABO-compatible with the mother and infant. However, many hospital blood banks issue only group O rhesus-compatible blood to neonates for top-up transfusion. This is particularly so where special modifications are being provided, for example CMV-negative blood or a mini-pack system. In this case, the donor serum should have a low titre of ABO isoagglutinins and must have no irregular antibodies. The blood should be rhesus-compatible and need only be rhesus-negative if the baby is rhesus-negative or if the transfusion is for haemolytic disease of the newborn due to rhesus-incompatibility. It is generally accepted that infants are immunologically compromised and do not produce antibodies until 3 months of age at the earliest. Any antibody present has been passively acquired from the mother and is often more readily detected in her serum. It is therefore considered unnecessary to cross-match neonates for simple transfusions until the infant reaches the age of immunocompetence. The British Society for Haematology and the British Blood Transfusion Society recently issued the following guidelines:

> For infants under 4 months, both baby and maternal blood samples should be ABO and Rh D grouped, the maternal serum screened for unexpected antibodies, and a direct AHG test done on the baby's cells. If a negative maternal antibody screen is obtained and the baby's direct AHG test is negative, blood of the same ABO and Rh D group as the infant may be issued without cross-matching, even after repeated transfusions, provided the ABO and Rh D groups of the donor units are checked before issue. Recent studies indicate that infants under the age of 4 months do not make red cell alloantibodies even after multiple transfusions.

This approach is only appropriate for top-up transfusions. Where blood is being provided for neonates with haemolytic disease of the newborn a full cross-match should be carried out for each transfusion. Similarly, infants who receive large transfusions for cardiac surgery should be fully cross-matched for surgery and subsequent transfusions. The British Society of Haematology and the British Blood Transfusion Society recommend the following (Waters *et al.*, 1987):

> If the infant is suffering from haemolytic disease of the newborn (HDN), or if unexpected antibodies are detected in the maternal serum, it is important to use the maternal serum for compatibility testing. This may dictate the use of group O blood, and if the infant is not group O, care should be taken to ensure donor units have low titre anti-A and anti-B. If ABO HDN is suspected, group

O blood of low titre anti-A and anti-B should be used. An alternative to low titre group O blood is O cells reconstituted in one-third volume of AB plasma. In the event of an exchange transfusion, plasma reduced blood is indicated.

GRAFT VERSUS HOST DISEASE

Graft-versus-host-disease (GVHD) has been described in the immunocompromised host following blood transfusion and can be prevented by the irradiation of blood products prior to infusion. The immune mechanism of the neonate is immature, particularly that of the pre-term infant. Although there are several reports of probable GVHD following intra-uterine and exchange transfusion this remains a real rarity (Naiman *et al.*, 1969; Parkmann *et al.*, 1974; Lauer *et al.*, 1982). The routine irradiation of blood products for simple blood transfusion to neonates is not indicated (Blajchman *et al.*, 1984), but blood for IUT should be irradiated as the recipient is of early gestation with an immature immune system. The need for irradiating blood for exchange transfusion is less convincing, but some feel it is justified, particularly in the pre-term infant (Cochran, 1978). It is, however, essential to irradiate all blood products before transfusion to any neonate suspected of being immunodeficient.

NECROTIZING ENTEROCOLITIS

The aetiology of necrotizing enterocolitis (NEC) is still not clearly understood, although it is thought that the interaction of a number of factors are important including:

(1) Disturbance of the mucosal integrity
(2) Presence of pathogenic bacteria
(3) Availability of substrate (e.g. enteral feeding) to promote the growth of bacteria (Eyal *et al.*, 1982).

The integrity of the intestinal mucosa may be breached by a number of events including asphyxia, shock, umbilical catheterization and exchange transfusion. Rogers and Dunn (1969) were the first to note the association between the increased incidence of NEC complicating exchange transfusion and the widespread use of pre-packed gamma-irradiated polyvinyl-chloride (PVC) exchange transfusion kits in place of the previously employed rubber, glass and metal giving sets. The plasticizers used in the treatment of such PVC bags and catheters can leach out and accumulate in the blood during storage. The phthalate ester diethylhexyl phthalate (DEHP) may have toxic effects in the neonate. Studies based on post-mortem evidence have shown that increased concentrations of DEHP are present in the tissues of neonates who have had umbilical catheterization compared with stillborns, with the highest concentrations being found in neonates with NEC (Hillman *et al.*, 1975). Experimental studies have also shown that human umbilical arteries lose their normal physiological responsiveness after perfusion using PVC equipment, which can be restored by using glass, silicone and rubber tubing (Rogers and Dunn, 1969). These data suggest that leached toxic substances in blood may be capable of producing NEC directly by a toxic effect on the intestinal mucosa, or indirectly via damage to the portal vasculature with resultant vasospasm of mesenteric vessels predisposing to necrosis of segments of bowel. Bacterial colonization in the ischaemic bowel wall with anaerobic bacteria may follow. The infusion of packed cells with a haematocrit in excess of 50–55% may result in polycythaemia, and the associated hyperviscosity may be an additional factor in the development of mesenteric thrombosis. Most paediatricians are aware of the association between exchange transfusion and NEC, although lack of knowledge of the precise pathogenesis makes it difficult to evaluate.

INFECTIONS TRANSMITTED BY BLOOD TRANSFUSION

All blood products carry some infectious risk, particularly those products derived from large volumes of pooled plasma. Hepatitis, CMV and HIV can all be transmitted by blood transfusion. All donations of blood in the United Kingdom are now screened for HBsAg and antibodies to HIV. Blood is not routinely screened for CMV, but special categories of patients, including neonates and bone marrow transplant recipients, who are regarded as being at increased risk of acquiring CMV infection, are usually transfused CMV-screened blood if at all possible. Neonates are immunologically compromised and screening of donor blood for potentially transmissible infection deserves special consideration. Blood which has been collected in the routine manner by the Regional Blood Transfusion Service will have undergone strict, standard screening procedures.

HIV infection

Neonates can become infected in two ways; horizontal transmission following transfusion of a contaminated unit of blood or blood product, or vertical transmission whilst *in utero*. The majority of infants infected by transplacental spread have been born to intravenous drug users. It is impossible in the neonate to differentiate true infection from maternally acquired antibody which may persist until 18 months of age. From international studies it would appear that about 25–30% of infants born to HIV antibody-positive mothers are truly infected with the virus. The first case in the USA of transfusion-associated AIDS was reported in 1982. Since October 1985 all donations of blood collected in the United Kingdom by the National Blood Transfusion Service have been screened for antibodies to HIV. From October 1985 to the end of February 1987 approximately 3.7 million donations were tested: 72 were confirmed anti-HIV positive, i.e. 0.002% (Gunson and Rawlinson, 1988). There are problems associated with screening donations. In particular there is a high incidence of false-positive results, and, although from the recipient's viewpoint, this is much more desirable than false negative results, it does involve a great deal of work for the transfusion service. All positive results have to be confirmed and the donor has to be recalled and counselled. False-negative results also occur occasionally. If a donor is tested during the period between infectivity and the development of antibody, he will be antibody-negative but still be capable of transmitting the disease.

Premature infants appear to be at particular risk from transfusion-acquired AIDS, because they are relatively more immunocompromised and are in a group more likely to be transfused. O'Duffy and Isles reported transfusion-associated AIDS in four premature infants with gestational ages of 28–33 weeks, all of whom had received blood from the same donor (O'Duffy and Isles, 1984). The pattern of presentation was similar with persistent moniliasis, failure to thrive, pneumonitis and hepatosplenomegaly. Two of the infants were shown to be HIV antibody-positive. This report highlights several interesting points other than the increased susceptibility of the premature infant. Firstly, three of the four infants were dead within 7 months of the transfusion, which is quite different from the long latent period seen between infection and clinical AIDS in adults. Secondly, the donor was homosexual and subsequently shown to be anti-HIV positive. He would now be excluded by proper screening. Each infant received only a single top-up transfusion; some hospitals would employ a 'walking donor' panel for such transfusions, and it must now be obvious that testing of the blood prior to transfusion is essential. Thirdly, on this occasion, the donation was subdivided into a number of small aliquots. Much is made of the wastage of blood when a whole unit is issued for use to a neonate and most of it discarded. However, if units are to be subdivided, there is an even greater responsibility to ensure that adequate screening has been completed because the potential for spreading infection is increased. Finally, O'Duffy and Isles recommended the use of female donors. Because of heterosexual spread of the virus, this is no longer a safe approach.

Wykoff *et al.* (1985) reported three infants who received blood from a common donor who was HIV-positive. All three infants had antibodies to HIV but demonstrated a spectrum of symptomatology, which is also common in adults infected with the AIDS virus. One infant developed classical AIDS with failure to thrive, pneumocystis, candidiasis, lymphadenopathy and hepatosplenomegaly; the infant died at 14 months of age. The second presented with weight loss, persistent lymphadenopathy and hyperglobulinaemia. The third developed an autoimmune disease with thrombocytopenia and a positive direct Coombs' test and positive antinuclear factor (ANF), in addition to candidiasis, lymph node enlargement and hepatosplenomegaly. This report emphasizes the need to exercise a high degree of suspicion in any infant with a history of blood transfusion in the neonatal period, if symptoms are unusual or response to treatment abnormal. Sadly, tests to exclude HIV-positivity must now be made in any infant presenting with symptomatology suggestive of one of the inherited immunodeficiencies.

Transfusion-associated hepatitis

Since 1974, in the United Kingdom, all donations of blood have been routinely screened for HBsAg. Before then, hepatitis B accounted for 30–40% of transfusion-associated hepatitis. With the introduction of screening the pattern has now changed and non-A, non-B (NANB) hepatitis poses the major problem.

The likelihood of missing hepatitis B antigenaemia on testing depends on which antigens and antibodies are included in the screen. Only HBsAg is routinely tested for in the United Kingdom and some infected units of blood will go undetected. In the natural history of hepatitis B infection there is a convalescent window, which occurs during recovery when HBsAg becomes undetectable and before antibody to surface antigen (anti-HBs) appears. During this time low levels of infectious virus can still be present in the absence of detectable HBsAg. This problem can be overcome by screening for antibody to hepatitis B core antigen (anti-HBc), which rises early during antigenaemia and persists during convalescence and recovery. If neither HBsAg or anti-HBc is present, the donor is unlikely to have been infected.

There are, at present, no well-established specific viral markers for NANB hepatitis. Some centres, particularly in North America have implemented donor screening for alanine aminotransferase (ALT) in an attempt to reduce post-transfusion NANB hepatitis. However, such screening is very expensive. There are many causes of a raised ALT other than NANB hepatitis and the rejection rate of donor blood high when this criteria is employed. Hepatitis C virus (HCV) antibody testing is under assessment and looks promising (van der Poel *et al.*, 1990). However, HCV is not the only cause of NANB hepatitis and therefore screening donor blood for HCV antibodies can at best only reduce, but not eradicate, post-transfusion NANB hepatitis.

Transfusion-associated cytomegalovirus (CMV)

Immunocompromised individuals, particularly kidney and bone marrow recipients, are at particular risk of transfusion-associated CMV infection and it is the special needs of these patients which has prompted renewed interest in this problem. Many include premature, low birth weight infants amongst high-risk recipients (Benson *et al.*, 1979; Yeager *et al.*, 1981; Adler *et al.*, 1984).

There are numerous possible routes by which a neonate may acquire CMV infection and in any one case it is difficult to identify the route responsible. Because of this, the risk of a neonate acquiring CMV infection from a blood transfusion has not been properly defined. CMV infection can be contracted from an individual who is excreting the virus. The virus has been isolated from urine, saliva, stool, tears, breast milk, semen and cervical excretions. Therefore, even in neonates who have been transfused, there are many other potential sources of infection. Yaegar reported on 106 infants with birth weights of less than 1500 g and born to seropositive mothers. Although these infants received blood exclusively from seronegative donors, 18 infants (17%) acquired CMV infection, presumably from maternal sources (Yeager *et al.*,1983).

The morbidity associated with transfusion-acquired CMV infection in neonates has been variably reported. CMV is known to cause pneumonia, hepatitis, thrombocytopenia and haemolytic anaemia in the newborn. Late sequelae include hearing defects and neurological abnormalities. Obviously a neonate excreting virus constitutes a risk to pregnant nursing staff. Yeagar

Table 7.1 Reported incidences and morbidity of transfusion-acquired CMV.

Author	Percentage of infants with acquired CMV		Mean birth weight (g)	Morbidity (%)
	Not transfused	Transfused		
Yaeger (1974)	11 (8/74)	25 (19/77)	2500	—
Tobin *et al.* (1975)	2.2	29*	—	—
Spector *et al.* (1979)	—	14 (13/93)	—	23
Ballard *et al.* (1979)	—	31 (16/51)	1058	—
Yaegar (1981)	—	13.5† (22/164)	2000	50
Rawls *et al.* (1984)	11	18.5	< 2000	—
Adler (1984)	—	28 (7/25)	< 1300—	

* Infants received exchange transfusion only.
† Infants of seronegative mothers only.

and colleagues (1981) reported serious or fatal symptoms in 50% of premature infants with transfusion-acquired CMV infection, who had seronegative mothers and lacked transplacentally acquired antibody. Premature infants of seropositive mothers did not develop symptomatology that could be definitely attributed to acquired CMV infection. However, few studies deal with the outcome of infected infants.

Table 7.1 lists the reported incidences of transfusion-acquired CMV with the morbidity, if stated, from several large studies. Interpretation is difficult and comparison impossible because the study conditions are very variable and not at all standardized. Few state the serological status of the mother and infant at birth or of the donor units. Furthermore, techniques for studying seroconversion and virus isolation vary. Details of other possible routes of infection are often omitted and the incidence of viral excretion in non-transfused neonates is not always available for comparison. With these reservations, it does appear that neonates who are transfused are more likely to acquire CMV infection than infants who are not transfused. Those infants most at risk are premature infants of low birth weight, who are also the group most likely to receive multiple transfusions. If blood of unknown CMV status is issued, the risk of transfusion-associated CMV increases with the number of units of blood given to the infant.

The risk of acquiring CMV infection from blood transfusion varies with the donor population, the type of blood product and the age of the blood. Throughout the world there is a marked variation in the prevalence of CMV antibody, from 40 to 100% of the adult population. Industrial countries have a lower incidence of seropositivity than underdeveloped countries. Blood products that are heavily contaminated with granulocytes, especially granulocyte transfusions, carry the highest risk and fresh blood carries a higher risk than stored blood.

Several studies have shown that transfusion-associated CMV infection can be prevented in neonates, if they are transfused only with blood from seronegative donors (Yeager *et al.*, 1981; Adler *et al.*, 1983). This would appear to be particularly important for infants born to seronegative mothers, because they are the infants with acquired CMV infection associated morbidity (Yeager *et al.*, 1981). Unfortunately, the CMV status of the mother is often not known. In order to be sure of not exposing susceptible infants to seropositive blood, it may be necessary to transfuse all infants with CMV-screened blood. To incorporate CMV screening into blood banking is an expensive and time-consuming exercise and it might be done most economically by subdividing units of seronegative blood into small aliquots for neonatal purposes — already the practice in some Regional Blood Transfusion Centres.

PREVENTION OF PERINATALLY TRANSMITTED HEPATITIS B INFECTION

Although the majority of infants who become HBsAg–positive are asymptomatic, the carrier state is strongly associated with the development of chronic active hepatitis, cirrhosis and primary hepatocellular carcinoma. The prevalence of the carrier state and the risk of infection varies from country to country. The carrier state is low (0.1%) in Northern Europe, North America and Australia, approaches 5% in Eastern Europe, the Mediterranean, Central America and parts of South America, and reaches 15–20% in South East Asia. More than 90% of adults clear a *de novo* hepatitis B virus (HBV) infection. The perpetuation of the carrier state is thought to be due to perinatal vertical transmission, the mother having acquired her infection in childhood. Several facts have been established about the transmission and risk of infection with HBV.

(1) Transmission of the virus probably occurs around the time of birth and is thought to be due to maternal-fetal haemorrhage during labour and delivery. Probably only 5–10% of carrier infants are infected *in utero*. The virus does not cross the placenta and therefore intra-uterine infection is rare and when it happens can best be explained by maternal-fetal haemorrhage *in utero*. The evidence for perinatal transmission is two-fold. Firstly, the serological data is consistent with this. HBsAg and HBeAg are detected in the cord sera of only a very small percentage of babies born to HBsAg-positive mothers, and in such cases cord blood titres are usually low and probably reflect contamination by maternal-fetal leakage occurring during labour or delivery. Secondly, hepatitis B immunoglobulin (HBIg) alone is effective in preventing the carrier state in approximately 70% of at risk neonates and is equally effective in cord blood negative and cord blood positive infants. If HBsAg or HBeAg in the cord blood represented *in utero* infection, HBIg would be ineffective since it has no value in elimination of the chronic HBsAg carrier state. In areas of high carrier rates, especially amongst Chinese, approximately 20–40% acquire the infection perinatally. In Africa vertical transmission is low and more infants are infected horizontally later in childhood.

(2) HBeAg is a measure of high infectivity, and it is the presence of HBeAg and HBV-DNA in the mother's serum which determines the risk to the fetus. About 90% of infants born to mothers with HBeAg will become infected and the majority will become carriers. The incidence of HBeAg positivity amongst HBsAg positive mothers has considerable geographical

variation. In South East Asia 30–50% of HBsAg mothers are also HBeAg positive. Infants born to mothers who develop acute hepatitis B during the third trimester or within 2 months of delivery are also at increased risk. The risk of perinatal infection for these infants is approximately 70% and most will become persistent carriers.

A number of studies have provided the information required to best prevent the perinatal transmission of HBV. Beasley and colleagues demonstrated that the administration of HBIg at birth, 3 months and 6 months of age protected 75% of babies born to HBeAg-positive mothers (Beasley *et al.*, 1981). These infants were followed up until 15 months of age and did not become chronic carriers. Even a single dose of HBIg given at birth prevented persistent antigenaemia in 45% of at risk infants. The carrier rate was 91% for the placebo group. Anti-HBs could be detected in the sera of many of the HBIg-treated babies at a time when passively acquired antibody should have been cleared. This suggests that HBIg protects the infant by delaying viral replication until active immunity develops when the baby becomes immunocompetent. The timing of the administration of HBIg is important. HBIg should be given within a few hours of birth and the protection is lost if administration is delayed beyond 48 hours.

Those infants born to HBeAg-positive mothers will remain at high risk from horizontal transmission because of continuing exposure from their mothers and other HBV positive contacts. Short-term passive immunization cannot protect against this. Approximately 25% of infants who receive HBIg fail prophylaxis and become chronic carriers. An additional 20% who appear to be protected as neonates become infected later by horizontal transmission when their anti-HBs levels fall. Beasley and his co-workers demonstrated that HBV vaccination given at birth, one month and 6 months was as protective as multiple HBIg doses (Beasley *et al.*, 1981, 1983). The dual approach of passive and active immunization has been shown to be the most effective at eradicating the high failure rate associated with the use of HBIg or vaccination alone. This combined approach has been demonstrated in a number of studies to be effective in protecting more than 90% of infants at high risk. The infant's antibody response to vaccination is uninhibited by the presence of passive antibodies. When HBIg is given at birth, the timing of the start of vaccination may not be important but for maximal compliance it is easiest to give the first dose of vaccine during the confinement.

The trials reported here employed a licensed plasma-derived vaccine. This HBV vaccine is made by harvesting only the excess surface antigen protein coat of the virus (non-infectious 22 nm HBsAg particles) from the plasma of asymptomatic HBsAg-positive carriers. After purification and inactivation, the vaccine is safe, efficient and highly immunogenic. Neonates show an excellent immune response which is not compromised by the presence of circulating immunoglobulins. The vaccine has not been associated with transmission of AIDS or other infectious agents. However, vaccines in current use have been produced by recombinant DNA techniques in eukaryotic cells, particularly yeast. They appear to be safe, antigenic and free from side-effects.

Two large studies have provided evidence for the efficacy of a dual approach. Beasley and his co-workers reported on 243 infants born to HBeAg mothers in Taiwan. Seventy-four out of eighty-four (88%) infants who received no treatment developed persistent HBs antigenaemia in the first 6 months of life. One hundred and fifty-nine infants were treated with 3 different HBIg/vaccine schedules. Only nine infants (5.7%) became chronically infected giving an overall protection rate for combined treatment with HBIg and vaccine of 93.6% (Beasley *et al.*, 1983). Antibodies developed in all infants who did not become antigenaemic. Wong and co-workers reported on 140 infants born to HBeAg mothers and followed up for 6 months (Wong *et al.*, 1984). These infants were randomised to receive one of four schedules: (1) vaccine only, (2) placebo only, (3) vaccine + one dose of HBIg, (4) vaccine + multiple doses of HBIg. The rate of development of a persistent carrier state was high (73.2%) for the placebo group. However, more than 90% of infants in both groups receiving combination therapy were protected, confirming that a combined approach is very efficacious. In this study, multiple doses had no statistical advantage over single doses of immunoglobulin. Furthermore, even repeated doses of HBIg did not interfere with the anti-HBs response of the vaccine.

The work of these groups has demonstrated several important points:

(1) Infants born to HBeAg-positive mothers should receive both passive and active immunization with HBIg and HBV vaccine. This should be initiated as soon after birth as possible and prophylaxis should be extended to babies born to mothers who are HBsAg-positive and HBe antibody negative.

(2) Infants born to HBsAg-positive, HBeAg-negative mothers in endemic areas and/or where the lifetime risk of exposure is high should also be treated.

(3) It could be recommended that, ideally, infants born to all HBsAg-positive mothers including these with e antibody, should be vaccinated, although it is appreciated that the risk of perinatal infection in this group is very small. However, unless these children are immunized they are at continuing risk of infection by horizontal transmission later in life.

(4) Caesarean section may reduce the incidence of infection but does not fully protect, and infants so delivered should also receive prophylaxis (Lee *et al.*, 1988).

(5) At present, if vaccination is started at birth, there is no statistically significant advantage of multiple over a single dose of HBIg.

(6) In countries with low carrier rates for HBeAg mothers who are in high risk groups should be screened, for example immigrants from endemic areas, drug addicts, patients receiving multiple transfusions of blood products, chronic haemodialysis patients, and mothers with occupational exposure and household contacts.

Infants born to HBeAg-positive mothers should receive:

(a) 50 i.u. kg^{-1} HBIg (approximately 0.5 ml kg^{-1}) and 20 μg HBV vaccine (Engerix B), both given within 4 hours of birth at different sites.

(b) Booster doses of HBV vaccine at 1 and 6 months of age.

At 6 months of age blood samples should be taken for hepatitis B marker studies to establish adequate protection.

HBIg given at birth does not appear to interfere with DTP immunization given in infancy. It may well be possible to employ smaller doses of vaccine without affecting the antibody response. However, the information on newborns of HBsAg and HBeAg positive mothers is limited because reported clinical trials have employed different doses, schedules and brands of vaccine. Enormous savings could be made by reducing the dose of vaccine, and this is of tremendous importance to the countries where the problem is greatest.

FRESH FROZEN PLASMA

Fresh frozen plasma (FFP) is prepared by separating plasma from whole blood within 6 hours of donation and then freezing the separated plasma. It contains all the procoagulant factors and may be transfused to a neonate for two basic reasons. Firstly, it may be given to correct a coagulopathy of any aetiology. Secondly, ABO-compatible FFP may be used to resuspend packed red cells before transfusion if volume expansion is required. The volume of FFP given for correction of a coagulopathy is small, i.e. 10–15 ml kg^{-1}. If plasma can be subdivided into small aliquots before freezing, wastage is minimized. Group-specific plasma should be used whenever possible. If the infant's blood group is not known or group-specific plasma not available, group A plasma should be infused as it will be compatible with almost 90% of recipients.

PLATELET TRANSFUSION

Neonates may receive platelet transfusions to arrest or prevent bleeding secondary to thrombocytopenia. One unit of platelet concentrate is enough to raise the infant's platelet count to a level sufficient to stop haemorrhage. Ideally, the platelets should be rhesus-compatible whenever possible, particularly for female neonates. However, although platelet concentrates are contaminated by small amounts of red cells, the risk of sensitization in the immune incompetent neonate is theoretical rather than real.

Platelets should also ideally be ABO-specific. However, many hospitals are supplied only with group O platelets by their Regional Blood Transfusion Centre. Those who advocate the transfusion of ABO-specific platelets are concerned that the plasma from an ABO-incompatible donor may cause red cell haemolysis. This is obviously dependent on the volume of plasma in which the platelets are suspended and the problem can be overcome by preparing them in a reduced volume of plasma. It is more important to transfuse platelets to the neonate which have been screened for hepatitis, CMV and HIV than to be primarily concerned with ABO specificity. This requirement can often only be met by the exclusive use of group O platelets. The use of ABO specific platelets may mean sacrificing CMV negativity, and this is not justified.

ALBUMIN

Human albumin solution, 4.5%, may be used to resuscitate neonates in shock due to sepsis or acute blood loss. Albumin can be given promptly to restore the circulating fluid volume until blood is available for transfusion. Albumin carries no risk of transmitting viral infection.

GRANULOCYTES

Bacterial sepsis is a major cause of morbidity and mortality in the newborn period. Severe neonatal sepsis with organisms such as group B streptococcus may result in profound neutropenia. This further compromises the neonate with co-existing impaired neutrophil function. The neutropenia may result from a reduction of granulocyte stem cells and reserves of mature granulocytes in the bone marrow such that, when infection develops, neutrophil production from stem cells may be limited. These infants may benefit from transfusion of white cells in addition to appropriate antibiotic therapy (Christensen *et al.*, 1982). Laurenti claims benefit from granulocyte transfusion in non-neutropenic, seriously ill neonates with antibiotic-resistant Gram-negative septicaemia (Laurenti *et al.*, 1981). Because of the small number of granulocytes required for a neonate, they can be prepared from freshly collected units of whole blood using an automated blood processor, without the need to leucapherese a donor. Granulocytes prepared in this manner appear to function normally (Goldfinger *et al.*, 1983). Granulocyte transfusions are more likely to produce GVHD than any other blood product and should be irradiated to 1500 rad before transfusion to the sick premature neonate. The donor should also be known to be hepatitis B-, CMV- and HIV-negative.

SUMMARY

The pattern of neonatal transfusion has changed. With the decrease in haemolytic disease of the newborn, fewer intra-uterine and exchange transfusions are required. However, due to outstanding advances in neonatology, large numbers of tiny premature infants are surviving and requiring multiple small volume transfusions and blood product support. The hospital blood bank has to gear itself towards providing safe products of appropriate volume in the most efficient way.

REFERENCES

Adler SP, Chandrika T, Lawrence L and Baggett J (1983) Cytomegalovirus infections in neonates acquired by blood transfusions. *Pediatric Infectious Disease* **2**: 114–118.

Adler SP, Lawrence LT, Baggett J *et al.* (1984) Prevention of transfusion-associated cytomegalovirus infection in very low-birthweight infants using frozen blood

and donors seronegative for cytomegalovirus. *Transfusion* **24**: 333–335.
Ballard RA, Drew WL, Hufnagle KG and Reidel PA (1979) Acquired cytomegalovirus infection in preterm infants. *American Journal of Diseases of Children* **133**: 482–485.
Beasley RP, Hwang LY, Lin CC *et al.* (1981) Hepatitis B immune globulin (HBIG) efficacy in the interruption of perinatal transmission of hepatitis B virus carrier state. Initial report of a randomised double-blind placebo-controlled trial. *The Lancet* **2**: 388–393.
Beasley RP, Hwang LY, Lee GC *et al.* (1983) Prevention of perinatally transmitted hepatitis B virus infections with hepatitis B immune globulin and hepatitis B vaccine. *The Lancet* **2**: 1099–1102.
Benson JW, Bodden SJ and Tobin JO (1979) Cytomegalovirus and blood transfusion in neonates. *Archives of Disease in Childhood* **54**: 538–541.
Blajchman MA, Sheridan D and Rawls WE (1984) Risks associated with blood transfusion in newborn infants. *Perinatology* **11**: 403–415.
Boggs TR and Westphal MC (1960) Mortality of exchange transfusion. *Pediatrics* **26**: 745–755.
Bowman JM, Chown B, Lewis M and Pollock JM (1978) Rh-issoimmunization during pregnancy: antenatal prophylaxis. *Canadian Medical Association Journal* **118**: 623–627.
Bursaux E, Freminet A, Brossard Y and Poyart CF (1973) Exchange transfusion in the neonate with ACD or CPD stored blood. *Biology of the Neonate* **23**: 123–132.
Chaplin H Jr, Cohen R, Bloomberg G and Kaplan HJ (1973) Pregnancy and idiopathic autoimmune haemolytic anaemia: a prospective study during 6 months gestation and 3 months post partum. *British Journal of Haematology* **24**: 219–229.
Christensen RD, Anstall HB and Rothstein G (1982) Review: Deficiencies in the neutrophil system of newborn infants, and the use of leukocyte transfusions in the treatment of neonatal sepsis. *Journal of Clinical Aphersis* **1**: 33–41.
Clarke CA, Mollison PL and Whitfield AG (1987) Deaths from Rh haemolytic disease in England and Wales in 1984 and 1985. *British Medical Journal* **294**: 1001.
Cochran WD (1978) Increasing safety of exchange transfusion. *Pediatric Research* **12**: 462.
Eldor A, Yatziv S, Hershko (1975) Relapsing Coombs-negative haemolytic anaemia in pregnancy with haemolytic disease in the newborn. *British Medical Journal* **4**: 625.
Eyal F, Sagi E, Arad I, Avital A (1982) Necrotising enterocolitis in the very low birthweight infant: expressed breast milk feeding compared with parenteral feeding. *Archives of Diseases in Childhood* **57**: 274–276.
Gabra GS, Frame D and Blue A (1983) Antenatal anti-D immunoglobulin. *The Lancet* **2**: 734.
Goldfinger D, Medici MA and Hsi R *et al.* (1983) Preparation and in vitro function of granulocyte concentrates for transfusion to neonates using the IBM 2991 blood processor. *Transfusion* **23**: 358–360.
Gunson HH and Rawlinson VI (1988) HIV antibody screening of blood donations in the United Kingdom. *Vox Sanguinis* **54**: 34–38.
Hillman LS, Goodwin SL, Sherman WR (1975) Identification and measurement of plasticizer in neonatal tissues after umbilical catheters and blood products. *New England Journal of Medicine* **292**: 381–386.
Koenig JM and Christensen RD (1989) Neutropenia and thrombocytopenia in infants with Rh haemolytic disease. *Journal of Pediatrics* **114**: 625–631.
Laurenti F, Ferro R, Isacchi G (1981). Polymorphonuclear leukocyte transfusion for the treatment of sepsis in the newborn infant. *Journal of Pediatrics* **98**: 118–123.
Lauer BA, Githens JH, Hayward AR *et al.* (1982) Probable graft-vs-graft reaction in an infant after exchange transfusion and marrow transplantation. *Pediatrics* **70**: 43–47.
Lee SD, Lo KJ, Tsai YT *et al.* (1988) Role of caesarean section in prevention of mother–infant transmission of hepatitis B virus. *The Lancet* **2**: 833–834.

Naiman JL, Punnett HH, Lischner HW *et al.* (1969) Possible graft-versus-host reaction after intrauterine transfusion for Rh erythroblastosis fetalis. *New England Journal of Medicine* **281**: 697–701.

O'Duffy JF and Isles AF (1984) Transfusion-induced AIDS in four premature babies. *The Lancet* **2**: 1346.

Parkman R, Mosier D, Umansky I *et al.* (1974) Graft-versus-host disease after intrauterine and exchange transfusions for haemolytic disease of the newborn. *New England Journal of Medicine* **290**: 359–363.

Phillips HM, Holland BM, Abdel-Moiz A *et al.* (1986) Determination of red cell mass in assessment and management of anaemia in babies needing blood transfusion. *The Lancet* **1**: 882–884.

Placzek MM and Gorst DW (1987) T activiation haemolysis and death after blood transfusion. *Archives of Disease in Childhood* **62**: 743–744.

Rawls WE, Wong CL, Blajchman M *et al.* (1984) Neonatal cytomegalovirus infections: the relative role of neonatal blood transfusion and maternal exposure. *Clinical and Investigative Medicine* **7**: 13–19.

Rogers AF and Dunn RM (1969) Intestinal perforation, exchange transfusion and P.V.C. *The Lancet* **2**: 1246.

Spector SA, Schmidt K, Ticknor W and Grossman M (1979) Cytomegalovirus in older infants in intensive care nurseries. *Journal of Pediatrics* **95**: 444–446.

Tobin JO'H, MacDonald H and Brayshay M (1975) Cytomegalovirus infection and exchange transfusion. *British Medical Journal* **4**: 404.

Tovey LA, Townley A, Stevenson BJ and Taverner J (1983) The Yorkshire antenatal anti-D immunoglobulin trial in primigravidae. *The Lancet* **2**: 244–246.

van der Poel CL, Reesink HW, Schaasberg W (1990) Infectivity of blood seropositive for hepatitis C virus antibodies. *The Lancet* **335**: 558–560.

Waters AH, Boulton FE, Bruce M *et al.* (1987) Guidelines for compatibility testing in hospital blood banks. A joint publication of the British Society for Haematology and the Blood Transfusion Service. *Clinical and Laboratory Haematology* **9**: 333–341.

Wong VC, Ip HM, Reesink HW *et al.* (1984) Prevention of the HBsAg carrier state in newborn infants of mothers who are chronic carriers of HBsAg and HBeAg by administration of hepatitis B vaccine and hepatitis B immunoglobulin. Double-blind randomised placebo-controlled study. *The Lancet* **1**: 921–926.

Wykoff RF, Pearl ER and Saulsbury FT (1985) Immunologic dysfunction in infants infected through transfusion with HTLVIII. *New England Journal of Medicine* **312**: 294–296.

Yam P, Wilkinson L, Petz LD and Garratty G (1980) Studies on haemolytic anaemia in pregnancy with evidence of autoimmunisation in a patient with a negative direct antiglobulin (Coombs) test. *American Journal of Haematology* **8**: 23–29.

Yeager AS (1974) Transfusion-acquired cytomegalovirus in newborn infants. *American Journal of Diseases of Children* **128**: 478–483.

Yeager AS, Grumet FC, Hafleigh EB *et al.* (1981) Prevention of transfusion-acquired cytomegalovirus infections in newborn infants. *Journal of Pediatrics* **98**: 281–287.

Yeager AS, Palumbo PE, Malachowski N *et al.* (1983) Sequelae of maternally derived cytomegalovirus infections in premature infants. *Journal of Pediatrics* **102**: 918–922.

8

Inherited disorders

B.E.S. Gibson

Royal Hospital for Sick Children and Queen Mother's Maternity Hospital, Glasgow

Inherited blood disorders may affect the production, survival or function of red cells, white cells, platelets and coagulation factors. Many of these problems are dealt with in other chapters of this book and therefore are not covered here. Some disorders, although inherited, do not present until after the first year of life, and these too are excluded from this chapter, which concentrates only on those inherited blood diseases that are known to present in the neonatal period. Some of these occur as an isolated haematological problem, whilst others are associated with congenital anomalies and form a well-defined clinical syndrome. I have attempted to divide them according to the cell line affected, but there is much overlap. For example, many inherited anaemias are also characterized by thrombocytopenia. In such cases the disorder will be classified according to the cell line predominantly affected in the neonatal period. A number of neutropenias co-exist with lymphopenia and others demonstrate an abnormality of neutrophil function. In such cases, the disorder will be classified according to the predominant characteristic.

INHERITED ANAEMIAS

Anaemia in the neonatal period may result from either impaired red cell production or increased red cell destruction. Impaired red cell production is an unusual cause of anaemia in the newborn and, at this age, is nearly always hereditary and not acquired. Although rare, Diamond–Blackfan syndrome is the commonest cause. Transcobalamin II deficiency and, very rarely, congenital dyserythropoietic anaemia also present in the first months of life. Increased red cell destruction may or may not result in anaemia, depending on the bone marrow's ability to compensate by increasing red cell production, but the newborn's immature liver has a limited ability to conjugate bilirubin and even mild haemolysis may produce icterus. The destruction of 1 g of haemoglobin results in the production of 35 μmol of bilirubin. Therefore, in the neonate, increased red cell destruction is generally associated with jaundice and variable degrees of anaemia. Hereditary disorders of the red cell membrane, red cell enzymes and haemoglobin synthesis may all present as a congenital haemolytic anaemia.

Impaired red cell production

Diamond–Blackfan syndrome

In 1938, Diamond and Blackfan described the syndrome that now bears their names and has the characteristic bone marrow findings of a complete or virtually complete absence of red cell precursors, whilst the granulocytic and megakaryocytic series remain normal. This rare disorder is known by a number of other terms including congenital pure red cell aplasia, erythrogenesis imperfecta and, most commonly, congenital hypoplastic anaemia. Approximately 75% of the reported cases appear to be sporadic, the remainder being familial. Both autosomal recessive and autosomal dominant forms have been described. Caucasians are most commonly, but not exclusively, affected. Anaemia is present in 25% of patients at birth. In the remainder the onset of the anaemia is insidious, 65 and 90% being affected by 6 months and 1 year, respectively (Alter and Nathan, 1979). Presentation after the first year of life is rare. The male:female ratio is 1.2:1.0.

Congenital malformations are found in 25–30% of affected infants. Short stature is particularly common, although this may not be apparent in the newborn period. The most common abnormality at birth involves the thumb (10% of reported cases), which may be either triphalangeal or duplicated. Other reported defects include cleft lip and palate, peculiar facies (two-coloured hair, snub nose, thick upper lip and wide-set eyes; Figure 8.1), ptosis, blue sclerae, cataracts, microphthalmia, retinopathy, short or webbed neck and ventricular septal defects. Hyocalcaemia and hypogammaglobulin-aemia have also been reported.

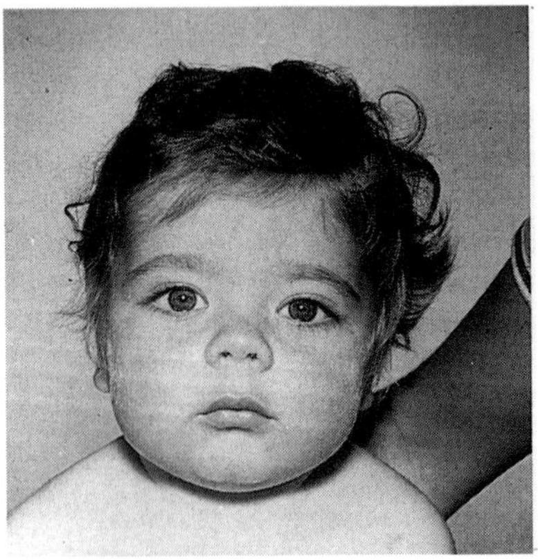

Figure 8.1 Facies of a child with Diamond–Blackfan anaemia showing snub nose, wide-set eyes and short neck (with permission of Salford Health Authority).

The classical laboratory findings include a normochromic, usually macrocytic, anaemia without an appropriate reticulocyte response in the presence of a normal white cell and platelet count. The mean corpuscular volume (MCV) is elevated for the gestational age and the macrocytosis persists even after a haematological remission is achieved. Fetal red cell characteristics continue past the normal period including the presence of 'i' antigen and raised levels of glucose-6-phosphate dehydrogenase (G6PD), glyceraldehyde-3-phosphate dehydrogenase and lactate dehydrogenase and increased HbF. These findings are, however, non-specific and they are not diagnostically helpful when presentation is in the immediate newborn period. The reticulocytopenia excludes haemolysis and points to a disorder of red cell production. The diagnosis is confirmed by the characteristic bone marrow findings of an absence or marked reduction of red cell precursors, with normal numbers of myeloid precursors and megakaryocytes. Vacuolation of the erythroid cells in the bone marrow has been reported.

The pathogenesis of the aplasia in this disorder has not been well identified and heterogeneity may exist. A defective microenvironment, abnormal red cell precursors and humoral or T-lymphocyte induced inhibition have all been implicated. Several facts concerning the erythropoiesis in Diamond–Blackfan anaemia have been established, whilst others remain very controversial. The aplasia is not due to a deficiency, quantitative or qualitative, of erythropoietin as levels of this hormone are increased in the plasma and urine. Antibodies to erythropoietin have not been identified, although there have been various reports of both serum- and cell-mediated inhibition of erythropoiesis. The existence of a serum inhibitor was initially reported by Ortega (Ortega *et al.*, 1975), but later refuted by other workers (Freedman *et al.*, 1975, 1976; Geller *et al.*, 1975). Similarly, investigators (Hoffman *et al.*, 1976) have detected evidence of cellular inhibition, but again T-lymphocyte induced inhibition of *in vitro* erythroid colony growth has not been a consistent finding. These descrepancies may reflect a heterogeneity of pathogenesis in the disorder. A defect in the erythroid progenitor cell is currently favoured, and erythroid culture experiments have shown an absence or decrease in numbers of erythroid colony forming units (CFU-E) and erythroid burst forming units (BFU-E) in patients with Diamond–Blackfan anaemia compared with normal individuals.

It is important that the diagnosis of Diamond–Blackfan syndrome is made as early as possible because prompt treatment with steroids may be required to achieve a response. Although steroid therapy is associated with improvement in approximately two-thirds of cases, Diamond reported the response to be better if there was only a short interval between the onset of anaemia and the instigation of steroid therapy (Diamond *et al.*, 1961). Variability of response may well reflect differences in pathogenesis rather than the importance of early therapeutic intervention. Prednisolone should be started at a dose of 2 mg kg^{-1} per day in three divided doses. If a response is obtained, it will generally happen within 1–4 weeks. The steroid dose should then be slowly tapered to the minimum that will maintain the haemoglobin. Many steroid-responsive children can be maintained on extremely small doses of corticosteroids. For those unresponsive to steroid therapy, regular transfusions will be necessary, with the risk of transfusion-related haemosiderosis unless intensive subcutaneous desferrioxamine can prevent this complication. Androgens have no proven role. Spontaneous remissions have been reported and steroid-unresponsive children successfully treated by bone marrow transplantation. Preliminary studies show that recombinant cytokines may be of value in steroid-unresponsive cases.

Hereditary transcobalamin II deficiency

Transcobalamin II is a β globulin that facilitates the absorption, transport and entry into cells of vitamin B_{12}. Deficiency of transcobalamin II is inherited as an autosomal recessive trait and results in an inability to transfer vitamin B_{12} into cells, giving the typical clinical picture of vitamin B_{12} deficiency. As transcobalamin I is present in normal amounts in these infants, serum vitamin B_{12} concentrations are normal, despite the presence of frank megaloblastosis.

Infants with transcobalamin II deficiency present with failure to thrive and diarrhoea. Anaemia becomes apparent in the first month of life and progresses to pancytopenia. Neurological complications can result. The bone marrow is hypercellular with frank megaloblastic features. The absence of anaemia at birth suggests that vitamin B_{12} transport has occurred normally *in utero*, and proposed mechanisms include a fetal type of transcobalamin, which normally disappears after the first few weeks of life, or transplacental transfer of maternal transcobalamin II. Transcobalamin II deficiency is usually associated with absence of the protein, but a functionally abnormal protein has also been described.

Treatment is with regular doses of vitamin B_{12}, as much as 1000 or 2000 μg weekly or twice weekly being recommended. Unbound vitamin B_{12}, when given at such a dosage, presumably enters cells by passive diffusion.

Congenital dyserythropoietic anaemia

The term 'congenital dyserythropoietic anaemia' was coined in 1968 by Heimpel and Wendt and now describes a group of hereditary disorders characterized by ineffective erythropoiesis. Congenital dyserythropoietic anaemia has been subclassified according to morphological features of the erythroid precursors in the bone marrow and specific serological tests. However, considerable overlap between subtypes is well recognized. Table 8.1 outlines the characteristics of the various subtypes presenting in the neonatal period.

Type II is by far the most common and merits special mention. It is commonly known by the acronym 'HEMPAS' — hereditary erythroblast multinuclearity with positive acidified serum lysis test. The red cells in this subtype are haemolysed by some acidified normal sera. The erythrocytes possess a specific surface antigen sensitive to lysis by an IgM anti-HEMPAS antibody, which is present in the sera of about 30% of normal people in sufficient amounts to induce lysis. This acidified serum haemolysis (Ham's) test is positive in only two conditions: congenital dyserythropoietic anaemia

Table 8.1 Characteristics of congenital dyserythropoietic anaemias.*

	Type I	Type II (HEMPAS)	Type III
Inheritance	Autosomal recessive	Autosomal recessive	Autosomal dominant
Age at diagnosis (range)	Birth to 32 years	Birth to 30 years	2 months to 72 years
Red cell morphologic features	Macrocytosis anisopoikilocytosis	Anisopoikilocytosis	Macrocytosis
Marrow erythroid features	Megaloblastic changes, internuclear chromatin bridges	Binuclearity, multinuclearity, karyorrhexis, pluripolar mitoses	Gigantoblasts, multi-nuclearity
Electron microscopy	Non-specific	Non-specific, 'double' cytoplasmic membrane	Non-specific
Serologic tests			
Acid haemolysis	Negative	Positive	Negative
Anti-I agglutination	Normal	Positive	Positive
Anti-i agglutination	Normal	Positive	Positive

* Adapted from Miller and Baehner, 1989, *Blood Diseases of Infancy and Childhood*, 5th edn: with permission of C.V. Mosby Company.

type II and paroxysmal nocturnal haemoglobinuria (PNH). HEMPAS can be distinguished from PNH by a negative sucrose lysis test and the absence of lysis (which occurs in PNH) by the patient's own acidified serum.

Despite the congenital nature of this disorder, diagnosis in the neonatal period is rare and is usually delayed until at least the second decade of life. If symptoms are present in the neonate they result from anaemia and hyperbilirubinaemia. The anaemia is variable in severity and the hyperbilirubinaemia due to an increase in unconjugated bilirubin. Hepatosplenomegaly may be present. The laboratory findings include an anaemia with an inappropriately low reticulocyte count. Increased unconjugated bilirubin and urobilingogen are evidence of increased red cell destruction. The low reticulocyte count is helpful in distinguishing this condition from causes of haemolytic anaemia in the neonatal period, which are associated with an appropriate reticulocyte response.

The specific red cell morphological features are given in Table 8.1. The erythrocytes of older patients retain features of fetal erythropoiesis including glycolytic enzymes in the same range as those of cord cells, an increased level of HbF, the γ-chain glycine:alanine ratio of fetal blood, the presence of 'i' antigen and a cord-blood lactic dehydrogenase isoenzyme pattern. These features are not specific but are seen in many dyserythropoietic states or refractory anaemias and are obviously not diagnostically helpful in the newborn period. Isotopic studies have shown the ferrokinetic pattern of dyserythropoiesis and a normal to moderately decreased red cell survival. The bone marrow findings are characteristic and include marked erythroid hyperplasia, binuclearity, multinuclearity and internuclear bridging (Figure 8.2). Distinguishing serological features are seen in types II and III congenital dyserythropoietic anaemia. The red cells in patients with both

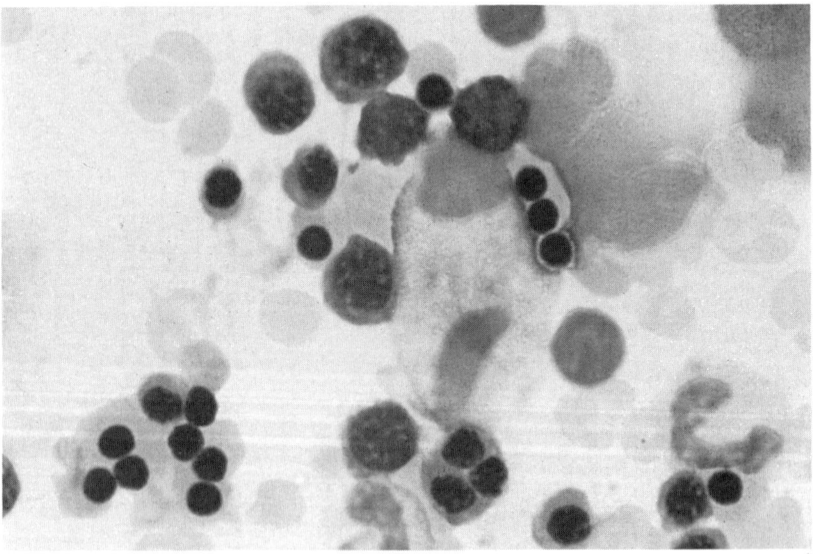

Figure 8.2 Characteristic bone marrow findings in congenital dyserythropoietic anaemia showing megaloblastic changes, binuclearity and multinuclearity.

these subtypes agglutinate and lyse with both anti-I and anti-i sera. The acidified serum lysis test is however only positive in type II.

The pathogenesis of congenital dyserythropoietic anaemia has not been established, although a variety of biochemical disturbances and defects of both the nuclear and plasma membranes have been described. Impaired DNA synthesis has been reported and electron microscopic studies have demonstrated a number of anomalies of the nuclear membrane, which might result in abnormalities in protein synthesis. A defect in the cytoplasmic membrane has been suggested by the presence of the HEMPAS antigen and increased agglutination with anti-i and anti-I sera.

There is no specific treatment, and corticosteroids and haematinics have no role. Transfusion may be necessary if the anaemia is sufficiently severe, but few patients are transfusion-dependent.

Anaemia due to bone marrow failure is recognized in a number of other familial disorders, including Fanconi's anaemia and dyskeratosis congenita. However, in these disorders, the onset is delayed until after the neonatal period.

Increased red cell destruction

A haemolytic process is characterized by shortening of the normal adult red blood cell (RBC) lifespan of 100–120 days. By this definition, virtually all term infants (RBC lifespan 60–80 days) suffer from haemolysis. The classical triad of anaemia, reticulocytosis and hyperbilirubinaemia is more variable in the neonate and, in particular, jaundice is more commonly the presenting feature. Congenital defects of the red cell associated with haemolysis fall into three groups: membrane defects, abnormalities of haemoglobin synthesis and enzyme abnormalities.

Hereditary red cell membrane defects

A number of the hereditary red cell membrane defects may present in the neonatal period. All are associated with morphological abnormalities of the red cell, which presumably reflect abnormalities of the cell membrane structure and function. In many instances the primary molecular defects have not been identified and indeed a specific red cell morphological abnormality appears to be the end product of a variety of molecular defects, which only have in common their localization in the cytoskeleton.

Hereditary spherocytosis. Hereditary spherocytosis (HS) is morphologically characterized by spherocytic red cells that have no central pallor because they have lost their biconcave disc shape (Figure 8.3). The cells are abnormally fragile under osmotic stress and susceptible to extravascular haemolysis in the spleen. In approximately 80% of affected individuals the inheritance of this disorder is clearly autosomal dominant, the remainder representing new mutations or an autosomal recessive form. HS is the commonest haemolytic anaemia in people of Northern European descent, in

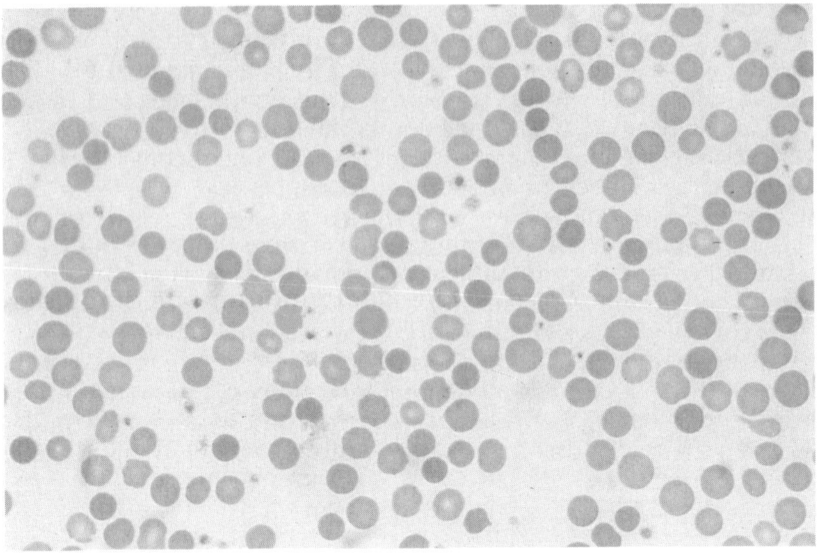

Figure 8.3 Peripheral smear of a patient with hereditary spherocytosis.

whom the incidence is 1:5000. Blacks and other racial groups are infrequently affected.

The characteristic triad of symptoms are anaemia, unconjugated hyperbilirubinaemia and splenomegaly. Hereditary spherocytosis is commonly symptomatic in the neonatal period, and a history of neonatal jaundice may be found in 50% of affected individuals. The haemolysis results in elevated levels of unconjugated bilirubin, the increment depending on the ability of the newborn's immature liver to conjugate the increased bilirubin load presented to it. The resulting degree of jaundice varies from mild to sufficiently severe to cause kernicterus. Jaundice is usually apparent in the first 2 days of life, but is delayed until after the first week in about 20% of affected neonates. An underlying red cell abnormality should always be considered in any neonate whose pattern of hyperbilirubinaemia does not fit with that typical of physiological jaundice of the newborn. This includes an early onset of jaundice within the first 24 hours of life, abnormally high levels of unconjugated bilirubin for the neonate's gestation and persistence of icterus beyond the first week of life. Anaemia is not a consistent finding and is generally mild. Schröter and Kahsnitz reported a haemoglobin of 15 g dl^{-1} or less in 10 of 23 neonates with hereditary spherocytosis (Schröter and Kahsnitz, 1983). Seven of 20 neonates had a reticulocytosis of greater than 10%. The unconjugated bilirubin is increased to variable degrees, and the same authors reported levels of greater than 20 μmol l^{-1} in 10 of 23 patients.

Spherocytes are seen on the blood film and the mean corpuscular haemoglobin concentration (MCHC) is generally greater than 36 g dl^{-1}. Spherocytes are, however, not diagnostic of HS and they are commonly seen in ABO incompatibility and neonatal sepsis. The classical laboratory finding in HS is an increased osmotic fragility. The osmotic fragility is always abnormal in incubated blood but, because of the increased osmotic resistance of neonatal erythrocytes, it may well be normal or only marginally increased if a non-incubated sample is tested. Because neonatal red cells are more resistant to osmotic lysis than these of older children or adults, it is important that each laboratory establishes its own normal values for the osmotic fragility of control infant erythrocytes. The autohaemolysis test is also abnormal and corrected by the addition of glucose. The diagnosis of HS is confirmed by a positive family history and the dual laboratory findings of spherocytosis and increased osmotic fragility in both the patient and a parent. In fact, because of the difficulty in obtaining adequate blood samples from neonates, it may only be possible to fully investigate the parents.

The disorder most likely to be confused with HS in the neonatal period is ABO incompatibility, which may be characterized by prominent microspherocytosis. However, in the latter disorder there is no abnormality in the parent's haemoglobin, reticulocyte count or blood film. A direct Coombs' test on the infant's red cells may be helpful but is often negative in ABO incompatibility and, in such instances, not useful in differentiating the disorders. However, serological tests will show the mother to be group O and the infant group A or B, with isohaemagglutinins present in the maternal serum. Elution studies may be informative. In the presence of spherocytosis, the osmotic fragility test will also be abnormal in ABO incompatibility; likewise the autohaemolysis test. The latter is corrected with the addition of glucose in HS but not in ABO incompatibility. If it is difficult to differentiate the disorders in the laboratory, the natural history will eventually clarify the situation.

The defect in hereditary spherocytosis remains elusive but appears to be intrinsic to the red cell membrane. Cross-transfusion experiments are consistent with this view. Red cells from patients with HS survive poorly in normal recipients but normal cells survive well in HS patients. The defect in the membrane results in a greater influx of Na^+ than is normal, but this is thought to be a secondary phenomenon, the primary abnormality being structural rather than metabolic. Both the lipid bilayer and protein component of the red cell membrane have been extensively studied, and although the principal molecular defect remains elusive it is considered to reside in the erythrocyte membrane skeleton. Patients with HS appear to be deficient in spectrin, the degree of deficiency correlating closely with the severity of the disease and with the degree of spherocytosis as measured by the osmotic fragility of the red cells. A defect of spectrin binding to protein 4.1 resulting in a defect of spectrin–actin 4.1 binding has been reported. It seems likely that HS is not a single disorder but a uniform manifestation of a variety of different molecular lesions of the erythrocyte cytoskeleton.

Most affected infants become relatively asymptomatic after the neonatal period and there is no evidence to suggest that children with HS who are symptomatic in the newborn period have a more severe form of the disease. Hyperbilirubinaemia is the most serious problem. Phototherapy may be sufficient, but exchange transfusion may be necessary. A simple transfusion may be required to correct anaemia and folate supplements should be given. Splenectomy should never be considered in this age group, although it will almost definitely be beneficial at a later date.

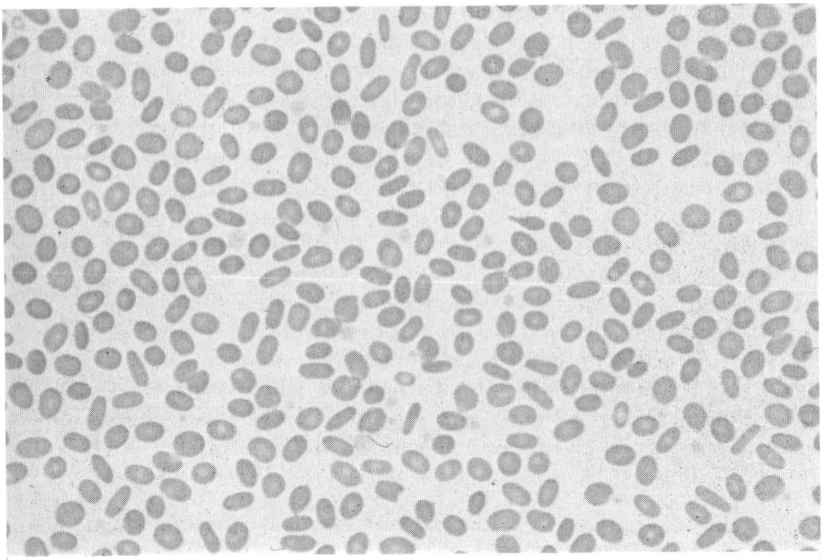

Figure 8.4 Peripheral smear of a patient with hereditary elliptocytosis showing numerous elliptocytes.

Hereditary elliptocytosis. This inherited disorder of the red cell membrane is a rare cause of haemolytic anaemia in the newborn period and is characterized by the presence of increased numbers of elliptical cells on the blood smear (Figure 8.4). Approximately 250–500 per million are affected by this disorder, which occurs in all races. Although spontaneous mutation is common, transmission is usually as an autosomal dominant trait, except in the case of the Melanesian autosomal recessive variant, which is confined to the aboriginal population of Melanesia and Malaysia.

The elliptocyte shape is not present in nucleated erythroblasts but first appears in reticulocytes and is fully evident in mature red cells. The defect is located in the membrane skeleton. Different molecular abnormalities of the membrane proteins have been described, including a complete or partial deficiency of protein 4.1, defective spectrin self-association related to abnormalities of the α- or β-chain, defective ankyrin-protein 3 interactions and defective binding of spectrin to ankyrin. It is accepted that a variety of molecular abnormalities can result in the red cell defect characteristic of hereditary elliptocytosis (HE). In some cases, the HE gene appears to be linked to the Rh locus on the short arm of chromosome 1, and such patients have a milder form of the disease. Another HE gene is located on the long arm of chromosome 1 in the region containing the spectrin α-chain gene.

Unlike patients with HS, most sufferers from HE are asymptomatic. Only about 12% of affected individuals have evidence of a haemolytic anaemia at any time during their life. However, presentation may be in the first weeks of life, with anaemia and jaundice. The diagnosis can be made easily by the finding of elliptocytes in sufficient numbers in the peripheral blood of the infant and one of the parents. There are two specific variants of HE which are particularly likely to present in the newborn period. Firstly, a few cases of homozygosity have been reported, producing severe haemolysis in the newborn period. The parents of such infants both have blood smears with classical features of hereditary elliptocytosis. Secondly, a variant (HE with infantile poikilocytosis) is recognized in which an initial poikilocytosis or pyknocytosis terminates in elliptocytosis as the percentage of elliptocytes increases in the first few months of life. Infants with this variant may present in the neonatal period with severe haemolytic anaemia. The blood film shows marked fragmentation, poikilocytosis and variable numbers of elliptocytes. Initially the disorder may be mistaken for infantile pyknocytosis or hereditary pyropoikilocytosis. During the first 6 months of life the haemolytic process declines and the number of elliptocytes increases, terminating in the classical picture of mild HE. Family studies are helpful for early diagnosis as one of the parents will have the typical blood film of HE. Infants with this variant are nearly always Black and their red cells are very heat-sensitive and fragment at a lower than normal temperature. The change in the course of the disorder appears to coincide with the conversion from fetal to adult haemoglobin, suggesting that some property of fetal red cells aggravates the basic defect in the membrane skeleton.

Treatment is rarely necessary and is dependent on the degree of anaemia and jaundice. Phototherapy or exchange transfusion may be required. If there is significant haemolysis, folic acid supplements should be given. For the rare, severe forms of hereditary elliptocytosis, splenectomy is beneficial but it should always be delayed until the child is older.

Hereditary pyropoikilocytosis. This rare cause of haemolytic anaemia, which has an autosomal recessive inheritance, is characterized by extremely bizarre red cell morphology (Figure 8.5). Microspherocytes, elliptocytes, red cell fragments and irregularly contracted red cells are striking on the blood smear. Most affected individuals have been Black. Hereditary pyropoikilocytosis (HPP) can present in early infancy as a moderate to severe haemolytic anaemia with an elevated level of unconjugated bilirubin and an appropriate reticulocytosis. Because of the large numbers of red cell fragments, the MCV is often low and the MCHC increased. Both osmotic fragility and autohaemolysis are markedly increased. The disorder derives its name from the finding that erythrocytes from affected individuals undergo fragmentation at a temperature of 46°C whereas normal red cells do not undergo such changes until the temperature reaches 50°C.

Hereditary pyropoikilocytosis is thought to be a subtype of HE as it shares many characteristics with homozygous HE. In many instances, other family members have mild hereditary elliptocytosis. The underlying biochemical defect appears to be a defect of spectrin self-association, due to abnormalities of the spectrin subunits. Individuals with hereditary pyropoikilocytosis are believed to be either double heterozygotes or homozygotes for mild HE. Many affected neonates require exchange transfusion and later become transfusion-dependent. Splenectomy lessens the degree of haemolysis but may not completely eliminate it and should be postponed as long as clinically possible.

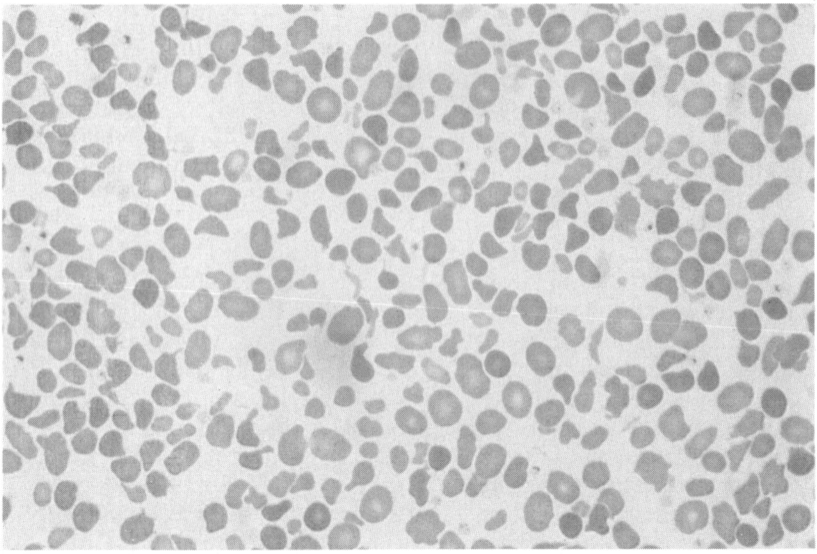

Figure 8.5 Blood smear of patient with hereditary pyropoikilocytosis.

Hereditary stomatocytosis. This disorder is characterized by red cells in which the central pallor of the biconcave disc is elongated to form a slit resembling a mouth. A number of disorders can produce this characteristic red cell appearance. However, hereditary stomatocytosis can be distinguished from the acquired forms by the greater number of stomatocytes and the presence of the same morphological finding in other family members. A clinically severe form inherited as an autosomal recessive and a mild form inherited as an autosomal dominant trait have been described.

The clinical picture is extremely variable. The severe form can present in infancy, when variable degrees of haemolysis result in anaemia, unconjugated hyperbilirubinaemia and an appropriate reticulocytosis. Stomatocytic red cells (10–50%) are seen on the blood smear. The osmotic fragility has been reported as increased or normal. The most striking defect of stomatocytic cells is their altered cation content and transport. Sodium influx and content are increased disproportionately to potassium loss. The erythrocytes progressively gain cations and water and become swollen and rigid. The underlying molecular defect responsible for the abnormal cation permeability has not been identified but presumably resides in the membrane skeleton. The variability in the clinical syndrome suggests heterogeneity in the pathogenesis. Transfusion may be required for those with sufficiently severe haemolysis, and in such patients splenectomy may be beneficial later in life.

Hereditary disorders of haemoglobin synthesis

Hereditary disorders of both haem and globin synthesis have been described in the newborn period. Amongst disorders of haem synthesis, congenital erythropoietic porphyria, a disorder of protoporphyrin synthesis, is discussed. Disorders of globin synthesis include both qualitative and quantitative defects. In the former an amino acid substitution in one of the globin chains results in the formation of an abnormal haemoglobin, and in the latter a decreased rate of synthesis of a normal globin chain produces a thalassaemia syndrome.

Congenital erythropoietic porphyria. This rare autosomal recessive disorder of protoporphyrin synthesis is characterized by mutilating cutaneous photosensitivity, haemolytic anaemia, red urine and reddish discolouration of the teeth. Although the haematological and dermatological problems tend not to develop until after the neonatal period, about one-third of patients present as newborns with red staining of their nappies due to excretion of excessive amounts of uroporphyrin I in their urine. The synthesis of excess uroporphyrinogen I in erythrocyte precursors and its subsequent excretion as oxidized porphyrin in the urine suggests that the defect in this disorder is in the haem biosynthetic pathway at the uroporphyrinogen III cosynthetase step (Figure 8.6); subnormal activity of the enzyme has been demonstrated. There is rarely a need for therapeutic intervention in the neonatal period. Later in life, avoidance of sunlight is important and the use of barrier creams helpful. Correction of the anaemia by blood transfusion temporarily suppresses erythropoiesis, resulting in a decrease in porphyrin production and excretion.

Abnormal fetal haemoglobins. Abnormal fetal haemoglobins involving both the α- and γ-globin chains have been reported, generally having been discovered by chance during routine population screening of cord bloods. Infants with α-globin chain variants are neither anaemic nor jaundiced. However, occasionally unstable haemoglobins resulting from α-chain mutations (e.g. Hb Hasharon) are clinically more significant in the neonatal period than in adult life, because of the lesser affinity between α- and γ-chains than between α- and β-chains. This results in an increased tendency to dissociation and haemolysis.

Electrophoretic studies on cord blood demonstrate two bands: one corresponding to normal HbF ($\alpha_2 \gamma_2$) and the other to the abnormal HbF ($\alpha^*_2 \gamma_2$). As β-chains replace γ-chains, normal ($\alpha_2 \beta_2$) and abnormal ($\alpha''_2 \beta_2$) HbA can be demonstrated electrophoretically. γ-Chain variants are rare, but both γ^G and γ^A variants have been described. These abnormal haemoglobins gradually disappear as HbF is replaced by HbA during the first few months of life. Their concentration in cord blood is between 10 and 40%, with higher levels being found when the abnormality occurs in the γ^G-chain, explained by the ratio of γ^G to γ^A chains in HbF of cord blood of 3:1. The γ-chain variants are not usually associated with any haematological abnormality. However, an infant has been reported presenting with haemolytic anaemia in the newborn period due to the presence of an unstable fetal

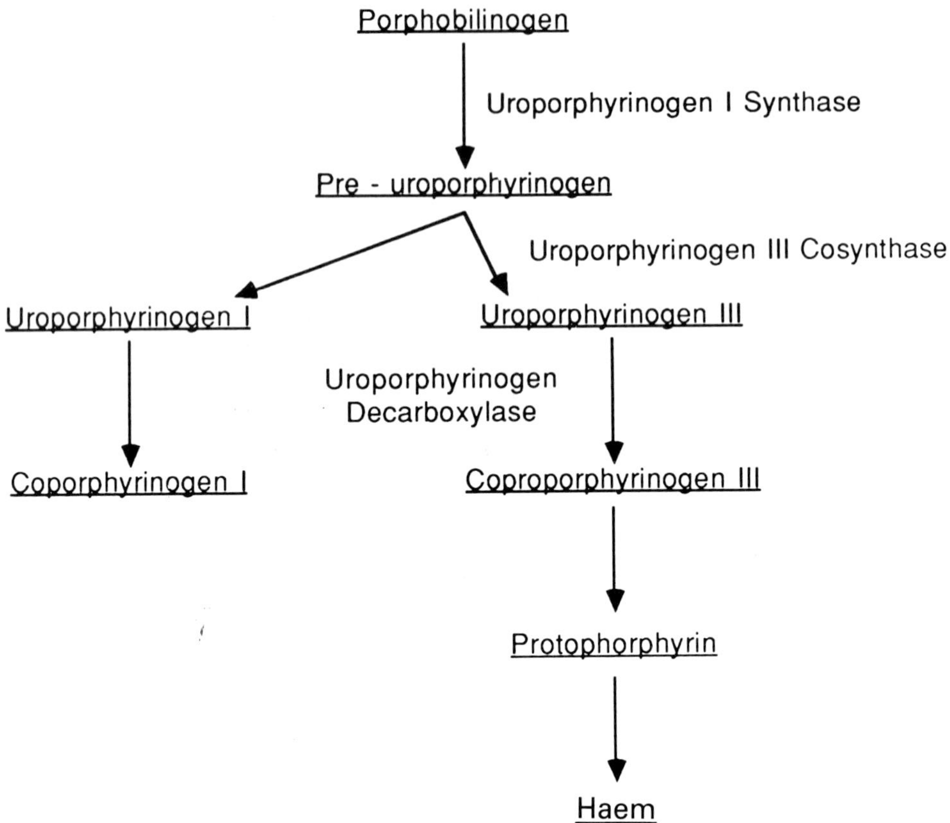

Figure 8.6 Schematic representation of the conversion of porphobilinogen to haem. The defect in congenital erythropoietic porphyria is thought to be a deficiency of the enzyme uroporphyrinogen III cosynthase. In the absence of this enzyme the pathway is diverted from the normal synthesis of uroporphyrinogen III to the production of uroporphyrinogen I from pre-uroporphyrinogen, which is not enzyme-controlled. Adapted from Kushner *et al.* 1982, *Blood* 59: 726, with permission of Grune and Stratton, Inc.

haemoglobin, HbF Poole. This γ^G-chain variant was undetectable by 6 weeks of age (Lee Potter *et al.*, 1975).

The α thalassaemia syndromes. The thalassaemia syndromes constitute a major world-wide health problem and as a group are probably the commonest single gene disorder. They are characterized by a reduced rate of synthesis of one or more of the globin chains. The disorders have a remarkably diverse molecular pathology and a wide clinical spectrum ranging from symptomless carrier states to intra-uterine death.

A reduced rate of α-globin chain synthesis characterises α thalassaemia. It predominantly affects South-east Asians and Blacks; Table 8.2 gives the frequency of the different genotypes seen in these ethnic groups. The α-

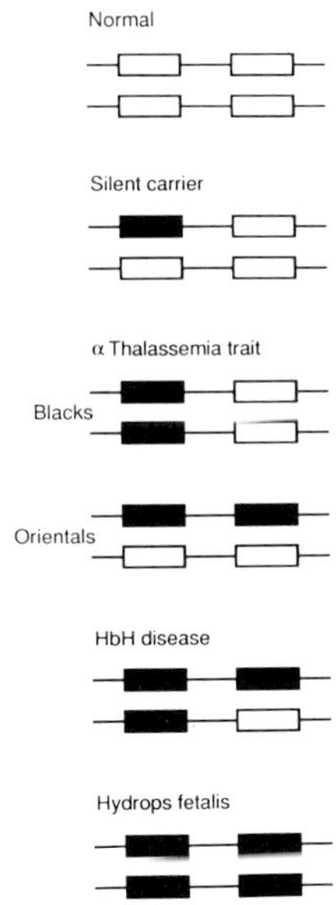

Figure 8.7 Different genetic patterns producing the various α thalassaemia syndromes.

globin genes reside on chromosome 16 and synthesis is under the control of four α-globin genes. There is a strong correlation between the severity of the clinical syndrome and the number of α-globin genes deleted (Figure 8.7).

Usually α thalassaemia is due to gene deletion, although point mutations also occur. Despite the genetic heterogeneity, four clinical α thalassaemia syndromes emerge, the characteristics of which are given in Table 8.3. Two heterozygote states exist; α^0 thalassaemia (α-thal-1 trait: two gene deletions) in which no α chains are produced and α^+ thalassaemia (α-thal-2 trait: 1 gene deletion) in which α chains are synthesized at a reduced rate. The clinical phenotype α-thal-1 trait occurs in two forms. Two α-genes can be deleted from the same chromosome (*cis* deletion) or one gene can be deleted from each of the pair of chromosome 16 (*trans* deletion). *Cis* deletion is common in people from Asia and the Mediterranean basin but not in Blacks,

Table 8.2 Estimates of α-thalassaemia genotypes in various ethnic groups. From Connor and Ferguson-Smith, 1984, *Essential Medical Genetics*: 142, with permission of Blackwell Scientific Publications.

Ethnic group	Genotype	Frequency (%)
Thais	-α/αα	5–8
	/αα	6
	--/--	0.4
Blacks	-α/αα	25
	--/αα	Rare

Table 8.3 Features of α thalassaemia syndromes.*

	Clinical features		Haemoglobin pattern			
Syndrome	Birth	Later life	Birth	Later life	β/α Ratio	Number of genes affected by thal mutation
Silent carrier (α-thal-2)	No anaemia or microcytosis	No anaemia or microcytosis	1–2% Hb Bart's (γ^4)	Normal	Synthesis index > 1	1
Thalassaemia trait (α-thal-1)	Mild anaemia and microcytosis	Mild anaemia and microcytosis	3–10% Hb Bart's (γ^4)	Normal	1.4–1.2:1	2
Hb H disease	Moderate microcytic hypochromic haemolytic anaemia	Moderate microcytic hypochromic haemolytic anaemia	20–40% Hb Bart's (γ^4)	5–30% Hb H (β^4)	2.5:1	3
Hb Bart's Hydrops syndrome	Severe hypochromic microcytic anaemia	Lethal	80% Hb Bart's 0–20% Hb H Small amount of Hb Portland	—	∞	4

* Adapted from Oski FA and Naiman JL, *Hematologic Problems in the Newborn*, 1982, 3rd edn: p 266, with permission of W.B. Saunders Co.

who show *trans* deletion. Hydrops fetalis (four gene deletions) results from the homozygous inheritance of the *cis* deletion of α-thal-1 trait, and HbH (three gene deletions) from the co-inheritance of the *cis* deletion of α-thal-1 trait and the α-thal-2 trait. This genetic pattern explains why hydrops fetalis and HbH are seen in Asians but not in Blacks.

In the fetus a deficiency of α-chains results in an excess of γ-chains or Hb Bart's (γ^4) and correspondingly, in adults, in an excess of β chains or HbH (β^4). Significant amounts of Hb Bart's or HbH, which can be measured electrophoretically, only occur in the red cells of individuals who have inherited two or more α thalassaemia determinants and have a relatively severe degree of α-chain deficiency. HbH is unstable and precipitates to form intracellular inclusion bodies in the red cells, which can be demonstrated by incubation with 1% brilliant cresyl blue. This instability results in a haemolytic anaemia. HbH and Hb Bart's do not give up oxygen at physiological tensions and therefore are useless oxygen carriers. Neither of the heterozygous states produce clinical symptomatology and they can be difficult to diagnose without resorting to the sophisticated technique of measuring the ratio of β- to α-chain synthesis by ^{3}[H]leucine incorporation into newly synthesized globin. This is normally balanced with a β:α ratio of unity, an imbalance reflecting the impairment of chain synthesis.

Silent carrier (α^+ thalassaemia or α thalassaemia-2 trait). This arises from the deletion of one α thalassaemia gene. Affected individuals are not anaemic and the red cell morphology is usually normal, although the red cell indices may be reduced. Globin chain analysis reflects the slight decrease in α-chain synthesis with a β:α ratio marginally exceeding one. However, even this is not a consistent finding. In the newborn period, small amounts (1–3%) of Hb Bart's (γ^4) can be detected, exceeding the tiny amounts found in many normal newborns (< 1%), which reflect the imbalance of globin chain synthesis. After the first few months of life Hb Bart's disappears, and therafter globin chain analysis is the only means of diagnosis. HbA_2 and HbF levels are normal.

Alpha-thalassaemia trait (α^0 thalassaemia or α thalassaemia-1 trait). The deletion of two α thalassaemia genes is associated with a mild hypochromic microcytic anaemia and reduced red cell indices. In neonates, 3–10% Hb Bart's can be detected. In adults the β:α synthetic ratio is between 1.2:1.0 and 1.4:1.0, and the diagnosis is made by excluding other causes of reduced red cell indices, in particular iron deficiency and β thalassaemia trait. Importantly, HbA_2 and HbF levels are normal or low in the α thalassaemia trait but raised in the β thalassaemia trait. The disorder is common in Orientals, with an incidence of about 20% in South-east Asia and between 2 and 5% in Blacks. Hydrops fetalis has not been described in Blacks, and HbH disease is rare; both are common in Orientals. The discrepancy in clinical severity of thalassaemia between the two ethnic groups can be explained by different α-gene deletion patterns. Blacks almost invariably have α thalassaemia gene mutations on different chromosomes, i.e. the abnormal gene is linked to a normal gene in the *cis* position. Consequently, children of a marriage between two Black α thalassaemia trait individuals will not inherit more than two α thalassaemia genes.

HbH disease. HbH disease results from the deletion of three α thalassaemia genes. Affected infants are the offspring of one parent with an α thalassaemia-1 trait, who will clinically have a mild microcytic anaemia, and another parent with an α thalassaemia-2 trait, who will be haematologically normal. The disease occurs predominantly in South-east Asians and occasionally in Mediterranean island populations and, for reasons already mentioned, rarely in Blacks. Affected infants have a moderately severe microcytic, hypochromic anaemia, haemolysis and splenomegaly. Microcytosis, hypochromasia and target cells are seen on the blood smear. Substantial amounts of Hb Bart's (20–40%) are present at birth. As β-chain synthesis increases, Hb Bart's is replaced by HbH, which eventually makes up 5–30% of the total haemoglobin. The severity of the anaemia is variable. HbH is unstable, forms intracellular inclusion bodies in the red cells and is seen as a fast moving band on electrophoresis. The β:α ratio is in the order of 2.5:1.0 reflecting the marked deficiency of α-chain synthesis. Both infection and oxidant drugs may increase the degree of haemolysis and, therefore, prompt treatment of infection is important and oxidant drugs should be avoided. Folic acid supplements are required and transfusion may be necessary.

Fetal hydrops syndrome. This disorder, which results from a total absence of any normal α genes, is incompatible with life and is a common cause of fetal death throughout South-east Asia. As the number of immigrants to the West from that part of the world increase, it is important to be aware of this problem, which may ultimately become more common than hydrops from rhesus incompatibility. The infants are stillborn or die soon after birth. Oedema and massive hepatosplenomegaly are present.

The haemoglobin ranges between 3 and 10 $g\ dl^{-1}$ (average 6–7 $g\ dl^{-1}$), with microcytosis and many nucleated red blood cells on the peripheral smear. Haemoglobin electrophoresis reveals predominantly Hb Bart's (γ^4) with small amounts of HbH and the embryonic Hb Portland. Because of absent α-chain synthesis, no HbF or HbA are produced. Hb Bart's is a high affinity haemoglobin releasing no oxygen at physiological conditions, resulting in severe tissue hypoxia. Hb Portland has a more favourable oxygen dissociation pattern and may improve tissue oxygenation until it disappears in the last trimester, which could explain why these infants do not die at an early gestation. Toxaemia of pregnancy is commonly found in women carrying infants with hydrops fetalis, and it should alert one to the possibility of hydrops fetalis in women of an at-risk ethnic background. It is of course now technically possible to transfuse such infants *in utero*. Should they survive they remain transfusion-dependant, and it is extremely questionable whether such an aggressive approach is justifiable in the long term.

The prenatal diagnosis of thalassaemia is discussed elsewhere in this book. Hydrops fetalis is universally fatal. Neither heterozygous carrier states require treatment. Infants with HbH disease may require transfusion for severe anaemia at birth but later the severity of the anaemia is very variable.

Haemoglobin Constant Spring syndrome (HbCS) ($d_2^{CS}\ \beta_2$). This heterogenous group, with four recognized variants, reflect different point mutations in the termination codon. HbCS is a structural defect of the α-chain, characterized by two elongated α-chains with either 28 or 31 amino acids at the C-terminal end. The β-chains are normal. The heterozygous state phenotypically resembles α thalassaemia-1 trait. The haemoglobin migrates slowly on electrophoresis and is found in minor amounts (1–2%).

β Thalassaemia does not present until after the first few months of life when β chain synthesis starts to dominate. However, a number of infants have been described with γβ thalassaemia. The anaemia in these infants is severe, with some terminating in neonatal death and others requiring exchange transfusion. Globin chain analysis has shown a reduction in synthesis of both γ and β chains. The severe anaemia has been self-limiting, and surviving children have progressed to a mild hypochromic, microcytic anaemia with normal levels of HbF and HbA_2. In some cases, DNA analysis has demonstrated a large deletion encompassing γ, β and δ gene regions on chromosome 11. In the newborn, γβ thalassaemia clinically resembles erythroblastosis fetalis and should be considered in the differential diagnosis of a hydropic baby.

Haemoglobin M disease. Five M haemoglobins have been described, all of which are exceedingly rare and have an autosomal dominant pattern of inheritance. HbM Boston and HbM Iwate result from single amino acid substitutions in the α-chain, present with cyanosis at birth and are associated with decreased oxygen affinity. A γ-chain variant, Hb Osaka, is also associated with methaemoglobinaemia in the neonatal period and disappears as β-globulin production increases. The β-chain variants HbM Saskatoon, HbM Hyde Park and HbM Milwaukee-1 do not present until several months of age. All but one of these M haemoglobins involve substitution of a tyrosine for a histidine residue. This substitution may stabilize the haem iron in the ferric form. The blood of affected individuals appears chocolate brown and does not turn red when exposed to oxygen. Diagnosis is made by spectrophotometric analysis and haemoglobin electrophoresis. In α-chain variants, the abnormal haemoglobin constitutes 20–30% of the total haemoglobin, and in β-chain variants 40–50% of the total. No treatment is required, although it is important to differentiate these disorders from more serious causes of cyanosis in particular pulmonary and cardiac problems. Ascorbic acid therapy is not effective.

Unstable haemoglobins. A number of unstable haemoglobins have been described, resulting from a single amino acid substitution in the α-chain. Occasionally, the fetal form of an α-chain mutation will be clinically more significant than the adult form of the mutation, for example Hb Hasharon. The unstable mutant haemoglobins have a greater tendency to dissociate into subunits, leading to haemolysis. This is accentuated in HbF, which is less stable than HbA because of the lesser affinity between α and γ chains than α and β chains. Hb Poole, a γ-chain unstable haemoglobin has been described in a newborn infant with clinically significant haemolysis and Heinz body formation. Unstable haemoglobins can be demonstrated by the heat instability and isopropanol precipitation tests, and identified by electrophoresis. Care with interpretation of the isopropanol precipitation test is required because HbF precipitates more readily than HbA. The pattern of inheritance is autosomal dominant and affected individuals are heterozygotes for the abnormal haemoglobin gene. Homozygosity would probably be incompatible with life.

Haemoglobin variants. The common structural haemoglobin variants HbS, C, D Punjab and E are all β-chain defects and, because they are not usually detectable before 3–6 months of age, do not generally cause problems in the newborn period.

Red cell enzymopathies

Red cell metabolic defects are an important cause of haemolytic anaemia in the newborn period. Jaundice is again the prominent clinical finding because of the limited conjugating capacity of the newborn's immature liver, and it may be sufficiently severe to require exchange transfusion. This will remove enzyme-deficient red cells, preventing further haemolysis, lower the bilirubin level and correct any anaemia. Examination of the blood smear should exclude other causes of haemolysis that are associated with characteristic morphology. Enzymopathies have no specific morphological features themselves, although basophilic stippling is seen in pyrimidine-5′-nucleotidase deficiency and occasional microspherocytes are seen in glucose-6-phosphate dehydrogenase (G6PD) deficiency during a haemolytic episode.

A red cell enzyme deficiency is often considered after other more common causes of haemolysis have been excluded by appropriate laboratory tests. It is important to enquire carefully into the infant's racial background, family history of blood disorders, evidence of haemolysis following exposure to drugs or infection, and neurological or muscular disease. Rapid screening tests are available for G6PD, pyruvate kinase, triosephosphate isomerase and glucose phosphate isomerase. Diagnosis of the other enzymopathies is dependent on quantitative enzyme assays or determination of metabolic intermediates.

When interpreting the results of red cell enzyme assays in the newborn it is important to compare with age-matched normal values as there are significant physiological differences between enzyme levels in the newborn and in the adult. Newborns have an increased proportion of young red cells, and, as might be expected, many enzymes of the glycolytic pathway and hexose monophosphate shunt have values in the same range as that of high-reticulocyte adult blood (Table 8.4). Not all the differences in the newborn enzyme levels can be explained on the basis of a younger cell population, as the activity of some enzymes is increased above the levels of high-reticulocyte blood. Equally, some enzymes have lower activity than is seen in normal adult red cells. The levels of enzyme activity are often gestation-dependent. The normal development of the enzyme pathways has already been described (see Chapter 1).

Glucose-6-phosphate dehydrogenase deficiency. Over 120 million people in the world are deficient in this enzyme, which is probably the most common inborn error of metabolism and the most common enzymo-

Table 8.4 Erythrocyte enzymes in newborns compared with normal and high-reticulocyte adults.*

Enzymes increased in comparison with normal adult or high-reticulocyte adult blood
Glucose phosphate isomerase
Glyceraldehyde-3-phosphate dehydrogenase
Phosphoglycerate kinase
Enolase
Enzymes increased in comparison with normal adult, but same as high-reticulocyte adult blood
Hexokinase
Aldolase
Triose phosphate isomerase
Phosphoglyceromutase
Pyruvate kinase
Lactate dehydrogenase
Glucose-6-phophate dehydrogenase
6-Phosphoglucose dehydrogenase
Glutathione reductase
Distal pentose shunt
Glyoxylase I and II
Galactokinase
Galactose-1-phophate uridyl-transferase
Enzymes decreased in comparison with normal adult and high-reticulocyte adult blood
Phosphofructokinase
Adenylate kinase
Glutathione peroxidase
Glutathione synthetase
Carbonic anhydrase
Catalase
Ribosephosphate pyrophosphokinase
Acetylcholinesterase
NADPH-methaemoglobin reductase

* From Matthay KK and Mentzer WC, 1981, *Clinics in Haematology 10(1)*: 35, with permission of W.B. Saunders Co.

pathy to cause neonatal haemolysis. It is particularly prevalent amongst Blacks and people from the Middle East, Greece and the Far East. Over 150 variants have been reported, each of which may well result from a single amino acid substitution. Haemolysis may be either chronic or episodic, but most common variants are associated with episodic haemolysis. The gene for G6PD is located on the X-chromosome. Males are affected, although carrier females can be identified. In the lyonization hypothesis, there is random inactivation of one of the X-chromosomes in the female embryo, such that a carrier of G6PD deficiency may or may not subsequently have low levels of G6PD. In parts of the world where G6PD deficiency is very common, homozygous G6PD-deficient females are not infrequently found.

Most of the variants described are unique to families or limited to small ethnic groups, but certain enzyme mutants are very frequent in some populations. Gd^{B} is regarded as the normal enzyme and represents the standard of normal activity. $Gd^{Mediterranean}$, an enzyme with normal electrophoretic mobility but almost no activity, is common in the Mediterranean areas and is also found in South-east Asia and in India. Two mutant enzymes with fast electrophoretic mobility are common in Africa: Gd^{A+} and Gd^{A-}. The latter is associated with decreased activity, whilst GdA^{+} has nearly normal activity.

The severity of the haemolysis and the recognized precipitating factors are dependent on the G6PD variant involved. The activity of normal G6PD declines exponentially; young red cells having higher levels than old. The instability of the G6PD variant, or rate of decline of activity, plays a major role in the severity of the haemolysis. For example the $Gd^{Mediterranean}$ variant loses its activity at such an accelerated rate that even newly circulating reticulocytes have reduced levels of activity; mature erythrocytes have nearly undetectable enzyme activity (0–5%) and symptoms are severe. In contrast, the other common mutant, Gd^{A-}, has an intermediate rate of loss of enzyme activity; mature erythrocytes have enzyme levels of 5–15% and symptoms are less severe. Haemolysis in Gd^{A-} is self-limiting, and normal levels of enzyme activity can be found during a haemolytic crisis because reticulocytes in these deficient males have the same enzyme activity as reticulocytes from normal individuals. The difference between this variant and the normal enzyme lies in the rate of decline of enzyme activity.

G6PD is required for the regeneration of reduced glutathione, which protects red cells from oxidative damage. It catalyses the first step in the pentose phosphate pathway in which NADP is reduced to NADPH by the oxidation of glucose-6-phosphate. An individual deficient in G6PD may have haemolysis following exposure to oxidant drugs, infection, acidosis or, in some variants, after ingestion of fava beans. There are several reasons why the neonate with G6PD deficiency is at particular risk of haemolysis. Firstly, the red cells of neonates are high in ascorbic acid, which has been shown to shorten survival of G6PD deficient erythrocytes. Secondly vitamin E levels and catalase activity are low, both of which predispose the red cell to hydrogen peroxide haemolysis.

Jaundice is usually apparent within 48 hours of life. The anaemia and reticulocytosis are usually mild. Microspherocytes may be seen on the blood film in severe cases, but usually there are no specific morphological findings. The degree of hyperbilirubinaemia is affected by prematurity, infection, acidosis, hypoxia, exposure to oxidant drugs and the G6PD variant involved. Significant hyperbilirubinaemia requiring exchange transfusion has been reported in G6PD deficient neonates from China, Thailand, Italy, Sardinia, Greece and Malaysia; in fact all areas where the more severe Mediterranean type of G6PD deficiency occurs. Significant neonatal hyperbilirubinaemia is rare in full-term American Blacks, but is seen in Black Africans, despite the fact that both have the same Gd^{A-} variant.

G6PD has an X-linked inheritance. It is probably justifiable to screen all male infants who are of an ethnic origin that has a high prevalence of G6PD deficiency. This allows avoidance of oxidant drugs in the infant and in the mother during future pregnancies and whilst she is nursing. It is important to treat hypoxia, sepsis and acidosis promptly. Phototherapy may be used to treat moderate icterus, and phenobarbitone has been given with success.

However, it has been suggested that phototherapy may accentuate haemolysis by reducing riboflavine, which can in turn result in a decrease in glutathione, further decreasing the anti-oxidant activity of the G6PD deficient individual. Exchange transfusion may be necessary to prevent kernicterus.

Other enzyme deficiencies involving the hexose monophosphate shunt are very rare and are listed in Table 8.5.

Pyruvate kinase deficiency. Pyruvate kinase (PK) catalyses the conversion of phosphoenolpyruvate to pyruvate in the penultimate step of the glycolytic pathway. The inheritance of this inborn error of metabolism is autosomal recessive, and it is the second most common enzyme deficiency causing neonatal haemolysis. However, it is very much rarer than G6PD deficiency, with only a few hundred reported cases, mostly in northern Europeans. Sporadic cases have been reported from other ethnic groups. Because of the position of the block caused in the glycolytic pathway by PK deficiency, phosphoenolpyruvate and, more importantly 2,3 diphosphoglycerate (2,3DPG) levels are increased. This leads to a decrease in oxygen affinity, which improves oxygen delivery to the tissues and helps to alleviate the clinical and biochemical effects of the anaemia. Clinical and biochemical heterogenity is recognized. Pyruvate kinase activity does not necessarily correlate with the severity of the haemolysis and can vary widely in affected individuals (0 50%), reflecting the genetic heterogeneity. There are many PK variants. Infants who are the product of consanguinity are usually homozygous for one deficient enzyme, whilst non-consanguineous affected infants are usually double heterozygotes for two deficient alleles. Variants have been reported with normal activity but abnormal enzyme kinetics, whilst others have decreased activity but normal kinetics.

The haemolysis associated with PK deficiency is chronic and variable in severity and can be particularly severe in the newborn. Significant neonatal hyperbilirubinaemia is common and the onset is within the first 24 hours of life and is associated with anaemia, reticulocytosis and splenomegaly. Infants who present at birth appear to have more severe haemolysis later in life. Exchange transfusion may be indicated to lower the bilirubin and correct the anaemia. Folic acid supplements should be given. Splenectomy may reduce transfusion requirements later in life but it is contraindicated in the newborn, because of the risk of infection.

Other enzyme deficiencies involving the glycolytic pathway are very much rarer and are listed in table 8.5.

INHERITED NEONATAL NEUTROPENIAS

Neutropenia is defined as a reduction in the absolute number of circulating neutrophils in the peripheral blood. Normal ranges vary according to age and race. At birth there is an excess of neutrophils, but by the end of the first week neutrophils and lymphocytes are present in equal numbers, and thereafter lymphocytes predominate for the first few years of life. The lower limit of a normal neutrophil count is 1.0×10^9 per litre for White infants

Table 8.5 Summary of neonatal features of erythrocyte enzymopathies associated with haemolytic anaemia.*

Enzyme deficiency	No. of cases	Inheritance	Neonatal manifestations			Special clinical features
			Frequency	Exchange transfusion	Death or kernicterus	
Defects in hexose monophosphate shunt and glutathione metabolism						
G6PD	$> 10^8$	X-linked	$>$ 5% except in full-term black infants where jaundice is rare	Yes	Yes	Onset jaundice at one to two days. Common variants have episodic haemolysis, may be precipitated by beans as well as oxidant drugs, infection, acidosis. May also have CNSHA†.
Glutathione synthetase	7	Autosomal recessive	0	–	–	Mild CNSHA.
Y-Glutamyl-cysteine synthetase	2	Autosomal recessive	1	–	–	Mild CNSHA. One family. Later cerebellar abnormalities.
Glutathione reductase	1	? Autosomal dominant and unknown	0	–	–	Episodic haemolysis after fava beans with complete deficiency. Partial deficiency does not cause haemolysis.

Defects in Embden–Meyerhof glycolytic pathway						
Hexokinase	19	Autosomal	5	1	0	Onset jaundice at one to three days. One jaundiced infant also G6PD deficient. One case with mental retardation, one with physical deformities, two with Fanconi's anaemia.
Glucose phosphate isomerase	35	Autosomal recessive	14	3	Yes (1)	CNSHA.
Phosphofructo-kinase	9	Autosomal recessive	0	0	0	Mild CNSHA; four patients with muscle weakness and pigmenturia after exercise.
Aldolase	1	?	0	0	0	Onset haemolysis at 6 weeks. Associated mental retardation, flat nose, epicanthal folds, lax skin, strabismus.
Triose phosphate isomerase.	11	Autosomal recessive	3	2	2	Onset of jaundice at birth, neurological abnormalities beginning at 6–12 months. Sudden death common.

Table 8.5 *continued.*

Enzyme deficiency	No. of cases	Inheritance	Neonatal manifestations			Special clinical features
			Frequency	Exchange transfusion	Death or kernicterus	
Phosphoglycerate kinase	8	X-linked	3	0	0	CNSHA. Later (age one to three) onset of mental retardation, tremor, ataxia, seizures.
Pyruvate kinase	176	Autosomal recessive	64	23	4	CNSHA. Onset of jaundice, usually day one.
Defects in purine and pyrimidine salvage pathways						
Pyrimidine-5′-nucleotidase	14	Autosomal recessive	1	0	0	Prominent basophilic stippling of erythrocytes
Adenosine deaminase overproduction	13	Autosomal dominant	0	0	0	Mild CNSHA.
Adenylate kinase	2	?	1	0	0	Onset jaundice and anaemia at age 2 weeks

* From Matthay KK and Mentzer WC, 1981, *Clinics in Haematology 10(1)*: 46–47, with permission of W.B. Saunders Co.
† CNSHA; congenital non-spherocytic haemolytic anaemia

between 2 weeks and 1 year of age; Blacks have lower neutrophil counts. Bacterial and viral infections are without doubt the most common cause of neutropenia in the newborn period, and such infants are generally clinically septic. Congenital neutropenia is rare and the increased risk of infection is often not apparent until the infant is several months old. If an underlying infection is confidently excluded, the mother should be investigated for disorders characterized by the production of anti-neutrophil antibodies capable of crossing the placenta and producing neutropenia in her infant, including alloimmune neutropenia. A careful drug history for both infant and mother is essential as drug-related neutropenia is common. Finally, a familial neutropenia may be obvious after determining the neutrophil counts of other family members or may be suggested by a history of unexplained deaths in the first year of life.

Cyclic neutropenia

Cyclic neutropenia is characterized by regular oscillation in the number of neutrophils in the peripheral blood from normal to neutropenic levels. It is a rare disease thought to have an autosomal dominant inheritance. A few cases presenting in the newborn period have been reported, although diagnosis is usually made well after this time. The defect lies in the stem cell line which periodically demonstrates decreased proliferation. The cyclic interval is generally 19–21 days, but may be as short as 11 days or as long as 35 days. Because the stem cell line is involved all haemopoietic cell lines are affected. Due to the relatively long half-life of red cells and platelets compared with neutrophils, anaemia and significant thrombocytopenia are not seen. However, reticulocytopenia and relative thrombocytopenia parallel the fluctuation of neutrophils. Serial bone marrow examinations show disappearance of granulocyte precursors preceding the onset of neutropenia, with their reappearance prior to the return of neutrophils in the peripheral blood. A monocytosis regularly precedes recovery, with parallel rises in serum muramidase. An absolute monocytosis and eosinophilia may be seen during the period of neutropenia. Neutrophil survival and function are both normal and neutrophil antibodies have not been demonstrated. The nature of this stem cell defect has not been identified.

Cyclic neutropenia is generally considered a benign disorder, although infection-related deaths have been reported. Neutrophils may disappear completely from the peripheral blood and the severity of the infections tends to correlate directly with the degree of neutropenia. Symptoms are rare until the neutrophil count falls below 0.5×10^9 per litre. Problems characteristic of the neturopenia include fever, oral ulceration, skin infections, peridontal disease and lymphadenitis. Cyclic neutropenia has been described in association with both agammaglobulinaemia and dysgammaglobulinaemia.

This disorder generally runs a benign course. Corticosteroids have produced a temporary improvement in the neutrophil count in some patients but have not been beneficial in the long-term. Supportive care with antibiotics should be vigorous. Cytokines such as granulocyte and granulocyte–macrophage stimulating factor (G- and GM-CSF) have shown great promise in those cases with significant problems.

Familial benign chronic neutropenia

This familial disorder with an autosomal dominant inheritance runs a very benign course and presentation in the newborn period is unusual. It is characterized by a chronic neutropenia in the range of 0.3×10^9 to 1.5×10^9 per litre and there is no accompanying anaemia or thrombocytopenia. Problems are few, although mouth ulcers, skin furuncles and gingivitis occur. This familial neutropenia can be thought of as similar to the mild neutropenia seen in black Africans, who commonly have neutrophil counts lower than those seen in other races.

The bone marrow morphology is variable but usually cellularity is normal, although a relative deficiency of the more mature granulocyte precursors has been described in some patients. Neutrophil antibodies and serum inhibitors of myelopoiesis have not been found. Familial benign chronic neutropenia requires no treatment except appropriate antibiotic therapy as clinically indicated.

Familial severe chronic neutropenia

This familial neutropenia has an autosomal dominant inheritance and is characterized by a more pronounced degree of neutropenia than familial benign chronic neutropenia and a monocytosis. The bone marrow is normocellular with a deficiency of mature granulocytes. Infections are usually more severe than in the benign condition, but survival to adult life can occur. Whether this disorder represents a more severe form of benign neutropenia or a distinct entity is not clear. Again, use of recombinant human cytokines such as G-CSF and GM-CSF has proved beneficial and abrogated the need for bone marrow transplant, which was previously often the only successful form of therapy.

Infantile genetic agranulocytosis

This disorder was first described by Kostmann in 1956 and is often referred to as Kostmann's syndrome. The inheritance is autosomal recessive. The neutropenia is severe ($< 0.3 \times 10^9$ per litre) and the clinical onset early. The predominant presenting features are fever, skin boils, umbilical sepsis, pneumonia, gingivitis, otitis media, perianal and urinary infections. Both Gram-positive and Gram-negative organisms are responsible and, later, deep-seated abscesses are common. A monocytosis and moderate eosinophilia frequently accompanies the neutropenia. Platelet numbers are normal. In older children, raised immunoglobulins reflect the chronic infection. The bone marrow cellularity is variable with maturation arrest at the promyelocyte–myelocyte stage. Promyelocytes are commonly vacuolated and myelocytes contain large azurophilic granules. Transfused neutrophils survive normally, pointing to a defect of granulocyte differentiation. Granulocyte colony formation is quantitatively normal, although qualitatively defective.

This disorder is frequently fatal and appropriate early antibiotic therapy may be life-saving. Agents that generally stimulate granulopoiesis, such as steroids and lithium, are ineffective. As the problem is thought to reside in the stem cell line, bone marrow transplantation has been employed. Recently the use of growth factors, in particular G-CSF, has been successfully reported and may abrogate the need for transplantation.

Schwachman's syndrome

This autosomal recessive disorder is characterized by pancreatic exocrine insufficiency, metaphyseal chondrodysplasia, dwarfism and variable neutropenia. The presentation is early and often within the first weeks of life. Failure to thrive, bulky foul smelling stools, eczema, otitis media and pneumonia are common manifestations. At a larger date short stature is a frequent finding.

Aggett *et al.* (1980) reported on 21 reviewed cases of Schwachman's syndrome. Sixteen out of 21 had problems in the neonatal period; 17 of 21 suffered recurrent severe infection and three patients (15%) died. The neutropenia of Schwachman's syndrome has been reported as chronic or less often intermittent. Aggett *et al.* found all evaluable patients to have intermittent neutropenia: 19 of 21 patients had neutrophil counts of less than 1.5×10^9 per litre, and 14 had neutrophil counts of less than 0.5×10^9 per litre. An appropriate neutrophil response to infection was observed in a number of patients.

Neutrophil mobility has been reported defective in this syndrome. Polymorphonuclear leucocyte chemotaxis depends upon microtubule and microfilament function. The surface distribution of concavalin-A receptors is a cytoskeleton-dependent function and Rothbaum studied three children with Schwachman's syndrome (Rothbaum *et al.*, 1982). Approximately a third of the neutrophils in each patient showed a patchy distribution of fluorescein-conjugated concavalin-A rather than the usual diffuse staining pattern. These findings suggest that a cytoskeletal defect exists which could contribute to the abnormal chemotaxis and frequent infections. The neutropenia is often not an isolated haematological finding. Aggett *et al.* (1980) reported 10 of 21 patients to be anaemic and 14 of 20 to be thrombocytopenic. Six patients had bone marrow aspirations and these all showed varying degrees of hypoplasia.

Immunoglobulins are usually normal, but both a slight decrease and dysgammaglobulinaemia have been reported. In this disorder the sweat test is normal. Duodenal juice lacks pancreatic trypsin, lipase and amylase. The faecal fat is high, but xylose excretion and jejunal biopsy are normal. Post-mortem examination of the pancreas shows replacement with adipose tissue with preservation of the islets and no fibrosis.

Approximately 15–25% of patients die during infancy or childhood. Treatment of the pancreatic insufficiency does not alter the haematological abnormalities. Recurrent infections continue, and disability from joint deformity may occur. Steroids have been reported to improve marrow function but are usually not warranted because of their associated risk of infection. Antibiotics should be given promptly and according to sensitivities from bacterial screening. Cytokines have now been used successfully in a few cases.

Cartilage–hair hypoplasia

This autosomal recessive disorder, which was initially reported in the Amish population, is characterized by short-limb dwarfism, sparse fine silky hair, hyperextensible joints and hypoplastic nails. Neutropenia, lymphopenia and defective cellular immunity have all been described. The neutropenia predisposes to recurrent bacterial infection, particularly otitis media, sinusitis and pneumonia. The defective cellular immunity is responsible for an increased susceptibility to viral infections, which may make the most significant contribution to morbidity. Bone marrow transplantation has been performed with some success, and recombinant cytokines are being tried out.

Reticular dysgenesis (alymphocytic neutropenia)

This disorder, which presents in the newborn period, is characterized by a virtual complete absence of white cells in the peripheral blood. The defect is at the level of the stem cell, and both neutrophils and lymphocytes of thymus and bone marrow origin are affected. Red cells and platelets are normal. The bone marrow shows an absence of myeloid precursor cells. The thymus is hypoplastic and lymphocytes are absent from the lymph nodes, tonsils, Peyer's patches and periarteriolar areas of the spleen. Agammaglobulinaemia is a consistent finding. Death is usually early and as a result of bacterial infection, although the infant is equally susceptible to viruses. The disorder is universally fatal, although as it is a stem cell defect, bone marrow transplantation may be effective.

Neutropenia with inherited immune disorders

Neutropenia may be associated with both humoral and cellular immunodeficiencies. About a third of boys with X-linked agammaglobulinaemia are neutropenic, and persistent and cyclical neutropenia have been reported with a number of other syndromes characterized by hypogammaglobulinaemia, particularly if IgM is raised.

INHERITED DISORDERS OF NEUTROPHIL FUNCTION WITH ONSET IN INFANCY

There are physiological functional differences between the neutrophils of neonates and those of older children and adults. Impaired neutrophil locomotion is undoubtedly the most important, and both chemotaxis and random neutrophil migration are abnormal. Decreased membrane deformability has been suggested as the underlying defect. Monocytes also demonstrate defective chemotaxis. Immune recognition is normal, but opsonization is impaired. Phagocytosis and intracellular killing of bacteria are both suboptimal under stress.

Many of the inherited disorders do not present until several months or years of age.

'Lazy-leucocyte' syndrome

This disorder may present in the newborn period, but more typically some time later. Neutropenia accompanies the impairment of both chemotaxis and random neutrophil movement. Infections are mild and generally involve the gums, skin, tympanic membranes and respiratory tract. Neutrophil migration into skin windows is defective. Despite the neutropenia, the bone marrow contains normal numbers of myeloid precursors and responds poorly to stimulation with standard agents, suggesting that the neutropenia may result from a failure of migration from marginated pools. Phagocytosis, bactericidal killing, humoral and cellular immunity are all normal.

Chédiak–Higashi syndrome

This disorder with autosomal recessive inheritance may present in infancy. It is characterized by the presence of large abnormal coalesced lysosomal granules, not only in the cytoplasm of neutrophils but also in many other tissues (Figure 8.8). The abnormal distribution of these giant granules in the hair, skin and eye leads to partial oculocutaneous albinism with photophobia and nystagmus. Frequent pyogenic infections and a mild bleeding diathesis are characteristic. A wide range of neurological abnormalities result from the presence of the same granules in neurological tissue.

Pyogenic infections, primarily involving the chest, skin and mucous membranes are frequent. Both Gram-positive and Gram-negative bacteria are common. Viral infections are dealt with normally, although fungal infections may be problematic.

Initially neutrophils are normal or low normal in number due to intramedullary destruction of abnormal myeloid precursors that already contain giant granules. Defects of chemotaxis, degranulation and bacterial killing have all been documented. The delayed killing of bacteria appears to be due to failure of the giant lysosomes of neutrophils containing ingested bacteria to transfer their peroxidative and lysosomal enzymes into the phagocytic vesicles. Neutrophils in this disorder exhibit impaired adherence to surfaces. Fluorescent concavalin-A capping, a technique used to study the cytoskeleton of the neutrophil, is defective. Capping is spontaneous in Chédiak–Higashi cells; normal cells only do this after colchicine treatment.

Although the basic defect in Chédiak–Higashi neutrophils has not been identified, it would appear to involve microtubule–membrane dependent

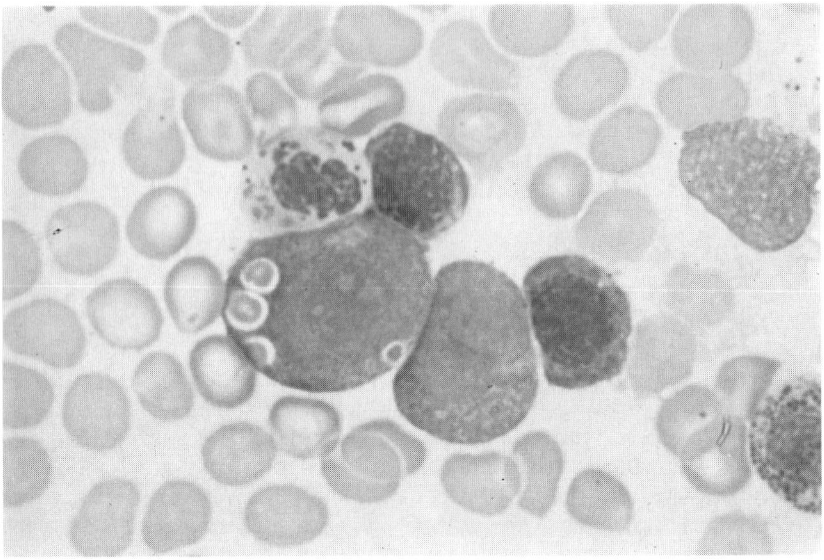

Figure 8.8 Bone marrow smear of Chédiak–Higashi syndrome showing the characteristic large eosinophilic coalesced granules in the myeloid percursors and a neutrophil with a pyknotic nucleus and large irregular cytoplasmic granules.

function. Microtubules are involved in the secretory and degranulatory function of cells. Raised levels of cyclic AMP have been reported in the neutrophils of a small number of patients with Chédiak–Higashi syndrome. Ascorbic acid lowers the level and corrects the defect of mobility, bacterial killing and concanavalin-A capping. Chédiak–Higashi neutrophils have also been reported to have increased membrane fluidity and a reduced ratio of polyunsaturated to saturated fatty acids, which is further evidence to support a basic membrane disorder. Lymphocytes may also contain giant cytoplasmic granules and natural killer cell function is diminished. On bone marrow examination, the giant lysosomal granules are seen to be present in granulocyte, eosinophil and monocyte precursors. As might be expected, immunoglobulin levels are often raised in older children as a result of chronic stimulation from repeated infections. Platelets may contain these large granules and aggregate abnormally, resulting in a prolonged bleeding time. Chédiak–Higashi platelets show impaired aggregation in keeping with a storage pool defect.

More than 85% of patients proceed to an accelerated phase that is rapidly fatal. It is characterized by widespread lymphocytic and histocytic infiltration of lymphoreticular organs, resulting in lymphadenopathy and hepatosplenomegaly. This transition can occur at any age and can be in the first year of life. When pancytopenia develops and thrombocytopenia co-exists with the platelet defect, bleeding can become problematic. High-dose corticosteroids may produce a temporary partial response during the accelerated phase, but generally cytotoxics have not met with success. A favourable outcome has been reported following bone marrow transplantation. Prior to the onset of the accelerated phase, high doses of ascorbic acid have been shown to correct the neutrophil dysfunction and decrease the severity of infections. Treatment is otherwise symptomatic, and appropriate antibiotic therapy is governed by results of bacterial surveillance. Prophylactic co-trimoxazole may be beneficial. Appropriate measures should be taken to protect against photophobia and skin sensitivity.

Chronic granulomatous disease

This disorder of neutrophil killing can present in the newborn period, although it rarely does so and more commonly presents later in the first year of life. The clinical problems result from a failure of neutrophils to undergo a respiratory burst, thereby reducing oxygen to the bactericidal product, hydrogen peroxide: the superoxide anion, hydroxyl radical and singlet oxygen are not formed.

The disorder is clinically characterized by chronic and recurrent bacterial and fungal infections (Figure 8.9). Chronic granulomata and abscesses develop in the skin, lymph nodes, lungs, liver and bones. Hepatic abscesses are a common presentation in the newborn period. Troublesome organisms

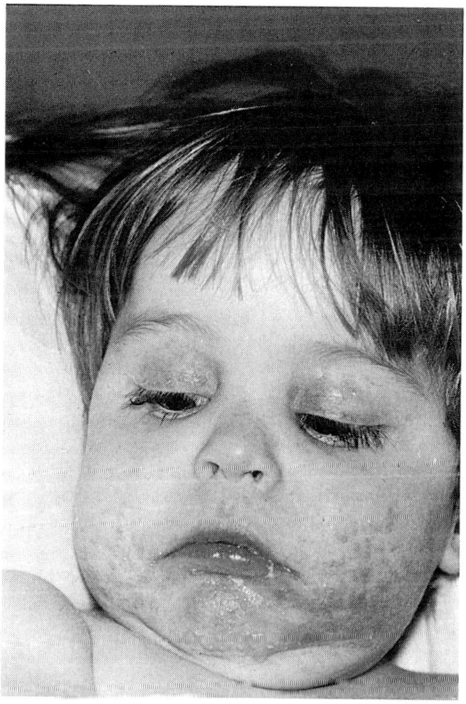

Figure 8.9 Infant with chronic granulomatous disease and infected facial eczema (with permission of Salford Health Authority).

include *Staphylococcus aureus, Serratia marcescens, Salmonella, Candida* and *Aspergillus*. Viruses do not present problems.

Neutrophils demonstrate normal chemotaxis and ingestion of bacteria, but catalase-positive organisms that don't elaborate their own hydrogen peroxide survive. Neutrophil fungicidal capacity is also impaired. The rate of reduction of oxygen to superoxide anion can be quantified by the reduction of nitroblue tetrazolium (NBT) to insoluble purple formazan. The ability of neutrophils to reduce NBT can distinguish normal individuals, patients with chronic granulomatous disease and carriers for the disorder. The NBT test has now been adapted for prenatal diagnosis.

There appear to be two modes of inheritance, X-linked and autosomal recessive, the former being far commoner. Failure to activate the respiratory burst can be due either to a defect of the oxidase enzyme system, which reduces oxygen, or to a more generalized abnormality of the membrane, leading to a failure of the activation pathway. NADPH oxidase in its active form catalyses the one-electron reduction of oxygen to superoxide. Cytochrome *b*-245 is considered to be a subunit of NADPH oxidase. Boys with X-linked chronic granulomatous disease have been shown to have an absence of the haemoprotein, cytochrome *b*-245. Segal *et al.* were unable to detect this cytochrome in the granulocytes of any of the 19 males he investigated who had X-linked chronic granulomatous disease (Segal *et al.*, 1983). Female heterozygotes had reduced levels. In contrast, he found the cytochrome to be present but non-functional in eight patients in whom the disorder had probably been inherited in an autosomal recessive manner, implicating an abnormality in the activation pathway and not a defect in the oxidase enzyme itself.

Neutrophils from normal individuals possess a Kell group antigen designated Kx, which is not present on the neutrophils of boys with X-linked chronic granulomatous disease who may be of the rare null blood group phenotype K_0, in which all antigenic products of the Kell antigen are absent. This association is not seen with the autosomal mode of inheritance and it is of interest because the Kell antigen is not located on the X-chromosome. The absence of a membrane antigen may be linked with the abnormal membrane function.

There is no specific therapy to correct the neutrophil defect, although there may be a role for bone marrow transplantation. Antibiotic therapy should be guided by sensitivity testing. Long-term prophylaxis with co-trimoxazole appears to be associated with a measurable reduction in infections. Sulphonamides, which generate free radical products of reduced oxygen, may have a special role. Granulocyte transfusions have been used in the presence of life-threatening sepsis with variable outcome. Although few children in the past reached their second decade, the prognosis appears to be improving, with some reaching adulthood. This probably reflects better antibiotic treatment and the heterogeneity of the disease, with milder forms being recognized.

MORPHOLOGICAL VARIANTS OF NEUTROPHILS

A number of inherited morphological variants have been described which can be detected in the neonatal period.

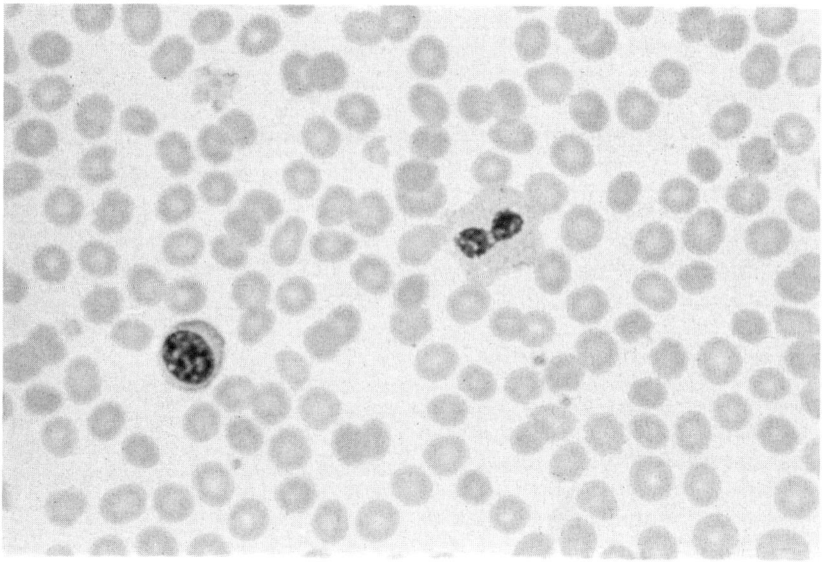

Figure 8.10 Blood film from a patient with Pelger–Hüet anomaly showing a bilobed and a round, unsegmented neutrophil.

Pelger–Hüet anomaly

This autosomal dominant disorder (Figure 8.10) has an incidence of 1:6000 and is characterized by a failure of normal nuclear segmentation. Neutrophils and eosinophils from affected individuals rarely have more than two lobes. Homozygotes have mature neutrophils with round nuclei, whilst heterozygotes have unsegmented, dumb-bell shaped or bilobed nuclei. In some cases, neutrophil migration has been reported as marginally impaired, but otherwise the neutrophils appear to function normally. The Pelger-Hüet anomaly may also occur as an acquired disorder, most importantly with myeloproliferative disorders.

Hereditary prevalence of nuclear appendages

Neutrophils with excessive numbers of thread-like nuclear projections may be seen as a familial condition or in trisomy 13–15 and in Turner's syndrome; it is important to distinguish these projections from drumsticks.

Hereditary hypersegmentation of neutrophils

The average number of lobes found in normal mature neutrophils is three, but in this autosomal dominant disorder it increases to four. This hypersegmentation is not associated with any abnormality but should be distinguished from vitamin B_{12} and folate deficiencies and myeloproliferative disorders.

Hereditary hypersegmentation of eosinophils

This inherited disorder of eosinophil hypersegmentation is characterized by an average eosinophil lobe number of three or four, compared with two or three for normal eosinophils. This anomaly has no adverse associations.

Hereditary giant neutrophils

This disorder is autosomal dominant and is characterized by both an increase in neutrophil diameter (50%) and hypersegmentation of the nucleus (6–10 lobes). This anomaly has no clinical significance and represents only a small percentage of neutrophils in affected individuals.

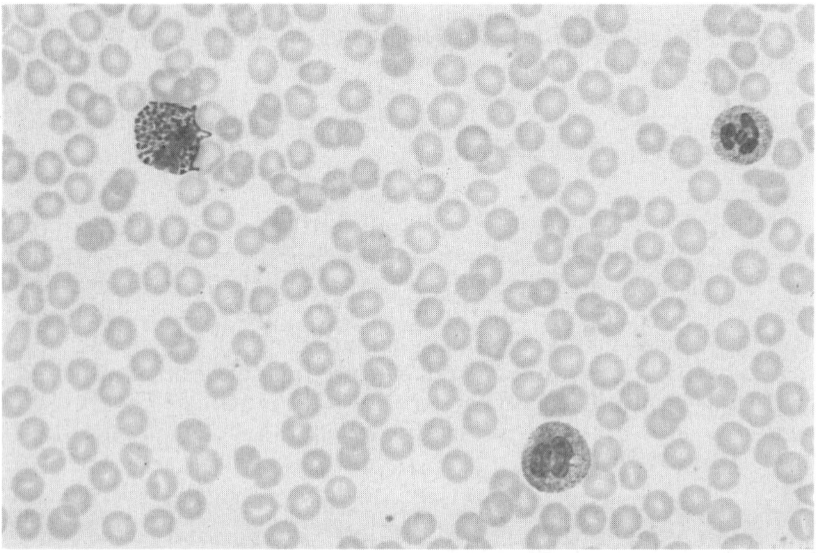

Figure 8.11 Blood film showing Alder–Reilly anomaly with characteristic dense granulation of the neutrophils (see Figure 8.12).

Alder–Reilly anomaly

This anomaly (Figures 8.11 and 8.12) describes the prominent azurophilic granules in neutrophils, lymphocytes and monocytes, which may be a feature of some types of mucopolysaccharidoses. The granules, which stain positively with metachromatic stains, have been reported in Hunter's syndrome, Hurler syndrome and Sanfilippo's syndrome.

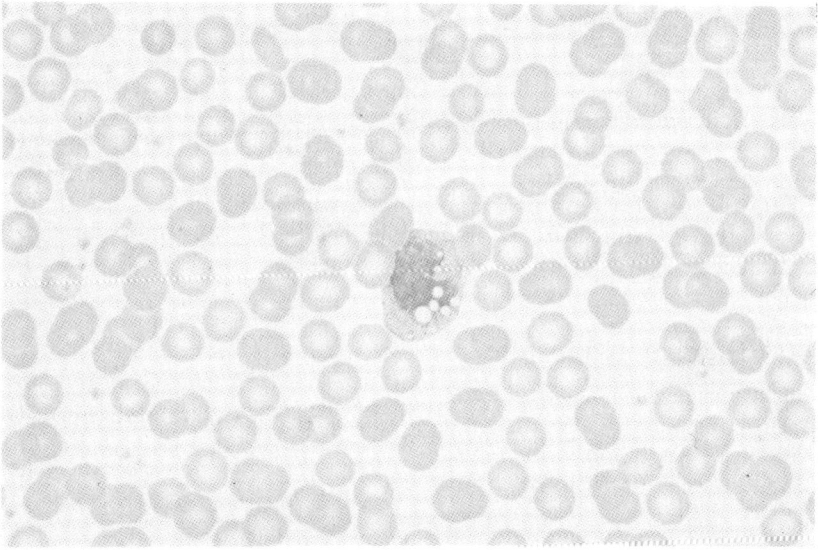

Figure 8.12 Alder–Reilly anomaly, with prominent lymphocyte vacuolation (same patient as in Figure 8.11).

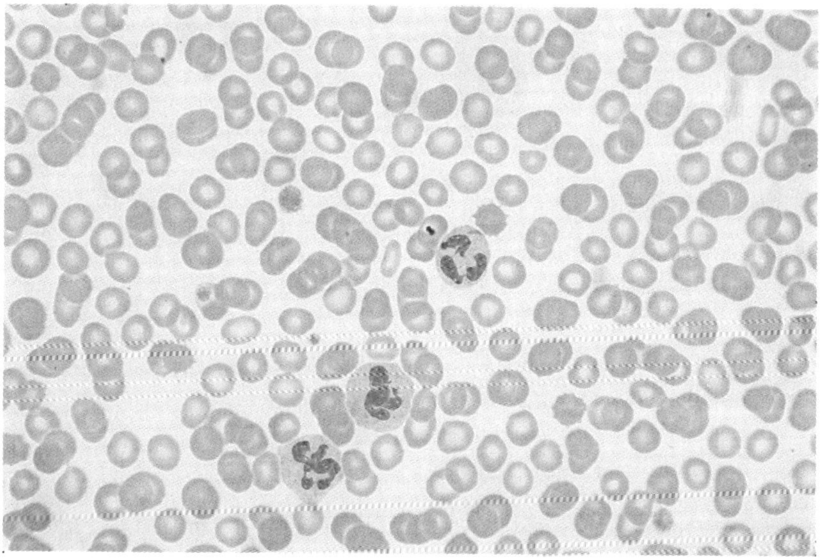

Figure 8.13 Blood film of May–Hegglin anomaly with characteristic giant platelets and Döhle bodies in the neutrophils.

May–Hegglin anomaly

This autosomal dominant disorder (Figure 8.13) is characterized by giant platelets, leucopenia and neutrophils which contain large cytoplasmic inclusions consisting of aggregates of ribosomal material resembling Döhle bodies. These inclusions are also found in eosinophils, basophils and monocytes. One third of patients have thrombocytopenia and defects of platelet function have also been described. There is no associated undue susceptibility to infection.

Chédiak-Higashi syndrome

This autosomal recessive disorder (Figure 8.8) is characterized by giant lysosomes in neutrophils and lymphocytes. These are associated with an increased susceptibility to infection.

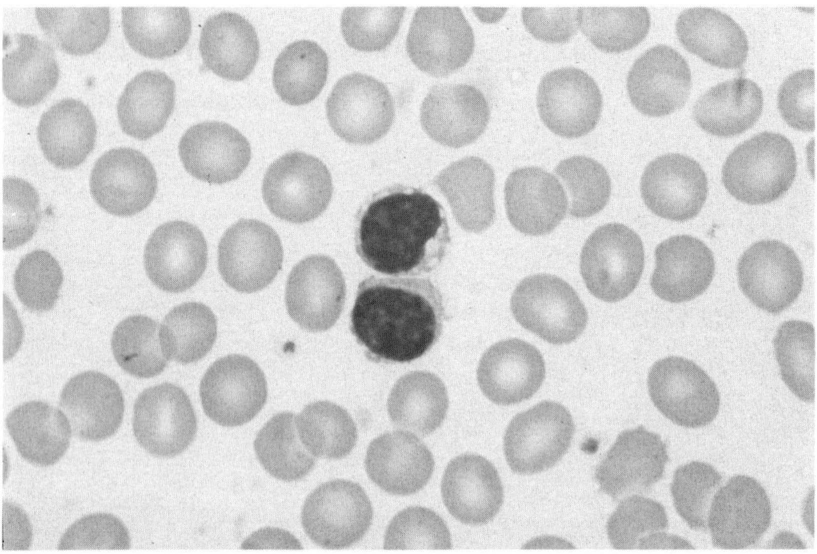

Figure 8.14 Blood film of Batten–Spielmeyer–Vogt disease showing vacuolation of the lymphocytes.

Batten–Spielmeyer–Vogt disease

This degenerative neurologic disorder is characterized by coarse azurophilic granules in neutrophils and lymphocytes which are not metachromic. Cytoplasmic vacuoles (Figure 8.14) have also been described.

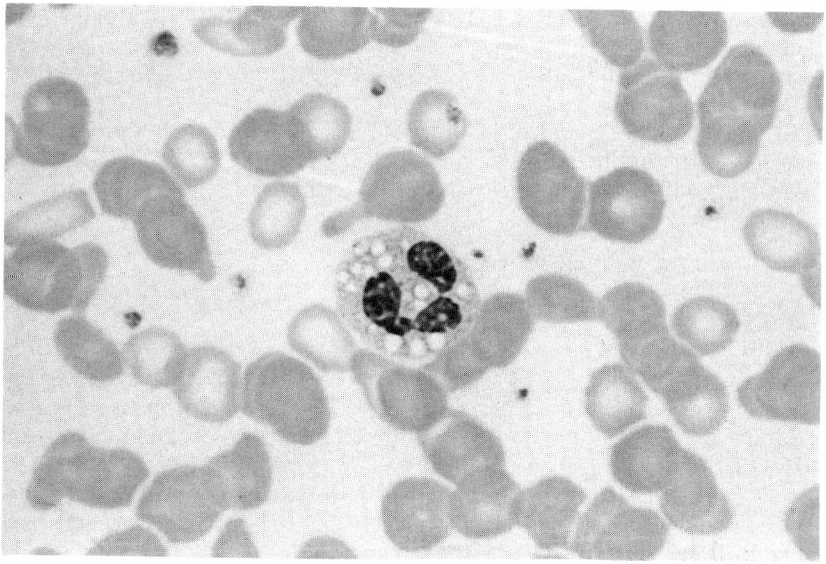

Figure 8.15 Blood film of Jordan's anomaly showing the characteristic prominent cytoplasmic vacuolation of the neutrophils.

Jordan's anomaly

This familial disorder (Figure 8.15) is characterized by lipid-containing vacuoles in the cytoplasm of granulocytes, monocytes and, less often, lymphocytes. Some affected individuals have had ichthyosis, whilst others have developed a progressive muscular disease.

NEONATAL LYMPHOPENIA

The lymphocyte count at birth is between 3.0×10^9 and 5.0×10^9 per litre and rises during the first few weeks of life. Large- and medium-sized lymphocytes dominate. In the newborn period most lymphopenias are hereditary. A lymphocyte count at birth of less than 1.5×10^9 per litre merits further investigation. Until such investigations have been completed and the nature of the immune deficiency determined, such infants should not receive live vaccines and should be transfused irradiated blood products, if required. At birth B lymphocyte numbers are normal, and the relative inability of the neonate to produce antibody is related to impaired helper T cell function. Neonatal T lymphocytes are less effective than those of adults. The B cell disorders of agammaglobulinaemia and dysgammaglobulinaemia generally do not present clinically in the neonatal period, although the characteristic recurrent bacterial infections may date from the second half of the first year of life. These disorders are not usually associated with undue susceptibility to viral infections. It is important not to confuse true immune deficiency with transient hypogammaglobulinaemia of infancy. Because the levels of immunoglobulins are normally low in the early months of life, it is difficult to be confident about the diagnosis of B cell defects by measuring immunoglobulin levels alone. Complete or partial B cell defects are not associated with such serious infections as T cell deficiencies, which frequently result in a profound inability to handle both viral and fungal infections and present early.

Severe combined immunodeficiency syndromes

This heterogeneous group of disorders, termed SCID, is characterized by severe impairment of both humoral and cell mediated immunity. Affected individuals may have no T or B lymphocytes, no T cells and variable numbers of B cells, or normal numbers of both T and B cells which are phenotypically abnormal or immature. The pathogenesis is controversial and probably also heterogenous. A defect of a common lymphoid stem cell has been postulated to explain the involvement of both T and B lymphocytes. Alternatively, a primary lack of T cells would result directly in the cell-mediated immune impairment and indirectly in the humoral component of the disease through lack of helper cell stimulation of B cells.

The infants generally present with infection in the first few months of life and these commonly affect the skin or respiratory tract. Opportunistic infections are frequent, in particular *Pneumocystis carinii* and *Candida* affecting both the mouth and nappy area can be problematic. Diarrhoea with failure to thrive is the commonest presenting symptom. A morbilliform rash is also characteristic. Infections with CMV, varicella, measles and adenovirus are usually life-threatening. If these babies are vaccinated they will develop disseminated vaccinia. If they are transfused blood that has not been irradiated, engraftment of the transfused cells may result in fatal graft-versus-host-disease (GVHD). Similarly maternal engraftment *in utero* may result in an exfoliative dermatitis of GVHD. Affected babies who are breast fed may do better than those who are not in the early months, because of antibodies acquired from human milk. However, these disorders are fatal within the first year or two of life and, to date, bone marrow transplantation holds the best hope for survival.

The infants are usually lymphopenic, and small lymphocytes are particularly depleted. These disorders are heterogenous in terms of lymphocyte characteristics, but T cells are usually absent or scarce and the lymphocytes present are B or null cells. Peripheral lymphocytes are completely unresponsive to phytohaemagglutinin or pokeweed stimulation. Skin test reactivity to recall antigens is negative. Immunoglobulins are low and, although this is physiological in the newborn, they remain low. However variants have been described in which immunoglobulin levels are normal (Nezelof's syndrome) or in which there is a selective immunoglobulin deficiency. Isohaemogglutinins and antibodies to previously administered vaccine antigens are absent. Lymphocytes and plasma cells are absent from the bone marrow and lymph nodes. Myeloid pecursors are normal in number and an eosinophilia is common. The thymus gland is absent on the chest X-ray, and aplasia of the thymus and lymphoid tissue is found at autopsy, despite chronic infection.

Autosomal and X-linked recessive inheritance is recognized. The male to female ratio is 3:1. The term SCID covers a heterogeneous group of disorders of immunodeficiency. About 20% of children with SCID have defects of enzymes necessary for the catabolism of purines, most commonly adenosine deaminase (ADA) deficiency, which is inherited as an autosomal recessive disorder and the structural gene located on chromosome 20. ADA is found in all cells of the body, and the severity of the immune defect correlates with the amount of residual ADA activity in lymphocytes. A second enzyme defect, purine nucleoside phosphorylase deficiency (PNP), results in profound T cell deficiency. The gene for this autosomal recessive condition is located on chromosome 14. Both enzyme defects lead to an inhibition of DNA synthesis through inhibition of ribonuceotide reductase. Whether this is the only mechanism leading to failure of normal development of the lymphoid system is unclear.

As already stated, bone marrow transplantation gives the best hope for these infants. However, few have a histocompatible sibling. Haplotype grafts, using a parent as the donor, are often the only option and these are associated with major graft-versus-host problems. ADA deficiency is found in donor red cells, and some infants with ADA deficiency have been reported to benefit temporarily from red cell transfusion as judged by a rise in lymphocyte numbers and immunoglobulin levels. Enzyme replacement may soon be a therapeutic option. The benefits of long-term germ-free nursing are arguable. Adequate nutrition, co-trimoxazole prophylaxis and breast-feeding may all play a worthwhile role. Intravenous immunoglobulin is beneficial, and specific infections should be treated vigorously with antibacterial and fungistatic drugs.

Prenatal diagnosis is now available by means of lymphocyte phenotyping or measurement of ADA or purine nucleoside phosphorylase levels in amniotic fluid, chorionic villi or fetal red cells.

The WHO classification of primary immunodeficiency diseases is given in Table 8.6.

NEONATAL THROMBOCYTOPENIA

Neonatal thrombocytopenia may be either acquired or inherited and can result from impaired platelet production or increased peripheral destruction. It is a common occurrence and is usually acquired and associated with specific stimuli operating at this time; for example, maternal antibodies, infection, hypoxia and exchange transfusion. However, both hereditary thrombocytopenia and qualitative platelet defects can present in this age group. The degree of thrombocytopenia is then generally less severe, especially when compared with immune-mediated thrombocytopenia. An inherited basis is suggested by co-existent congenital anomalies (although these may also occur with infection, e.g. rubella) and a positive family history.

Table 8.6 Classification of primary immunodeficiency diseases.*

Designation	Serum Ig and antibodies	Circulating B cells	Circulating T cells	Presumed pathogenesis	Inheritance	Associated features
Predominantly antibody defects						
X-linked agammaglobulin-aemia	All isotypes decreased	Usually absent	–	Intrinsic defect pre-B- to B-cell differentiation	XL	–
X-linked hypogamma-globulinaemia with growth hormone deficiency	All isotypes decreased	Usually absent	–	Unknown	XL	Short stature
Autosomal recessive agammaglobulin-aemia	All isotypes decreased	Decreased	–	Unknown	AR	–
Ig deficiency with increased IgM (and IgD) ('hyper-IgM syndrome')	IgM and IgD increased or normal, other isotypes decreased	IgM- and IgD-bearing cells normal, others absent	–	Isotype switch defect	Various: XL, AR, unknown	–
IgA deficiency	IgA_1, with IgA_2 decreased, with or without IgG_2, IgG_3, or IgG_4 decrease	Normal	–	Failure of terminal differentiation	Various: AR, unknown	Frequent in families with CVID

	IgA_1 or IgA_2 decreased	Normal	–	Chromosomal deletion at 14q32 in some patients	AR	–
Selective deficiency of other Ig isotypes	Decrease in one or more isotype, other isotypes normal or increased	Unknown	–	Defects of isotype differentiation	Unknown	–
k-chain deficiency	Ig(k) decreased; antibody response normal or decreased	Normal or K^+ decreased	–	In some patients point mutations at chromosome 2p11	Unknown	–
ID with thyoma	All isotypes decreased	Absent or very low	–	Unknown	Unknown	Thymoma, anaemia, eosinopenia
Transient hypogamma-globulinemia of infancy	IgG and IgA decreased	Normal	–	Terminal differentiation maturation defect; delayed maturation of helper function in some	Unknown	Frequent in families with other IDs
Common variable immunodeficiency						
Predominant antibody deficiency	Various decreases of multiple isotypes	Normal or decreased	Usually normal	Intrinsic B-cell defect; low B-cell number; defective helper function; antibodies to B cells	AR, AD, or unknown	

Table 8.6 *continued.*

Designation	Serum Ig and antibodies	Circulating B cells	Circulating T cells	Presumed pathogenesis	Inheritance	Associated features
Predominant CMI defect	Various decreases of multiple isotypes	Normal	Normal or decreased	Activated suppressor-T-cell function; markedly reduced T-cell numbers; autoantibodies to T cells	Unknown AR	Autoimmune phenomena
Severe combined immunodeficiency						
Reticular dysgenesis	Decreased	Decreased	Decreased	Defective differentiation of T and B cells; lymphomyeloid maturation defect	AR	Pancytopenia
Low T- and B-cell numbers	Decreased	Decreased	Decreased	Maturation defect of both T and B cells	AR or XL	–
Low T-, normal B-cell numbers	Normal or decreased	Normal	Decreased	Lymphoid maturation defect of both T and B cells	AR or XL	–
Adenosine deaminase deficiency	Progressive disease	Decreased	Decreased	T-cell (and B-cell) defects from toxic metabolites due to enzyme deficiency	AR	Dysostosis in some

Purine nucleoside phosphorylase deficiency	Progressive decrease	Normal	Progressive decrease	T-cell defect from metabolites due to enzyme deficiency	AR	Anemia, mental retardation
MHC class I deficiency ('bare lymphocyte syndrome')	Normal or decreased	Normal	Normal (CMI defective)	Defect of gene transcription	AR	–
MCH class II deficiency	Decreased or normal	Normal	Normal (CMI defective)	Defect of gene transcription	AR	Intestinal malabsorption
Immunodeficiency associated with other major defects						
Wiskott–Aldrich syndrome	Decreased IgM, antibody to polysaccharides particularly decreased	Normal	Progressive decrease	Cell membrane defect affecting haemopoietic stem cell derivatives	XL	Thrombocytopenia, small defective platelets, eczema, lymphoreticular malignancy
Ataxia telangiectasia	Often decreased IgA, IgE, and IgG; increased IgM (monomers); antibodies variably decreased	Normal	Decreased	Unknown; defective T-cell maturation	AR	Ataxia, telangiectasia, defective chromosomal repair, raised α fetoprotein, lymphoreticular malignancy
3rd and 4th pouch/arch syndrome (DiGeorge)	Normal or decreased	–	Decreased	Embryopathy: abnormal thymus with resultant T-cell defects	None or unknown	Hypoparathyroidism: cardiac outflow tract malformation,

Table 8.6 *continued.*

Designation	Serum Ig and antibodies	Circulating B cells	Circulating T cells	Presumed pathogenesis	Inheritance	Associated features
						abnormal facies, mental defect (some), GI tract malformation (some)
Transcobalamin 2 deficiency	All isotypes decreased	Normal	Normal	Defect in B_{12} transport resulting in defective cell proliferation, B cell to plasma cell differentiation	AR	Megaloblastic anaemia, intestinal villous atrophy; defective granulocyte bactericidal activity
ID with partial albinism	Decreased	Normal	Decreased or normal	Unknown	AR	Cerebral atrophy, pigment clumping in melanocytes, defective NK cells
ID following hereditary defective response to EBV	Decreased only after EBV infection	Decreased only after EBV infection	Decreased only after EBV infection; NK cells increased	Unknown	XL, AR	Fatal EBV infection, aplastic anaemia, lymphoproliferative disease in some

* Report of a WHO Scientific Group. XL = X-linked, AR = autosomal recessive, CVID = common variable immunodeficiency, AD = autosomal dominant, GI = gastrointestinal, ID = immunodeficiency, NK = natural killer, EBV = Epstein Barr virus.

Decreased production of platelets

Thrombocytopenia due to decreased platelet production is nearly always associated with obvious congenital anomalies in the affected infant. Several distinct syndromes have emerged from classification of the patterns of associated anomalies, the thrombocytopenia with absent radii (TAR) syndrome and Fanconi's anaemia being the best examples. The inheritance of some congenital thrombocytopenias has not been clearly defined and the probability of a genetic origin hinges on reports of more than one child in a family being affected. In such cases an autosomal recessive mode of transmission seems likely.

Fanconi's anaemia

Fanconi's anaemia is an uncommon autosomal recessive disorder characterized by bone marrow failure, resulting in pancytopenia. It is associated with a wide spectrum of congenital anomalies, primarily involving musculoskeletal and genitourinary systems. Approximately 75% of affected individuals have abnormal patchy pigmentation, which is usually central in distribution. Short stature will become apparent in about the same percentage. The majority have skeletal malformations, which most commonly affect the thumbs or radii. About a quarter of infants have renal anomalies, most often an absence of one kidney.

Although the congenital anomalies are evident at birth, pancytopenia typically is delayed for 5 or more years. This contrasts with the TAR syndrome, in which haemorrhagic problems manifest themselves within the first few days of life. Examination of the bone marrow initially shows erythroid hyperplasia and megaloblastosis, but progressive hypoplasia later develops. Thrombocytopenia is usually the first expression of the progressive marrow failure and there have been a few reports of this occurring in the neonatal period. At the author's laboratory one infant has presented at birth with thrombocytopenia, and increased chromosomal fragility confirmed the diagnosis. Anaemia has also been reported in the newborn.

The disorder appears to be very heterogenous. In addition to classical Fanconi's anaemia, one family member may have the congenital anomalies without the haematological manifestations, whilst another has the haematological manifestations without the congenital anomalies. Acute non-lymphoblastic leukaemia is a common complication and both affected and non-affected family members have an increased incidence. DNA repair is defective. Chromosomal defects seen in mitomycin-C stimulated peripheral blood lymphocytes include chromatid and chromosomal breakages, gaps and constrictions. This increase in mitomycin-C induced chromosomal breaks is diagnostic for Fanconi's anaemia and distinguishes it from other forms of aplastic anaemia. Prenatal diagnosis is possible by demonstrating an increase in spontaneous and diepoxybutane-induced chromosomal breaks, and the technology can be applied to cultured fetal amniotic fluid cells or chorionic villus samples, the latter having the advantage of allowing termination of pregnancy in the first trimester. Although the inheritance is

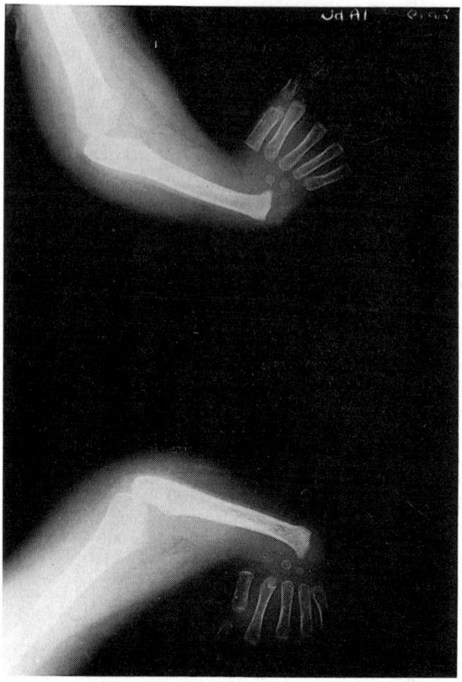

Figure 8.16 An X-ray of an infant with TAR syndrome showing bilateral absence of the radii (with permission of Salford Health Authority).

probably autosomal recessive, the heterogeneity between members of an affected family suggests that a second, perhaps environmental factor, is involved.

Bone marrow transplantation has been employed with success. Androgens are widely used but are generally more effective in improving erythropoiesis than thrombocytopoiesis. Haemorrhage, particularly intracranial, is a major cause of death.

Thrombocytopenia with absent radii (TAR syndome)

This disorder is characterized by thrombocytopenia and bilateral absence of the radii (Figures 8.16 and 8.17) and is the commonest familial thrombocytopenia to present in the neonatal period. Both thumbs are present, which helps to distinguish the disorder from Fanconi's anaemia. Megakaryocytes are absent or decreased in the bone marrow, and in the latter case are small and immature. The platelet count is commonly in the range of 10×10^9 to 30×10^9 per litre. A platelet-function defect resembling storage pool disease has been reported. Bone marrow culture studies suggest that other cell lines are not involved. In the first few months of life a leukaemoid reaction is common. The white cell count is greater than 30×10^9 and may exceed 100×10^9 per litre and be left-shifted. Although leukaemia has been

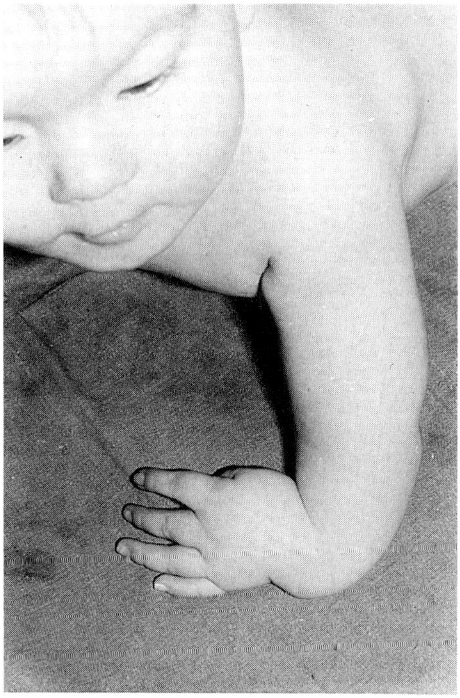

Figure 8.17 An infant with TAR syndrome showing the classical forearm deformity; the thumb is present, distinguishing the disorder from Fanconi's anaemia (with permission of Salford Health Authority).

reported in the past, it is likely that it was mistaken for the leukaemoid reaction associated with this disorder. Haemorrhagic manifestations are usually apparent within the first few days, or at best weeks, of life. Petechiae and melaena are common. Intracranial haemorrhage poses the greatest risk to life in the newborn period. Anaemia may be present and is usually secondary to blood loss, but a decreased red cell survival has been reported. Bilateral absence of the radii are evident at birth and there may be other associated congenital deformities. Variants with complete phocomelia have been reported. Some affected families have been described as having members with absent radii but a normal platelet count.

About 30% of affected infants die in the first year of life from haemorrhage. It is important to prevent fatal intracranial haemorrhage during the first months of life, when bleeding may be particularly severe, as the outlook may be favourable if the infant survives the first year. Single donor units of platelets are preferable to minimize the chance of sensitization. Gradual improvement in the platelet count usually takes place towards the end of the first year, when low normal levels may be achieved. Life expectancy thereafter normalizes. Orthopaedic procedures should be delayed until the platelet count has attained an acceptable level. Corticosteroids and splenectomy have no role. If there is already an affected infant in the family, genetic advice may be possible. Assuming an autosomal recessive inheritance, the chance of a subsequent pregnancy being affected is one in four. Absent radii have been detected by fetal ultrasonography and appropriate counselling about termination given. If necessary the fetal platelet count can be measured on a sample obtained by fetoscopy at 18–20 weeks.

Other congenital hypoplastic thrombocytopenias

Fanconi's anaemia and TAR are the best established familial amegakaryocytic thrombocytopenias. Congenital hypoplastic thrombocytopenia associated with microcephaly has been reported in three infants, two of whom were brothers (Eisenten, 1966; Hoyeraal *et al.*, 1970). The thrombocytopenia persisted into the second year of life, making an infectious cause such as rubella unlikely. Amegakaryocytic thrombocytopenia is an uncommon finding in both trisomy 13 and 18. Some cases of trisomy 18 have been associated with absent radii.

Increased destruction of defective platelets

Wiskott–Aldrich syndrome

This rare X-linked disorder is characterized by eczema (Figures 8.18 and 8.19), chronic thrombocytopenic purpura and an increased incidence of recurrent infection due to both viruses and bacteria. Combined humoral and cellular immunodeficiencies result in frequent infections of variable severity. Presentation is usually in the first few months of life and symptoms due to thrombocytopenia generally present first. Melaena and purpura are common. An increased risk of lymphoreticular malignancy is well documented. A forme fruste of the disorder is recognized in which thrombocytopenia is the predominant problem, with little or no evidence of eczema or immunodeficiency. However, these infants may become immune deficient at a later date and should be carefully monitored.

Examination of the blood smear shows small, infrequent platelets (Figure 8.20). Adequate numbers of megakaryoctyes are present, but a variety of bizarre nuclear anomalies may be seen. The thrombocytopenia is thought to result from the dual mechanisms of decreased production and increased destruction. The small abnormal platelets also have a functional defect resembling storage pool disease. A 115 000 Da glycoprotein has been reported to be absent from T cell membranes and glycoprotein Ib from platelets of affected individuals. Lymphopenia is usual and progressive, and lymphocyte function becomes increasingly impaired. IgG and IgA are usually normal, but IgM levels are low and isohaemagglutinins not produced.

More than half of affected boys die in the first decade of life. Death results from infection, haemorrhage or a lymphoid malignancy. Treatment is supportive; antibiotics for infection and platelet infusions for bleeding

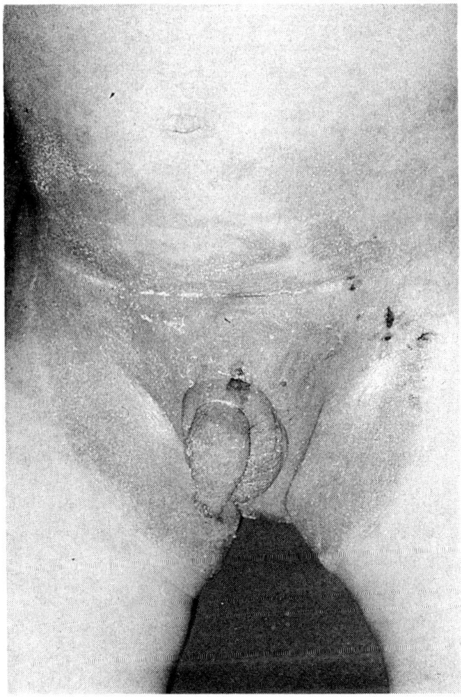

Figure 8.18 Severe eczematous nappy rash with haemorrhagic areas in an infant with Wiskott–Aldrich syndrome (with permission of Salford Health Authority).

episodes. Steroids have not been beneficial in correcting the thrombocytopenia and splenectomy is contraindicated at this age because of infection, but it may be worthwhile later. The increased risk of infection post-splenectomy in an already immunocompromised individual must be balanced against the benefit of increasing platelet survival and decreasing the risk of haemorrhage. Children with the forme fruste of Wiskott–Aldrich syndrome, characterized primarily by thrombocytopenia, may well benefit from splenectomy with less risk of post-splenectomy infection if they show no evidence of co-existent immune incompetence. Bone marrow transplantation has been employed successfully to correct both the thrombocytopenia and immunodeficiency (Kapoor *et al.*, 1980). Supportive blood products should be irradiated to prevent GVHD, particularly in older children with severely compromised cellular immunity.

INHERITED THROMBOCYTOPATHIES

Glanzmann's disease commonly presents in early infancy, but Bernard–Soulier syndrome, although inherited, usually presents after the neonatal period. These disorders are of interest because both can now be diagnosed in infancy by monoclonal antibody techniques.

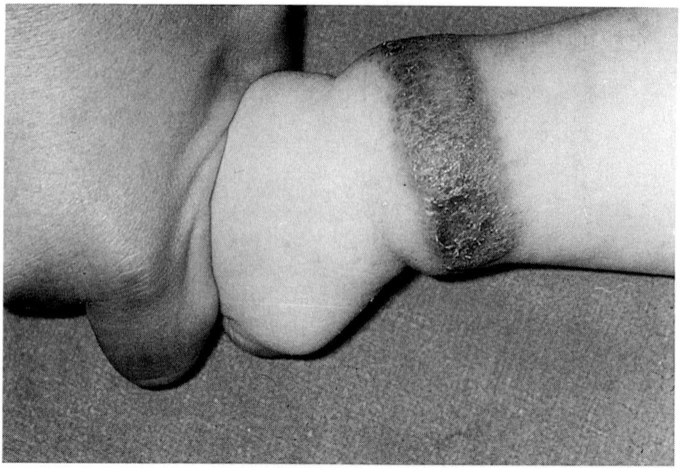

Figure 8.19 Severe allergic reaction to a plastic name-tag in an infant with Wiskott–Aldrich syndrome (with permission of Salford Health Authority).

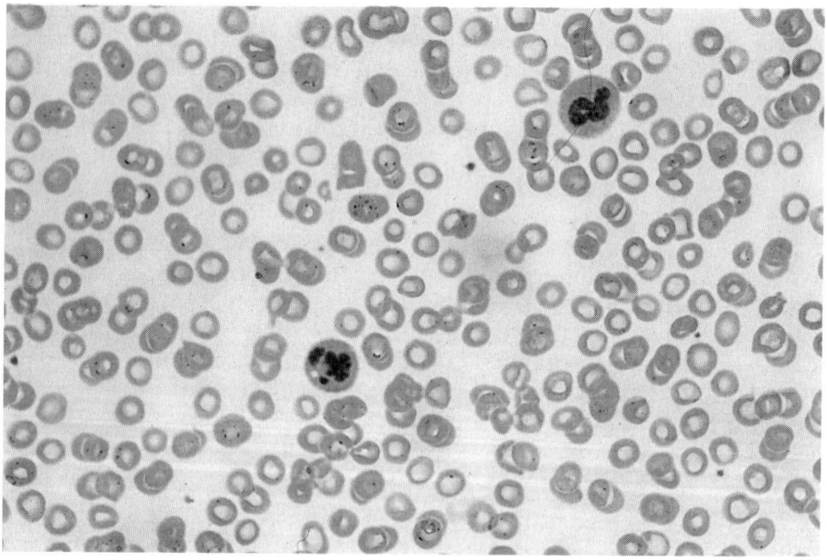

Figure 8.20 Blood film of Wiskott–Aldrich syndrome showing infrequent small platelets.

Bernard–Soulier syndrome

This rare disorder with an autosomal recessive inheritance is characterized by mild to moderate thrombocytopenia and giant platelets on the blood smear (Figure 8.21). The bleeding time is prolonged and platelet adhesion is defective. Platelet aggregation with ristocetin is abnormal, but normal with all other agonists. The defective platelet function results from absence of specific platelet membrane glycoproteins. In Bernard–Soulier syndrome platelets lack platelet membrane glycoproteins Ib, V and IX. Glycoprotein Ib is the receptor site for von Willebrand factor, which is essential for normal platelet adhesion. Ristocetin induces the binding of von Willebrand factor to platelets, and ristocetin-induced platelet aggregation requires intact platelet membrane glycoprotein Ib. Monoclonal antibodies are now available which will detect the absence of glycoprotein Ib and clinch the diagnosis.

Corticosteroid therapy and splenectomy are of no benefit. Platelet transfusions should be limited to serious bleeding. Individuals with Bernard–Soulier syndrome may rapidly become sensitized to random platelets with intact glycoprotein Ib. Although this may not be a problem in the neonatal period, it may present problems later.

Glanzmann's disease

This autosomal recessive disorder has a normal platelet count but prolonged bleeding time due to deficient or absent clot retraction and defective platelet aggregation. Platelet adhesion is normal. Platelets fail to aggregate with ADP, collagen, thrombin and adrenaline, but they do aggregate normally

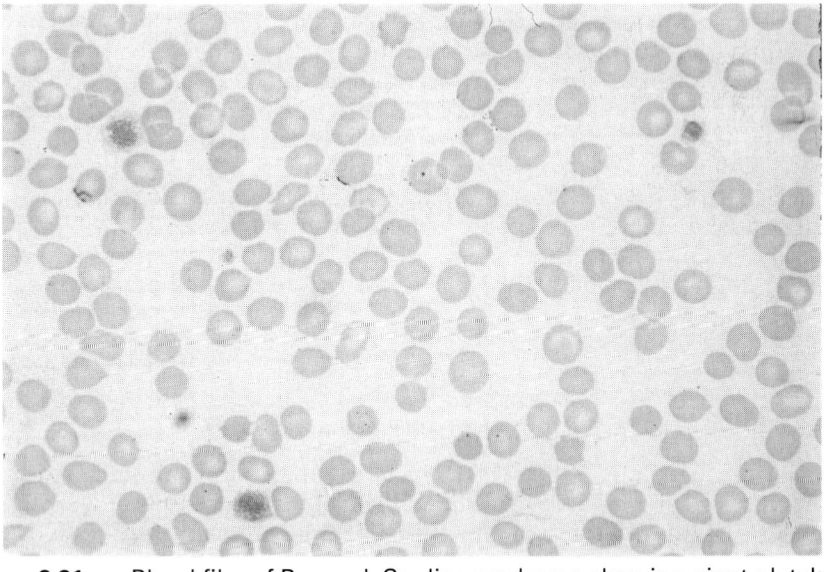

Figure 8.21 Blood film of Bernard–Soulier syndrome showing giant platelets which are almost the same size as the erythrocytes.

with ristocetin. Platelets from affected individuals lack the membrane receptors, glycoprotein IIb and IIIa. The failure of aggregation is not due to defective binding of the aggregating agents to the platelet surface, but instead to defective platelet–platelet interaction, which is mediated by the bridging of platelets at the glycoprotein IIb–IIIa complex, usually by fibrinogen.

Haemorrhagic manifestations are generally apparent from infancy and may be mild through to severe. As with Bernard–Soulier syndrome, corticosteroids and splenectomy have no beneficial role. Supportive therapy with platelet infusions should be kept to a minimum to avoid sensitization. These glycoproteins carry a number of platelet-specific alloantigens, Pl^{A1} on glycoprotein IIIa and Bak^{a} antigen on glycoprotein IIb, which are potent immunogens.

NON-HAEMATOLOGICAL DISORDERS AFFECTING THE HAEMOPOIETIC SYSTEM

Disorders affecting the reticuloendothelial system may present in infancy. These are rare and cannot be dealt with in detail in this chapter. Only familial erythrophagocytic lymphohistiocytosis and the infantile variants of the lysosomal storage diseases are briefly described.

Familial erythrophagocytic lymphohistiocytosis

Langerhans' cell histiocytosis is discussed in Chapter 9. A related disorder, familial erythrophagocytic lymphohistiocytosis presents in infancy with fever, pancytopenia and hepatosplenomegaly. The inheritance is autosomal recessive. The lesions consist of accumulations of active histiocytes and lymphocytes; the histiocytes are not Langerhans' cells, and varying degrees of haemophagocytosis are seen. Lesions have a predilection for the bone marrow, lymph nodes, spleen, liver and meninges. Bone and skin lesions do not occur. Hepatic dysfunction may predispose to a coagulopathy. The pathogenesis is unknown but the condition is not malignant. Hyperlipidaemia and immunodeficiency are associated with this disorder (Ladisch *et al.*, 1982), which is usually fatal, and responses to chemotherapy have been rare.

Lysosomal storage diseases

The lysosomal storage disorders have in common an inherited deficiency of an enzyme involved in lipid metabolism. Products of cellular metabolism, ordinarily degraded by this enzyme, remain undigested and overload the lysosomes. Circulating white blood cells have a high metabolic rate and the capacity to phagocytose non-degraded material and are therefore particularly vulnerable. This explains the cytoplasmic inclusions, vacuolation and other morphological changes seen in leucocytes from platelets with storage disease. Macrophages similarly act as scavengers and accumulate distinctive intracellular lipids associated with specific storage disorders. Consequently, examination of the bone marrow and other tissues of the reticuloendothelial system is important in the diagnosis of these diseases. Biochemical studies are usually required to reach a definitive diagnosis. Affected children may have pancytopenia, leucocyte inclusions, vacuolation of mononuclear cells, characteristic storage cells in the bone marrow, hepatosplenomegaly and lymphadenopathy. Other organs may be affected particularly the central nervous system. The clinical features primarily reflect the pattern of distribution of the non-degradable products. In Gaucher's disease and Niemann–Pick disease this occurs in the bone marrow and reticuloendothelial tissue. The central nervous system is the site of predominant pathological changes in disorders of ganglioside metabolism.

Gaucher's disease

Gaucher's disease is characterized by the storage of cerebrosides in the reticuloendothelial system. The majority of cases have an autosomal recessive inheritance. Three clinical forms have been described. Type 1 disease is the most common and is a non-neuropathic, chronic disorder characterized by hypersplenism and bone involvement. Type 2 disease is a much rarer disorder, characterized by hepatosplenomegaly, central nervous system involvement and death during infancy. Presentation is between birth and 6 months of age, with failure to thrive, hepatosplenomegaly and severe neurological deterioration. Death occurs before the age of 2 years. Because of the early onset and fatal outcome, prenatal diagnosis is recommended. Type 3 disease is defined by the onset of neurological symptoms in childhood, adolescence, or even adulthood, rather than in infancy (Beaudet, 1987).

Gaucher's cells are present in the bone marrow and reticuloendothelial tissue. Glucocerebroside levels are increased in reticuloendothelial tissue, and the activities of serum acid phosphatase and angiotensin-converting enzyme are elevated. Gaucher's disease is caused by a deficiency of lysosomal glucocerebrosidase, the evidence indicates that the various forms of the disease represent allelic disorders with different mutations in the structural gene for the enzyme. The three clinical forms may represent a somewhat arbitrary segmentation of a spectrum of phenotypes resulting from different mutations at the glucocerebrosidase locus, with a minimum effect from modifier genes or non-genetic factors. The glucocerebrosidase gene has now been cloned and a specific mutation, ^{444}leucine–proline, described (Tsuji *et al.*, 1987). Additional mutant alleles will probably be reported in the future. Therapeutic options explored include enzyme infusion and bone marrow transplantation. The limited data available suggests that bone marrow involvement may be improved by bone marrow transplantation, but the central nervous system involvement is unlikely to be prevented.

Niemann–Pick disease

Niemann–Pick disease is a rare autosomal recessive disorder found most commonly in Jewish people, as is the case for Gaucher's disease. Spingomyelin accumulates primarily in reticuloendothelial tissue and the central nervous system. At least five variants have been described. Type A clinically resembles type 2 Gaucher's disease. The disorder dates from birth and is characterized by massive hepatosplenomegaly and progressive physical and neurological deterioration. A cherry-red macula is a common finding and death occurs in infancy. The diagnosis is easily made by examination of the bone marrow which shows the presence of the foam cells characteristic of Niemann–Pick disease. Similar storage cells are present in the liver, spleen and lymph nodes. Enzymatic assays demonstrate sphingomyelinase deficiency. Antenatal diagnosis is possible. Effective enzyme replacement therapy is not available.

A number of storage disorders are characterized by foam cells in the bone marrow, and the presence of Reilly bodies in the polymorphonuclear leucocytes and vacuoles in the lymphocytes and monocytes can aid in their diagnosis and in diagnosis of some of the mucopolysaccharidoses.

REFERENCES

Aggett PJ, Cavanagh NP, Matthew DJ *et al.* (1980) Schwachman's syndrome — A review of 21 cases. *Archives of Disease in Childhood* **55**: 331–347.

Alter BP, Nathan DG (1979) Red cell aplasia in children. *Archives of Disease in Childhood* **54**: 263–267.

Beaudet AL (1987) Gaucher's disease. *New England Journal of Medicine* **316**: 619–621.

Connor JM and Ferguson-Smith MA (1984) *Essential Medical Genetics*, p 142. Oxford: Blackwell Scientific Publications.

Diamond LK and Blackfan KD (1938) Hypoplastic anaemia. *American Journal of Diseases of Childhood* **56**: 464.

Diamond LK, Allen DM and Magill FB (1961) Congenital (erythroid) hypoplastic anaemia. A 25-year study. *American Journal of Diseases of Children* **102**: 403–415.

Eisenstein EM (1966) Congenital megakaryocytic thrombocytopenic purpura. *Clinical Pediatrics* **5**: 143.

Freedman MH, Amato D and Saunders EF (1975) Haem synthesis in the Diamond–Blackfan syndrome. *British Journal of Haematology* **31**: 515–520.

Freedman MH, Amato D and Saunders EF (1976) Erythroid colony growth in congenital hypoplastic anaemia. *Journal of Clinical Investigation* **57**: 673–677.

Geller G, Drivit W, Zalusky R *et al.* (1975) Lack of erythropoietic inhibitory effect of serum from patients with congenital pure red cell aplasia. *New England Journal of Medicine* **292**: 98–201.

Heimpel H and Wendt F (1968) Congenital dyserythropoietic anaemia with karyorrhexis and multinuclearity of erythroblasts. *Helvetica Medica Acta* **34**: 103–115.

Hoffman R and Zanjani ED (1976) Diamond-Blackfan syndrome: lymphocyte-mediated suppression of erythropoiesis. *Science* **193**: 899.

Hoyeraal HM, Lamvik J and Moe PJ (1970) Congenital hypoplastic thrombocytopenia and cerebral malformations in two brothers. *Acta Paediatrica Scandinavica* **59**: 185–191.

Kapoor N, Kirkpatrick D, Blaese RM *et al.* (1981) Reconstitution of normal megakaryocytopoiesis and immunologic functions in Wiskott–Aldrich syndrome by marrow transplantation following myeloablation and immunosuppression with busulfan and cyclophosphamide. *Blood* **57**: 692–696.

Kostmann R (1956) Infantile genetic agranulocytosis. A new recessive lethal disease in man. *Acta Paediatrica Scandinavica* **105**: 45.

Kushner JP, Pimstone NR and Kjeldsberg CR (1982) Congenital erythropoietic porphyria, diminished activity of uroporphyrinogen decarboxylase and dyserythropoiesis. *Blood* **59**: 725–737.

Ladisch S, Ho W, Matheson D *et al.* (1982) Immunologic and clinical effects of repeated blood exchange in familial erythrophagocytic lymphohistiocytosis. *Blood* **60**: 814–821.

Lee Potter JP, Deacon-Smith RA, Simpkiss MJ *et al.* (1975) A new cause of haemolytic anaemia in the newborn: A description of an unstable fetal haemoglobin: F Poole, alpha 2-G-gamma 2 130 tryptophan yields glycine. *Journal of Clinical Pathology* **28**: 317–320.

Matthay KK and Mentzer WC (1981) Erythrocyte enzymopathies in the newborn. *Clinics in Haematology* **10**: 33–55.

Ortega JA, Shore NA, Dukes PP (1975) Erythropoietic inhibitory effect of serum from patients with congenital hypoplastic anaemia. *Blood* **45**: 83 (Abstr.).

Oski FA and Naiman JL (1982) *Hematologic Problems in the Newborn*, 3rd edn, 266. W.B. Saunders Company, Philadelphia.

Rothbaum RJ, Williams DA and Daugherty CC (1982) Unusual surface distribution of concanavalin A reflects a cytoskeletal defect in neutrophils in Schwachman's syndrome. *The Lancet* **2**: 800–801.

Schroter W and Kahsnitz E (1983) Diagnosis of hereditary spherocytosis in newborn infants. *Journal of Pediatrics* **103**: 460–463.

Segal AW, Cross AR, Garcia RC *et al.* (1983) Absence of cytochrome b-245 in chronic granulomatous disease. A multicentre European evaluation of its incidence and relevance. *New England Journal of Medicine* **308**: 245–251.

Tsuji S, Choudary PV, Martin BM *et al.* (1987) A mutation in the human glucocerbrosidase gene in neuronopathic Gaucher's disease. *New England Journal of Medicine* **316**: 570–575.

9

Neonatal tumours and leukaemia

I.M. Hann
The Hospitals for Sick Children, London

It is not within the scope of this book to discuss neonatal tumours and leukaemia in detail; in particular, the difficult clinical and ethical problems that arise are left to textbooks of oncology. This chapter gives a brief description of those problems, inherent in the subject, that rarely confront neonatologists and haematologists.

Most neonatal tumours are embryonic in origin, but transplacental seeding with metastases from mother to fetus have been recorded rarely in cases of choriocarcinoma and melanoma (Strauss, 1964). Tumours at this time of life are often more benign than their counterparts in later life and they also often undergo spontaneous regression or maturation. The Children's Cancer Research Group in Oxford has provided the most accurate assessment of their incidence within the United Kingdom (Table 9.1). Their rarity is emphasized by the overall incidence of 1.7 per 100 000 live births. Or, put another way, a very busy obstetric unit with 5000 deliveries per year would only see one case approximately every 12 years.

Table 9.1 Malignant tumours in the neonatal period in the United Kingdom 1970–1971.*

Tumour type	Males	Females	Total
Neuroblastoma	18 (0.59)	9 (0.3)	27 (0.45)
Acute leukaemia	10 (0.32)	7 (0.24)	17 (0.3)
Malignant teratoma	4 (0.13)	12 (0.42)	16 (0.27)
Sarcoma	5 (0.16)	8 (0.28)	13 (0.22)
Brain tumours	6 (0.2)	6 (0.2)	12 (0.2)
Wilms' tumour	5 (0.16)	3 (0.1)	8 (0.13)
Hepatoblastoma	0	3 (0.1)	3 (0.05)
Other	2 (0.07)	3 (0.1)	5 (0.08)
Totals	50 (1.63)	51 (1.8)	101 (1.7)

* Figures in parentheses represent the rate per 100 000 live births. Incidence based on cancer registrations, Childhood Cancer Research Group, Oxford; courtesy of Dr C. Stiller.

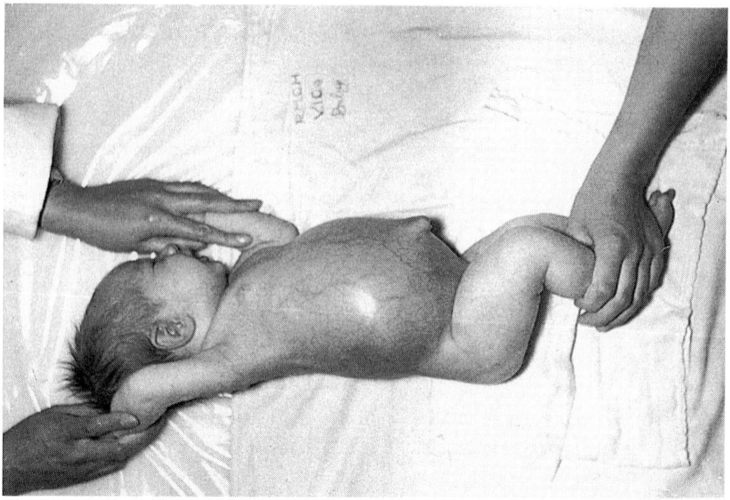

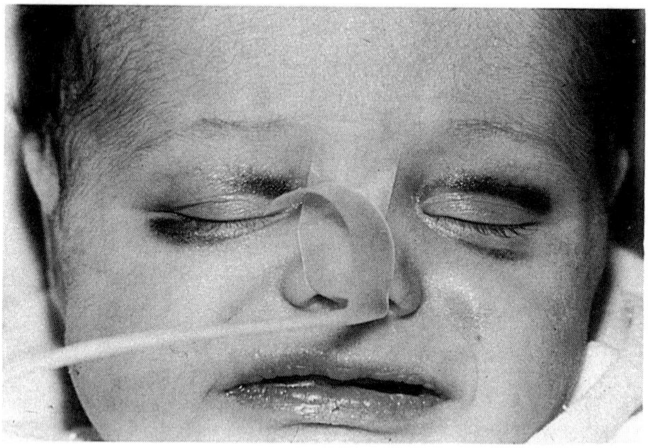

Figure 9.1 Neuroblastoma in the neonate. Massive abdominal swelling due to neuroblastoma (upper), and neonatal neuroblastoma presenting with typical periorbital ecchymoses (lower).

NEUROBLASTOMA

This is the commonest malignancy, accounting for about 25% of all neonatal tumours. More than half present as a mass in the abdomen and pelvis (Figure 9.1). Posterior mediastinal tumours are also common and can cause respiratory obstruction or superior vena cava obstruction. One-third of cases present with bluish subcutaneous nodules (Figure 9.2). Other modes of presentation are with spinal cord compression and bone marrow involvement. Rare cases are described of neuroblastoma metastasizing to the placenta and causing maternal hypertension due to catecholamine excretion.

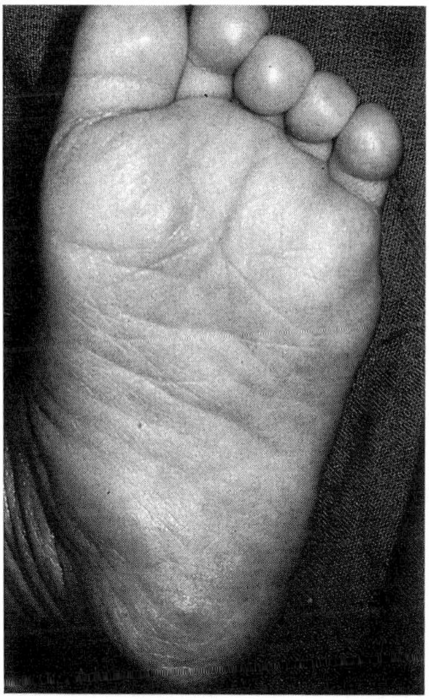

Figure 9.2 Plantar skin nodules in a case of neonatal stage IVS neuroblastoma.

In fact 95% of these tumours will be catecholamine-secreting.

Neonatal neuroblastoma usually has a very good prognosis because of the predominance of IVS cases – localized primary tumours but with remote soft tissue disease involving liver, skin (Figure 9.2) and minimal bone marrow disease but no bone disease. The overall 5-year disease-free survival (DFS) for all ages is: stage I, 97%; stage IVS, 83%, stage II, 90%; stage III, 63%. Stage IV disease, with bony metastases, is very rare in neonates but has a better outlook than the 20% DFS that is seen in older children.

ACUTE LEUKAEMIA

Most cases of neonatal leukaemia are of non-lymphoblastic or 'null cell' type and a quarter are associated with Down's syndrome. There is a particular problem with the latter as these children have a predisposition to exhibit 'leukaemoid' reactions, as well as myelofibrosis and occasionally other myeloproliferative disorders such as megakaryoblastic leukaemia. It is important to establish the diagnosis very carefully and to seek the opinion of a paediatric haematologist, as there is no doubt that so-called 'congenital leukaemia' has been over-diagnosed in the past.

Clinically, the liver and spleen may be palpable at birth with widespread skin and mucosal bleeding phenomena. Typical raised blue nodular skin plaques (Figure 9.3) are frequently seen and other unusual features are respiratory distress due to lung infiltration, and the opisthotonic position which may be adopted because of bone pain. A bulging fontanelle can signal intracranial bleeding or leukaemia.

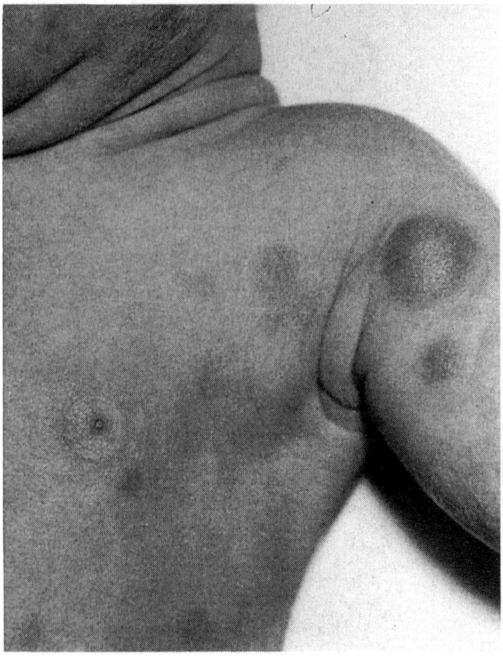

Figure 9.3 Typical (blue) nodular plaques of acute non-lymphoblastic leukaemia in a baby.

Diagnosis is made on the basis of bone marrow morphology, immunology, cytochemistry and cytogenetics, as for leukaemias occurring in later life. At present this disorder is regarded as being uniformly fatal and untreatable, but no doubt improvements will be made.

Recently the literature on congenital leukaemia in stillbirths has been expanded with three more cases (Gray *et al.*, 1986) to add to the four already reported. It seems very likely that the infrequency of published cases is due to the low autopsy rate in stillbirths and the generally poor standard of histopathological examination accorded to them. The three most recently reported cases were thought to be in one case acute monocytic and in the other two acute lymphoblastic. The acute lymphoblastic case was in a trisomy-21 stillbirth; chromosomal analysis was not available for the other two. In each case there was a moderate degree of hydrops, probably related to cardiac failure and widespread visceral involvement. However, unlike the reports of neonatal leukaemia, there was no evidence of skin involvement. No doubt more cases will come to light now that perinatal pathology is receiving the attention that it deserves.

TERATOMA

These are germ-cell tumours occurring usually in the midline or the gonads. The striking feature in neonates is the female to male preponderance (3:1), it

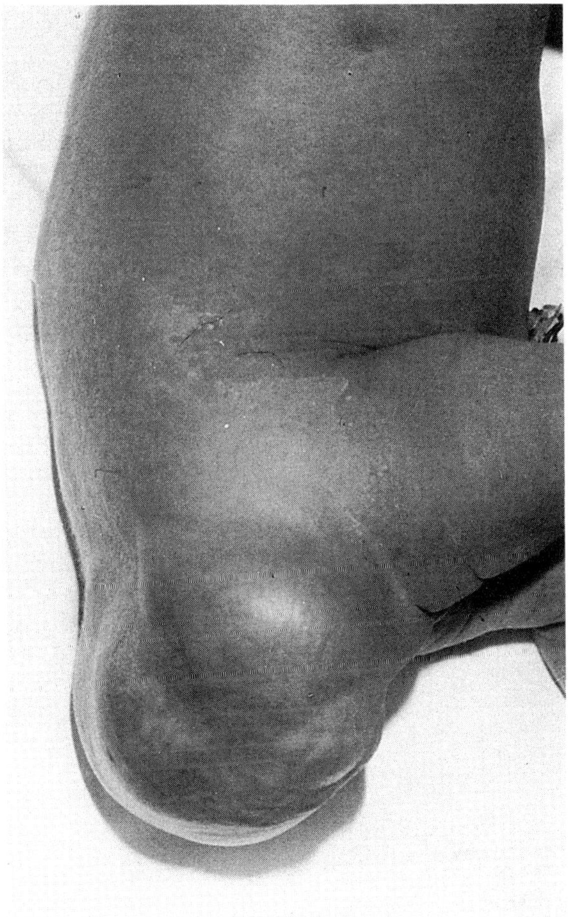

Figure 9.4 A massive sacrococcygeal teratoma presenting in the classical position behind the anus and between the buttocks.

should be noted that only 10% of the total are malignant. Most present between the buttocks and behind the anus (Figure 9.4) and are of greatly variable size from a small blip to a tumour equalling the size of the baby and interfering with delivery. Some will extend intra-abdominally and can be palpated as arising from the pelvis, in which case the chance of malignancy is about 20% (Altman, 1974). Other less common sites are the head and neck, where the teratoma can cause airways obstruction at delivery. Apart from the usual investigations, α-fetoprotein (αFP) is raised in two-thirds of malignant cases and can be used as a tumour marker. In a similar way, β human chorionic gonadotrophin can be used.

Benign tumours are removed, but malignant ones require a multimodal approach.

BRAIN TUMOURS

These are rare and account for only 10% of neonatal tumours. The UK study of cases showed a variety of types: two medulloblastoma; two ependymoma; one each of oligodendroglioma, craniopharyngioma, glioma, medulloepithelioma and meningeal sarcoma; two tumours of unknown type. One case (craniopharyngioma) survived. Treatment is very problematic because of the severe morbidity associated with radiotherapy to the neonatal brain.

WILMS' TUMOUR (NEPHROBLASTOMA)

Until recently there has been a great deal of confusion over the distinction between the two main types of neonatal renal tumours; mesonoblastic nephroma and Wilms' tumour. They both present as abdominal masses, usually without haematuria. A unique feature is the presentation of Wilms' with hydrocephalus due to cerebral secondaries (Kalousek, 1977). Wilms' tumour is associated with a wide variety of congenital abnormalities; the commonest are Beckwith's syndrome, aniridia, hemihypertrophy and genitourinary abnormalities. Mesoblastic nerhroma is the commonest neonatal renal tumour and is not a true malignancy.

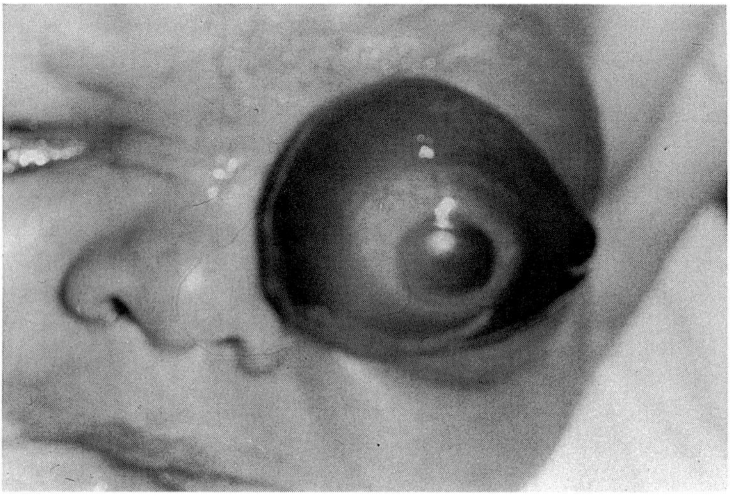

Figure 9.5 A grotesque orbital rhabdomyosarcoma causing proptosis in a neonate.

Wilm's tumour of the types with unfavourable histology (bone metastasizing and rhabdoid) have not been found in the neonatal period and the prognosis overall in babies is good. Six of the eight cases in the UK series have survived, although it is possible that some of these patients may actually have had mesoblastic nephroma.

LANGERHANS' CELL HISTIOCYTOSIS

This is a non-malignant 'reactive' disorder in which cells with the characteristics of epidermal Langerhans' cells are found in the dermis and other organs. Neonates usually present with a rash, which may be present from birth or within the first few days of life. The typical distribution of the brownish-red, slightly raised, pinhead plaques is in the skin folds of groins and axillae, behind the ears and in the 'necklace' area and trunk. The scalp may also be involved and this tends to look like 'cradle-cap'. Lung involvement, leading to respiratory distress, and liver, spleen and bone marrow infiltration can all occur. Another form of neonatal presentation is with congenital self-healing histiocytosis of the Hashimoto–Pritzer type, and a discrete nodular rash found in the trunk and limbs as well as face, feet and hands. However, treatment is only required for constitutional upset or significant impairment of organ function.

HEPATOBLASTOMA AND OTHER TUMOURS

Rare cases of hepatoblastoma occur in neonates and are of either fetal or embryonal form. The prognosis is uncertain, but there is now more effective chemotherapy, which renders some cases surgically curable. Hepatoblastomas may cause considerable abdominal swelling and splinting of the diaphragm sufficient to cause respiratory embarrassment. Other tumours occur rarely, including rhabdomyosarcoma (Figure 9.5).

SUMMARY

Malignancy in the neonatal period is thankfully a great rarity. Generally the prognosis of the malignant tumours that are not surgically resectable is not good, and treatment of certain malignancies (e.g. brain tumours) is made almost impossible by the age of the patient. Thus, it is still often a difficult ethical decision as to whether therapy is worthwhile for those malignancies for which the outcome is extremely poor. Nevertheless, the report of Campbell *et al.* (1987) has documented 102 cases over 60 years in Toronto and reported an overall mortality of 41% from malignant tumours; another encouraging aspect of this report was the apparent lack of long-term major handicaps, despite the frequent use of multimodal therapy. Furthermore, there was only one case of second malignancy, which was a thyroid cancer within the radiation field. Isaacs, also in 1987, reviewed the Los Angeles Children's Hospital series covering the period 1938–1985, when neonatal tumours accounted for 2.5% of the total recorded in pathology records. Remarkably, they also showed a 41% survival for malignant tumours. Only one of the 13 leukaemic neonates was known to have survived, and prognosis for brain tumours, Wilms' tumours and retinoblastoma was apparently worse than in older children.

Finally, a recent report (Crom *et al.*, 1989) has detailed neonatal tumours

Table 9.2 Childhood malignancies seen at St Jude Children's Research Hospital.*

Malignancy	Total no. of patients (%)	No. of neonates (%)
ALL	2036 (35.6)	4 (11.7)
AML	533 (9.7)	2 (5.8)
Neuroblastoma	409 (7.2)	19 (55.9)
Retinoblastoma	132 (2.3)	3 (8.8)
Wilms' tumour	294 (5.1)	2 (5.8)
Germ cell tumours	127 (2.2)	2 (5.8)
Melanoma		2 (5.8)
Hodgkin's disease	410 (7.2)	
Osteosarcoma	242 (4.2)	
Ewing's sarcoma	170 (3.0)	
Rhabdomyosarcoma	287 (5.0)	
Other malignancies	1056 (18.5)	

* Figures in parentheses are percentages. ALL = acute lymphoblastic leukaemia, AML = acute myeloid leukaemia.

at St Jude Children's Research Hospital between 1962 and 1988. Table 9.2 shows the overall numbers and percentage of children with tumours compared with the neonatal tumours. Twenty-three of this group of babies (68%) were alive and free of disease 2 months to 24 years after diagnosis. Thus, modern series appear to be showing a more hopeful outlook for certain categories of patient.

REFERENCES

Altman RP, Randolp JG and Lilly JR (1974) Sacrococcygeal teratoma. *Am Ac Paed Surg Survey J Paed Surgery* **9**: 389–398.

Bolande RP (1974) Congenital infantile neoplasia of the kidney. *The Lancet* **2**: 1497–1499.

Campbell AN, Chan HSL, O'Brien A *et al.* (1987) Malignant tumours in the neonate. *Archives of Disease in Childhood* **62**: 19–23.

Crom DB, Wilimas JA, Green AA *et al.* (1989) Malignancy in the neonate. Medical and Paediatric Oncology **17**: 101–104.

Gray ES, Balch NJ, Kohler H, Thompson WD and Simpson JG (1986) Congenital leukaemia: an unusual cause of stillbirth. *Archives of Disease in Childhood* **61**: 1001–1006.

Isaacs H Jr (1987) Congenital and neonatal malignant tumours: a 28-year experience at Children's Hospital of Los Angeles. *American Journal of Pediatric Haematology/Oncology* **9**: 121–129.

Kalousek DK, de Chadarerian JP, Mackie GC and Bolande RP (1977) Metastatic infantile Wilms' tumour and hydrocephalus. *Cancer* **39**: 1312–1316.

Strauss L and Driscoll G (1964) Congenital neuroblastoma involving the placenta. Report of 2 cases. *Paediatrics* **34**: 23–31.

10

Prenatal diagnosis of haematological disorders

D.J. Weatherall
Institute of Molecular Medicine, John Radcliffe Hospital, Oxford

Until the mid-1970s intra-uterine diagnosis of inherited haematological disorders was restricted to fetal sexing by examining the chromosomes of amniotic fluid cells of mothers at risk of carrying fetuses with X-linked disorders such as haemophilia. However, with the development of fetal blood sampling and, more recently, the application of recombinant DNA technology to the analysis of fetal DNA obtained from amniotic fluid cells or chorion biopsy, the whole scene has changed and many genetic disorders of the blood are now amenable to prenatal diagnosis.

In this chapter, an extended and updated version of a previous review of the topic (Weatherall, 1985), we shall examine the methods which are now available for prenatal diagnosis of inherited blood diseases and summarize what is known about their safety and reliability. For more general accounts of the diagnosis of genetic disease by DNA analysis, and its application to prenatal detection of inherited disorders, the reader is referred to several recent reviews and monographs (Davies and Robson, 1987; Davies and Reid, 1988; Antonarakis, 1989; Weatherall, 1990).

METHODS FOR PRENATAL DIAGNOSIS OF HAEMATOLOGICAL DISORDERS

Cells or tissue for prenatal diagnosis can be obtained by fetal blood sampling, amniocentesis or chorion villus sampling (Rodeck and Nicolini, 1989). Fetal blood sampling can be used for the diagnosis of genetic disorders of red cells, white cells or platelets, and for the identification of clotting factor deficiencies. The haemoglobin disorders can be identified by measuring the relative rates and patterns of globin chain synthesis; other conditions are diagnosed using micromethods for the assay of enzymes or clotting factors. Amniotic fluid cells can be used for cytogenetic or biochemical analysis, and as a source of fetal DNA. Chorion villus sampling is used to obtain cells for cytogenetic or biochemical analysis and to isolate fetal DNA.

Fetal blood sampling

Fetal blood can be obtained towards the end of the second trimester by two methods (Alter, 1984). The first involves aspiration of blood from the placenta under ultrasound guidance (Kan *et al.*, 1974). This usually produces a mixture of fetal and maternal cells. The relative contribution of each can be determined by analysing their size distribution using a Coulter Channelyzer. It is often necessary to take multiple samples until an adequate number of fetal cells has been obtained.

There are several approaches to the isolation of fetal cells from fetomaternal mixtures; the most useful is the Orskov procedure, which is based on the principle that adult cells, because they contain carbonic anhydrase, lyse in the presence of NH_4Cl and NH_4HCO_3, whereas fetal cells remain intact under these conditions (Alter *et al.*, 1979). More pure fetal blood samples can be obtained by fetoscopy (Hobbins and Mahoney, 1974; Rodeck, 1980). When this approach was first introduced, blood was obtained from fetal vessels on the chorionic plate, but subsequently blood was aspirated directly from the umbilical vein at the placental insertion of the cord. Such samples contain pure fetal blood, with no contamination by maternal blood or amniotic fluid, and hence are suitable for analyses requiring cells, serum or plasma. However the use of the fetoscope is associated with pre-term labour, amniotic fluid leak and an overall fetal loss rate of 6–7%. With the development of techniques of fetal blood sampling using a 20 gauge needle under ultrasound guidance first reported by Daffos *et al.* (1983) the use of the fetoscope has been largely abandoned and most centres have adopted this new technique.

Procedure related fetal losses associated with this method of fetal blood sampling are no more than 1% in skilled hands. More recent modifications and other techniques for fetal blood sampling are reviewed by Rodeck and Nicolini (1989).

Haemoglobin disorders

Although fetal blood samples have been used for prenatal identification of many haematological disorders, by far the most experience has been gained in the diagnosis of the structural haemoglobin variants and thalassaemias. Fetal cells are incubated with [^{3}H]leucine-labelled globin chains, separated by carboxymethylcellulose chromatography, and the relative amount of radioactivity incorporated into each chain determined (Clegg *et al.*, 1965; Weatherall *et al.*, 1965; Figure 10.1). For the prenatal diagnosis of β thalassaemia, the ratio of β- to γ-chain production is determined. The ratio increases slowly during the first and second trimesters in normal fetuses, and is 0.11 ± 0.05 at 16–24 weeks' gestation (Cividalli *et al.*, 1974; Alter, 1980). If a fetus is homozygous for β^0 thalassaemia there is no β chain synthesis; if it is homozygous for β^+ thalassaemia, or is a compound heterozygote for β^0 and β^+ thalassaemia, there is a reduced β/γ synthesis ratio, usually less than 0.035. The precise diagnostic ratios have to be established for individual laboratories. Remarkably, the overall error rate in

Table 10.1 Some of the disorders that can be identified by fetal blood sampling.

Haemoglobinopathies	*Other red cell disorders*
Structural haemoglobin variants S, C, E, Lepore	Rhesus haemolytic disease
β thalassaemia	Specific enzyme defects
α thalassaemia, Hb Bart's hydrops	Hereditary erythroblastic multinuclearity with a positive acidified serum lysis test (HEMPAS)
Coagulation and related disorders	
Haemophilia	*White cell and related disorders*
Christmas disease	Chronic granulomatous disease
von Willebrand's disease	Genetic neutropenia
Other factor deficiences	Immunodeficiency states
Thrombocytopenia	
Wiskott–Aldrich syndrome	*Cytogenetic analysis*
α_1-antitrypsin deficiency	Fanconi's anaemia
	Bloom's syndrome
	Xeroderma pigmentosum

experienced laboratories is only about 0.08% (Alter, 1981, 1984, 1989), and may be even lower (Old *et al.*, 1989). The main source of error is maternal cell contamination or poor chromatographic technique. With an incomplete separation of γ and β chains it is difficult to distinguish homozygous from heterozygous β^+ thalassaemia. This technique can also be used for the diagnosis of the homozygous state for α^0 thalassaemia (haemoglobin Bart's hydrops syndrome), and structural haemoglobin variants such as haemoglobins S, C, E, O-Arab, and Lepore, the synthesis of which can be detected because of the charge difference of the abnormal globin chain (Figure 10.1).

Other inherited haematological disorders

A variety of haemostatic and coagulation disorders can be identified *in utero* by fetal blood analysis (Table 10.1). Factors $VIIICA_g$, $VIIIRA_g$ and IXA_g can be assayed by immunological techniques even in the presence of amniotic fluid, thus allowing the prenatal recognition of haemophilia, von Willebrand's disease and Christmas disease (Firshien *et al.*, 1979; Hoyer *et al.*, 1979; Mibashan *et al.*, 1980; Ljung *et al.*, 1982; Mibashan *et al.*, 1982). Rare haemostatic disorders that have been identified *in utero* include autosomal recessive thrombocytopenia (Luthy *et al.*, 1979), and the Wiskott–Aldrich syndrome (Holmberg *et al.*, 1983). For a recent comprehensive review of prenatal diagnosis of haemostatic disorders see Mibashan *et al.* (1989).

Potentially, many other red cell disorders can be identified by fetal blood sampling. Normal values, during fetal life, of several red cell enzymes have been established by Lestas *et al.* (1982). For example triose phosphate isomerase deficiency has been identified in fetal blood (Rosa *et al.*, 1984). It is also possible to grow erythroid colonies from fetal blood as an approach to the prenatal diagnosis of stem-cell disorders (Linch *et al.*, 1982b).

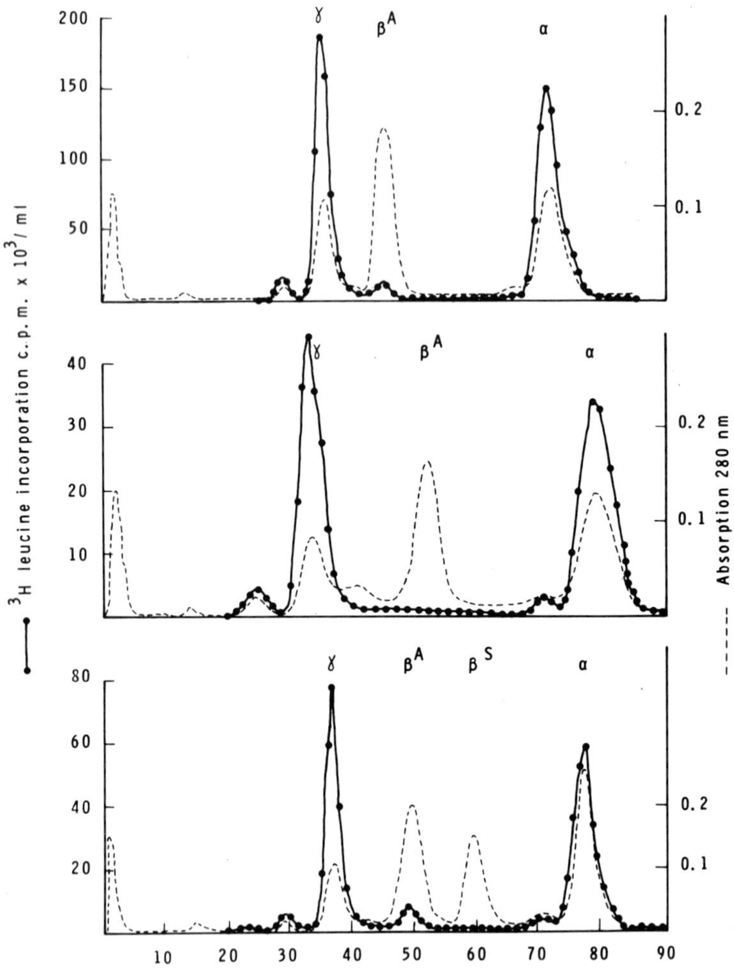

Figure 10.1 Prenatal detection of haemoglobin disorders by fetal blood sampling and radiolabelling of globin chains. The chains have been separated by carboxymethyl cellulose chromatography. The protein profile is shown by a broken line and radioactive profile by a continuous line. Upper: normal fetal blood. Middle: a case of β^0 thalassaemia. Lower: a normal profile in a fetus at risk for carrying the sickle cell trait or disease.

Fetal white cells can also be used for prenatal diagnosis. Chronic granulomatous disease can be diagnosed by the inability of the white cells of affected fetuses to reduce nitroblue tetrazolium (Newburger *et al.*, 1979; Borregard *et al.*, 1982). Fetal cells have also been used for the prenatal diagnosis of the inherited immunodeficiency syndromes (Linch *et al.*, 1982a). For example, adenosine deaminase (ADA) deficiency has been identified *in utero* (Simmonds *et al.*, 1983) and severe combined immunodeficiency has been diagnosed by analysing T and B lymphocyte subsets (Durandy, 1982; Levinsky *et al.*, 1982). Fetal white cells are particularly useful for cytogenetic studies; chromosomal analysis can be carried out within 72 h, much quicker than is the case when cultured amniotic fluid cells are used.

Amniocentesis

Although the main value of amniocentesis for the prenatal diagnosis of genetic disorders of the blood is for obtaining cells for DNA analysis (see below), cytogenetic and biochemical analysis of amniotic fluid cells can also be used for identifying haematological disorders. For example, patients with Fanconi's anaemia have increased chromosome fragility, which is magnified after culture of their cells with diepoxybutane (DEB), a DNA cross-linker. Prenatal recognition of this condition has been carried out in this way using amniotic fluid cells (Alter, 1984) and chorionic villus samples (Auerbach *et al.*, 1990). If the fetus proves not to have inherited Fanconi's anaemia and is HLA-compatible with the affected sibling, successful marrow transplantation is possible using blood retrieved from the umbilical cord of the unaffected neonate at delivery (Gluckman *et al.*, 1989, Auerbach *et al.*, 1990). This is because of the presence in normal human cord blood of haemopoietic stem cells and multipotential (CFU-GEMM) erythroid (BFU-E) and granulocyte-macrophage (CFU-GM) progenitor cells (see Chapter 1). Other fragile-chromosome syndromes that can be identified *in utero* include ataxia telangiectasia, Bloom syndrome and xeroderma pigmentosum (Halley *et al.*, 1979; Shaham *et al.*, 1982; Alter, 1984). Several conditions can be identified by enzyme analysis of amniotic fluid cells. These include glucose phosphate isomerase deficiency (Whitelaw *et al.*, 1979), congenital methaemoglobinaemia due to NADH-linked methaemoglobin reductase deficiency (Junien *et al.*, 1981) and recessive erythropoietic porphyria (Deyback *et al.*, 1980).

The diagnosis of metabolic disorders using amniotic fluid cells depends on the demonstration of reduced enzyme activity or the accumulation of a metabolite due to an enzyme deficiency. This approach is thus feasible for red or white cell enzyme deficiencies only if these are expressed in other tissues, such as fibroblasts. Hecht and Cadien (1984) provide an extensive review of conditions that can be identified prenatally by biochemical analysis of amniotic fluid cells; a partial list of disorders of particular interest to haematologists is given in Table 10.2. Valentine and Paglia (1984) have reviewed the increasing list of red cell enzyme defects that, as well as causing haemolytic anaemia, are associated with multi-system diseases. These deficiencies are expressed widely in tissues other than the haemopoietic cells; at least some of them should be amenable to identification *in utero* by analysis of amniotic fluid cells.

It seems likely that, in the future, cells obtained by chorion biopsy will be equally useful for cytogenetic and biochemical analysis.

Table 10.2 Some of the metabolic disorders that can be identified by biochemical analysis of amniotic fluid cells (Hecht and Cadien, 1984).

Condition	Enzyme
Acatalasaemia	Catalase
Combined immunodeficiency disease	Adenosine deaminase
Glutathione synthetase deficiency	Glutathione synthetase
Glucose isomerase deficiency	Glucose isomerase
α-glutamylcysteine deficiency	α-glutamylcysteine synthetase
Methyltetrahydrofolate reductase deficiency	Methyltetrahydrofolate reductase
Tetrahydrofolate reductase deficiency	Tetrahydrofolate methyl transferase
Orotic aciduria	Orotate phosphoribosyl transferase Orotine 5-phosphate decarboxylase
Erythropoietic porphyria	Uroporphyrinogen synthetase
Coproporphyria	Coproporphyrinogen oxidase
Intermittent porphyria	Uroporphyrinogen 1-synthetase
Protoporphyria	Haem synthetase
Methaemoglobinaemia	NADH-linked diaphorase
Gaucher's disease	Ceramidase
Lesch–Nyhan syndrome	Hypoxanthine-guanine phosphoribosyl transferase (HGPRT)

Fetal DNA analysis

The development of techniques for DNA analysis has already revolutionized the prenatal diagnosis of genetic disease. So far this approach has been applied mainly to the prenatal diagnosis of the haemoglobin and coagulation disorders; this will not be the case for long.

Sources of fetal DNA

Fetal DNA can be obtained either from amniotic fluid cells or chorion villus sampling (CVS). Unfortunately, the yield of DNA from a conventional amniotic fluid tap is usually too small for DNA analysis, though this problem may be overcome by the new techniques for amplifying DNA (see below). If the precise defect is known and can be identified by one restriction enzyme analysis (see below), it may be possible to obtain enough DNA by simply spinning down the amniotic fluid cells. If more extensive DNA analysis is required, the cells must be grown in culture for several weeks. In the latter case, a prenatal diagnosis cannot be made until late in the second trimester.

Recently, CVS has been widely explored as an approach to obtaining fetal DNA in the first trimester. The history of the development of this method and the various techniques used have been reviewed by Rodeck and Morsman (1983). The chorion is composed of an outer layer or trophoblast, an inner mesodermal layer, and fetal blood vessels supplying the villi that extend all over the gestation sac until the end of the second month of pregnancy. As development proceeds, continuing growth of the gestation sac causes thinning of the decidua capsularis until, by 14 weeks, the extra-placental chorion is denuded of villi. Thus the ideal time to carry out CVS is 9–11 weeks' gestation. Currently, the optimum method for obtaining chorionic tissue is not absolutely certain. Several have been explored, including blind aspiration, ultrasound-guided needle aspiration, the use of biopsy forceps, endoscopy combined with ultrasound guidance, and others. There is an increasing interest in the use of the trans-abdominal approach, which can be used up to 13–14 weeks' gestation.

It is too early yet to be certain about the safety of CVS. Several large, multicentre clinical trials have been set up to compare the relative safety of CVS with amniocentesis. Quite recently the first report of this type, the Canadian Collaborative CVS–Amniocentesis Clinical Trial Group (1989), has been published. The results are encouraging, particularly as each group (CVS and amniocentesis) consisted of over 1000 pregnancies. The total fetal losses (made up of spontaneous and induced abortions and late losses) in the CVS group was 7.6% and in the amniocentesis groups 7.0%. Mean birth weights for each week of gestation were similar in both groups. Perinatal mortality was slightly greater in the CVS group. There was no evidence of an excess of intra-uterine growth-retarded babies in the CVS group, and maternal morbidity was similar in both groups. Comparable results were obtained in a large multicentre trial carried out in the USA (Rhoads *et al.*, 1989). Although in both trials there were no obvious deleterious effects on infants in the pregnancies that had undergone CVS, it must be emphasized that not until there have been some years of careful follow-up will it be absolutely certain that CVS has no side-effects on development. However, from data currently available, it appears that CVS is likely to be a safe and acceptable procedure for prenatal diagnosis of serious genetic disease.

The yield of DNA from chorion biopsy varies from 2 to 100 μg with an average of about 20–30 μg. There is good linear correlation between the weight of trophoblast tissue and the yield of DNA.

Methods for DNA analysis

The methods that can be used for analysing fetal DNA have been reviewed extensively (Old and Higgs, 1983; Orkin, 1984; Emery, 1984; Davies, 1988; Weatherall, 1990). So far, most experience has been obtained using restriction endonuclease mapping, although there have been several recent technical developments, which promise to revolutionize the rapid prenatal detection of genetic disease.

The principle of gene mapping is as follows. DNA is prepared from chorionic biopsy tissue or amniotic fluid cells and is cut up into small fragments with restriction enzymes. The latter are bacterial enzymes that cleave DNA at very specific sequences. The resulting fragments are separated by gel electrophoresis, blotted onto nitrocellulose papers and immobilized. The appropriate gene or gene fragments are identified by hybridization with radioactive gene probes (lengths of DNA with sequences identical to those of the gene, or related sequences, under study). Probes of this kind can be made from cloned genomic DNA or by making a complementary DNA copy (cDNA) from the messenger RNA (mRNA) of the particular gene for which the probe is required.

To appreciate fully the applications of gene mapping of this type — or its more recent modifications — for the diagnosis of single gene disorders it is important to understand their molecular pathology. Much of this information has been obtained from studies of the haemoglobinopathies. The structural haemoglobin disorders, such as sickle cell anaemia, result from single base changes in specific DNA codons, which lead to the substitution of a single amino acid in one or other of the globin chains. The thalassaemias, all of which are characterized by a reduced rate of synthesis of one or more globin genes, have a much more complex molecular basis (Orkin *et al.*, 1982, 1983; Orkin and Kazazian, 1984; Thein and Weatherall, 1988; Higgs *et al.*, 1989). The common forms of α thalassaemia result from loss of one or both linked α-globin genes on chromosome 16. In addition, there are less common non-deletion forms of α thalassaemia in which point mutations or deletions of a few bases cause either a partial or complete lack of function of one of the linked α-globin genes. The molecular pathology of the β thalassaemias is different. Deletions are the exception, and most β thalassaemias result from single base changes or loss of one or more bases, which either partially or completely inactivate the β-globin genes. They include nonsense and frameshift mutations, single base changes within introns or exons that interfere with processing of mRNA, and point mutations in promoter boxes. Over 60 mutations of this type have now been described and the disease appears to be very heterogeneous even within the same population. The δβ thalassaemias result from long deletions of the β-globin gene cluster.

The molecular pathology of other genetic haematological disorders seem to follow the same pattern as that which has been found for the thalassaemias. For example there is a wide variety of mutations that involve the fibrinogen genes and give rise to different structural forms of fibrinogen, resulting in defective coagulation, an increased tendency to thrombosis, or defective wound healing. It is becoming apparent that both haemophilia and Christmas disease are highly heterogeneous at the molecular level; not surprising perhaps, considering that many cases represent new mutations. Like the thalassaemias they include deletions of part or the whole of the factor VIII or factor IX genes and a variety of point mutations that interfere with transcription or translation of the mRNA products of these genes (Tuddenham, 1989; Giannelli, 1989).

The different approaches to the prenatal diagnosis of mutations by fetal DNA analysis are shown in Table 10.3.

Direct identification of mutant genes with restriction enzymes

Major gene deletions or rearrangments can be identified directly by gene mapping using appropriate DNA probes. For example, the homozygous state for α^0 thalassaemia (haemoglobin Bart's hydrops), or the Indian form

Table 10.3 Prenatal diagnosis by DNA analysis.

Direct
Deletions and rearrangements by Southern blotting
Point mutations that are identified by restriction enzymes; Southern blotting
Oligonucleotide probes and Southern blotting
Polymerase chain reaction (PCR)
Identification with oligonucleotide probes
Electrophoresis or dot blot
Amplification refractory mutation system
Indirect (Southern blotting or PCR)
RFLP linkage — flanking or intragenic
Allele-linked RFLP

of β^0 thalassaemia due to a deletion at the 3′ end of the β-globin gene, can be identified in this way. Some of the single base mutations giving rise to structural haemoglobin variants or thalassaemia actually alter restriction enzyme sites and hence can be identified directly with the appropriate enzyme. For example, the difference between sickle cell haemoglobin and normal haemoglobin is a glutamic acid → valine substitution in the sixth position of the β-chain, due to an A → T change in the DNA of the β-globin gene. This substitution changes a sequence normally recognized and cleaved by three different restriction enzymes, *Dde* I, *MnI* I, and *Mst* II; for technical reasons, the latter is the most useful.

Other common haemoglobin variants and thalassaemias that can be analysed in this way are summarized in Table 10.4; rare structural variants that might be amenable to diagnosis by the same approach are reviewed by Trent *et al.* (1985). However, apart from the deletion forms of α thalassaemia, two types of non-deletion α thalassaemia, the Indian variety of deletion β^0 thalassaemia and a few other varieties of β^0 and β^+ thalassaemia (Table 10.4), most of the common forms of β thalassaemia are not amenable to diagnosis directly by restriction enzyme analysis because the mutations causing them do not change the site of cleavage of any known enzyme.

RFLP linkage analysis

Scattered throughout human DNA every few hundred bases or so there are single base changes that produce either new restriction enzyme sites or remove previously existing ones (Jeffreys, 1979; Antonarakis *et al.*, 1982; Orkin *et al.*, 1983). These harmless polymorphisms, which are inherited in a simple Mendelian way, provide a wealth of genetic markers that, with appropriate gene probes, can be identified easily by gene mapping (Figures 10.2 and 10.3). A restriction fragment length polymorphism (RFLP) of this type, which is close enough to a gene for the RFLP and the gene not to be separated during meiosis, can be used as a linkage marker to determine which chromosome carries the thalassaemia mutation in a particular family. Alternatively, the polymorphism may be within the gene itself. The

Table 10.4 β thalassaemia mutations directly detectable by restriction analysis.

Mutation	Restriction enzyme
β⁰ thalassaemia	
1. Indian deletion	Various enzymes — 619 bp
2. American Black deletion	Various enzymes — 1.35 kb
3. Dutch deletion	Various enzymes — 10 kb
4. Czech deletion	Various enzymes — 4.2 kb
5. Turkish deletion	Various enzymes — 300 bp
6. −1 codon 6	*Mst* II
7. IVS 2 splice junction	*Hph* I
8. IVS 1 (−25 bp)	*Fnu* 4H, *Mst* II
9. IVS 1 (−17 bp)	*Fnu* 4H, *Mst* II
10. IVS 1-position 116	*Mae* I
11. IVS 1 position 6	*Sfa* N1
12. IVS 2 3′ end AG → GG	*Alu* I
13. β^0 39	*Mae* I
14. β^0 17	*Mae* I
15. β^0 37	*Ava* II
16. β^0 121	*Eco* RI
β⁺ thalassaemia	
17. IVS 2 position 745	*Rsa* I
18. −87 C → G	*Avr* II
19. Hb E	*MnI* I

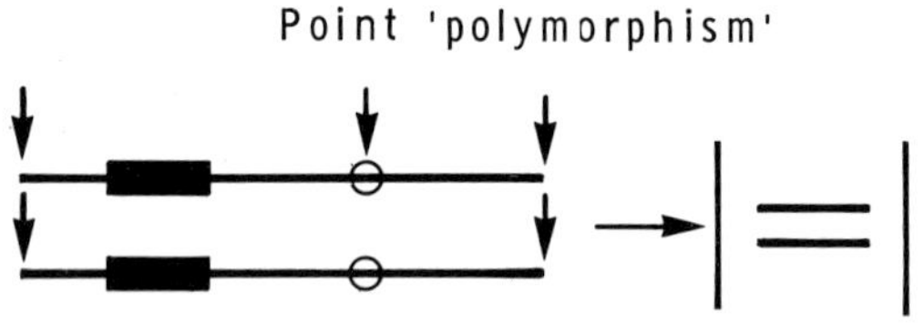

Figure 10.2 Mechanisms for the production of restriction fragment length polymorphisms.

principle of this approach is shown in Figure 10.4. The idea is to study the parents and previously born children or other relatives using several restriction enzymes and gene probes to see if an RFLP can be found on the chromosome carrying the mutant gene in each parent. If so, and if the fetus is homozygous for the particular RFLP, then it must also be homozygous for the particular mutation.

The problem with this method is that, to establish a linkage, a previously born child or other family members are required, and hence a considerable amount of laboratory work must be done before the diagnosis can be made. Furthermore, the frequency of different RFLP markers varies between different racial groups. For example, studies in Britain suggest that this approach for the prenatal diagnosis of β thalassaemia will be feasible in about four-fifths of Cypriot and Asian families (reviewed by Old *et al.*, 1989).

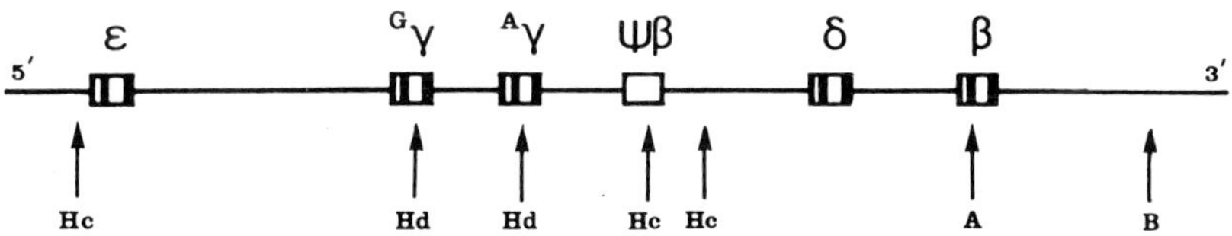

	Hc	Hd	Hd	Hc	Hc	A	B
I	+	−	−	−	−	+	+
II	−	+	+	−	+	+	+
III	−	+	−	+	+	+	−
IV	−	+	−	+	+	−	+
V	+	−	−	−	−	+	−
VI	−	+	+	−	−	−	+
VII	+	−	−	−	−	−	+
VIII	−	+	−	+	−	+	−
IX	−	+	−	+	+	+	+

Figure 10.3 The restriction fragment length polymorphisms of the β-globin gene cluster. The + or − indicates the presence or absence, respectively, of a cutting site. Rather than a random arrangement of these polymorphisms they fall into a number of subgroups, designated by Roman numerals.

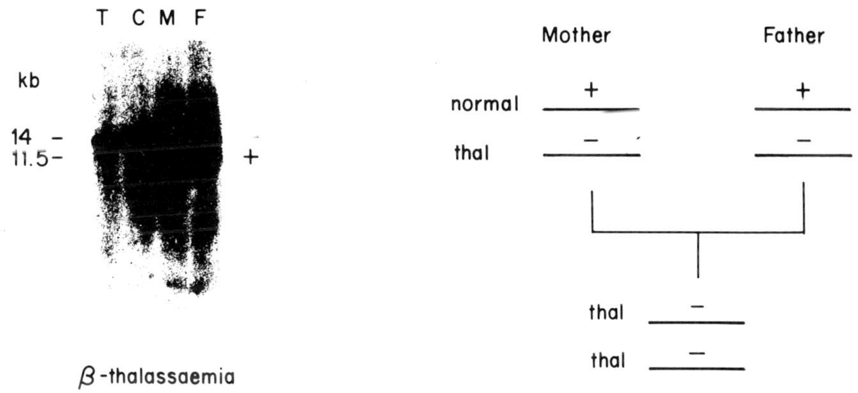

Figure 10.4 Prenatal diagnosis, using restriction enzyme analysis in a family study, of β thalassaemia using a *Pvu* II polymorphism close to the β-globin genes. T, trophoblast; C, child with β thalassaemia major; M, mother; F, father.

Allele-linked RFLPs

The arrangement of RFLPs along the α- and β-globin gene clusters is not random; they exist in a series of patterns, called haplotypes, within individual populations (Antonarakis *et al.*, 1982; Orkin *et al.*, 1983). Thus, within any particular racial group, it is usual to find particular β thalassaemia mutations associated with a specific RFLP haplotype. However, this phenomenon cannot be used for prenatal diagnosis, since the same haplotypes occur in *normal* members of the same population. Occasionally mutations may be in so-called linkage disequilibrium with particular polymorphic sites. For example, it has been found that an *Hpa*I polymorphism is strongly associated with the β^S mutation in West Africans (Kan and Dozy, 1978), and a *Bam* H1 polymorphism is associated with the common β^0 thalassaemia mutation in Sardinia (Kan *et al.*, 1980). However, examples of linkage disequilibria of this type are uncommon, and it is usually necessary to establish linkages between a particular β-globin mutation and an RFLP within an individual family.

Polymorphisms of this type may be useful, nevertheless. For example, a polymorphism for the restriction enzyme *Ava*II in the ψβ gene of the β-globin gene cluster is found in Mediterranean populations. This polymorphic site is absent from over 50% of chromosomes carrying the β thalassaemia mutation but absent from only 2–3% of normal chromosomes. This difference in frequency in these populations greatly increases the feasibility of prenatal diagnosis of β thalassaemia by DNA analysis (Wainscoat *et al.*, 1984). Indeed, Wainscoat *et al.* have estimated that, using the frequency difference together with other RFLPs, it should be possible to carry out prenatal diagnosis in over 90% of families which have the common (Mediterranean; IVS1 110) β thalassaemia mutation.

Oligonucleotide probes

The long DNA probes used for standard gene mapping analysis are not able to detect single base changes of the kind that cause many forms of thalassaemia and other single-gene disorders. However, under appropriate conditions, short synthetic DNA fragments (oligonucleotides or oligomers) can be constructed which hybridize to their homologous sequences but not to heterologous sequences, i.e. to those with *any* mismatch, even a single base difference (Wallace *et al.*, 1981, Conner *et al.*, 1983). For example, it is possible to construct short probes consisting of 19 nucleotides (19-mers), which contain the sequence of the normal β-globin gene in the region of the β^S mutation, and which hybridize efficiently with the normal gene but not with DNA that contains the sickle cell mutation. Using high-specific-activity labelling of these synthetic probes, normal and sickle sequences can be distinguished after hybridization of restriction-enzyme-digested total human DNA. Two 19-mers are made, one directed against the normal sequence, the other against the sequence with the altered base. Using both probes, the genotype of an individual with respect to a specific mutation can be established.

As well as a specific oligonucleotide probe against the β^S mutation, similar probes have been made against all the common β thalassaemia mutations (Piratsu *et al.*, 1983; Orkin, 1984; Old *et al.*, 1989) and are now used widely for the prenatal diagnosis of β thalassaemia (see below).

Recent technical developments

The 'classical' methods of gene analysis by Southern blotting take up to a week or more for diagnostic purposes. Recently, however, several new methods have been developed which have facilitated DNA analysis such that a diagnosis can easily be achieved in the same day. Most of the recent advances in this field have resulted from the development of a technique called polymerase chain-reaction (PCR), which allows the amplification of any short DNA sequence over a period of a few hours (Saiki *et al.*, 1985, 1988; White *et al.*, 1989).

The principle of PCR is to attach short DNA primers to the region containing a gene or part of a gene, one on each of the opposite ends of the two pairs of homologous strands. These primers are used to direct the enzyme DNA polymerase to copy each of the strands in opposite directions. Repeated cycles of enzymatic amplification increase the quantity of the targetted DNA region more than 2000-fold. By the development of a heat stable DNA polymerase it has been possible to carry out repeated rounds of DNA synthesis at an elevated temperature, thus greatly improving the amplification of targetted DNA over background DNA.

The PCR technique permits the direct visualization of stained DNA fragments on gels, and thus radioactive probes are not needed to define specific gene fragments. Furthermore, it is possible to amplify DNA from blood or tissue samples without previous purification. By combining PCR amplification with the use of specific oligonucleotide probes, as described above, it is possible to identify single base mutations very rapidly and, since

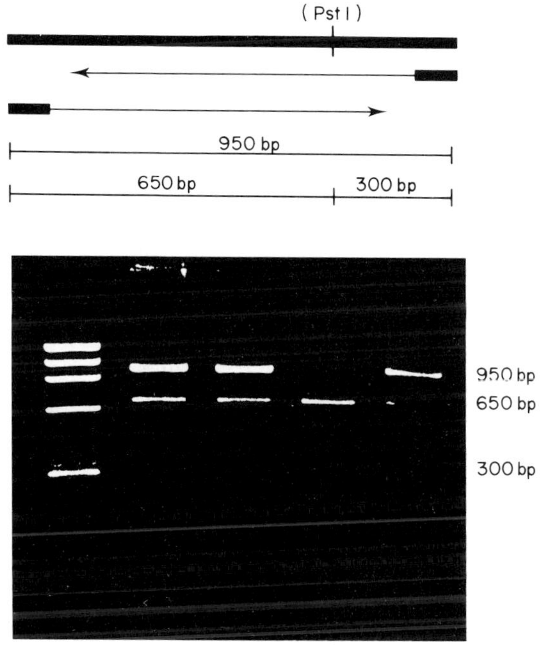

Figure 10.5 Identification of a *Pst* I polymorphism close to the gene for cystic fibrosis by polymerase chain reaction and direct identification of the fragments on electrophoresis. The solid black line indicates the total size of the DNA fragment and the solid lines with arrows the PCR primers used. The expected fragments with or without the *Pst* I cutting site are indicated.

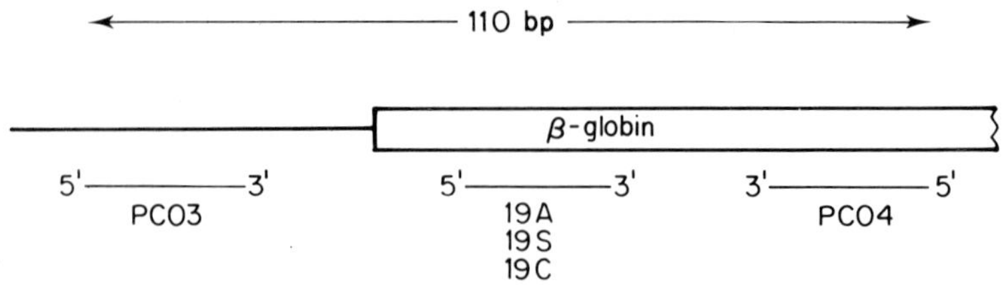

PCR primers

PCO3: ACACAACTGTGTTCACTAGC
PCO4: CAACTTCATCCACGTTCACC

ASC probes

19C: CTCCTAAGGAGAAGTCTGC
19A: CTCCTGAGGAGAAGTCTGC
19S: CTCCTGTGGAGAAGTCTGC

Figure 10.6 Oligonucleotide probe analysis of mutations of the β globin gene following the use of PCR. The sequence and sites of the two PCR primers (PCO3, PCO4) are shown together with the sequence of the three oligonucleotide probes used to identify haemoglobins A, S and C.

sufficient DNA can be amplified for direct visualization on gels, it is possible to identify any of the RFLPs that cause alterations in restriction enzyme patterns without needing to use radioactive probes (Figures 10.5 and 10.6).

The development of PCR has also led to a variety of new approaches for rapid sequencing of human genes, all of which bypass the need to clone the particular gene of interest. Thus it is now becoming possible to identify mutations in individual families for diagnostic purposes (reviewed by Caskey *et al.*, 1988, and White *et al.*, 1989).

Another recent approach for the identification of mutations using PCR is the amplification refractory mutation system (ARMS) (Newton *et al.*, 1989). This is based on the observation that, in many cases, oligonucleotides with a 3′ mis-matched residue will, under appropriate conditions, not function as primers in the PCR. Hence this method makes use of two primers. The normal form is refractory to PCR on mutant template DNA, while the mutant form is refractory to PCR on normal DNA. The difference between normal DNA and DNA with a particular mutation is identified by size differences of the amplified fragments. This technique has a wide variety of applications for prenatal diagnosis and is turning out to be particularly useful for diagnosing compound heterozygosity for two different mutations in fetal DNA.

Hitherto the gene probes that we have described for isolating and studying human genes, or fragments thereof, have been radioactively labelled. This has several disadvantages. In particular it is expensive and, in the case of oliginucleoitide probes, requires very high-specific-activity radioactive isotopes. These problems are being overcome by the use of non-radioactive sources of probe labelling. For example, biotinylated nucleotides can be used as non-radioactive probes. Biotin-labelled analogues of TTP and UTP can be enzymatically incorporated into DNA or RNA. The biotin incorporated into the probe can be coupled to avadin, and antibodies that identify the biotin–avadin complexes can be raised and labelled by immunofluorescence, immunoperoxidase or immunocolloidal gold. A variety of other ingenious approaches are being used for non-radioactive labelling of gene probes.

Finally, it is becoming feasible to amplify DNA so rapidly, and to quickly define single point mutations in the amplified DNA by using ologinucleotide probes, that it is now possible to analyse point mutations without the necessity of running DNA on gels. The DNA is simply blotted onto a nylon filter and probed with appropriate oligonucleotides. Such 'dot-blot' technology, if combined with non-radioactively labelled probes, provides a very rapid and simple laboratory approach to the diagnosis of genetic disease. This procedure can be automated, and it seems very likely that diagnostic genetics will move in this direction during the next few years.

Preimplantation prenatal diagnosis

The development of increasingly sophisticated microsurgical techniques, together with the availability of PCR, has raised the possibility that in the future it may be possible to identify genetic disease by biopsy procedures following *in vitro* fertilization. The idea would be to obtain a number of fertilized ova and analyse them for a particular genetic disease before replacing one of the unaffected ones into the uterus. Couples with a one in four or one in two chance of producing a baby with a serious genetic disorder, particularly if they find abortion unacceptable, would benefit particularly from this approach. Experimental studies have shown that it is possible to obtain cells for PCR amplification of DNA at about the eight-cell stage and also a little later at the blastocyst stage of development (Handyside *et al.*, 1989).

Clearly much more work will need to be carried out to determine the safety of this approach, particularly with respect to the further development of pre-embryos that have been manipulated in this way. Furthermore, the technical problems of DNA analysis from one or two cells should not be underestimated. Although PCR can undoubtedly produce enough DNA for a satisfactory analysis, the problems of preventing contamination of the sample are not inconsiderable. For example, it would only require the presence of a single cell from the skin or mucous membrane of an operator to confuse a diagnosis of this type. Thus it will be very important to build in techniques for defining the parental origin of cells. Nevertheless, there seems little doubt that this new approach will have an increasingly important place in clinical practice over the next few years.

OVERALL RESULTS OF PRENATAL DIAGNOSIS FOR HAEMATOLOGICAL DISORDERS

Fetal blood sampling

Up to the end of 1982 there were 3959 reports of prenatal diagnosis for the major haemoglobinopathies, mainly β thalassaemia and sickle cell anaemia (Alter, 1984). The overall fetal loss rate was 6.2%, with 1.6% maternal complications and 6.5% premature deliveries. The error rate was 0.8%. Perhaps most encouragingly, over the period covered by the report, the birth-rate of infants with β thalassaemia major declined to between 10 and 50% of the expected figures in north Italy, Cyprus, Greece and Sardinia, and among British Cypriots. Thus, fetal blood sampling for prenatal diagnosis of β thalassaemia has already made a major contribution to the public health burden posed by this disease. The results for prenatal diagnosis of other genetic blood diseases, though based on smaller numbers, are equally encouraging (Alter, 1984). The majority of diagnoses were for coagulation disorders: 208 cases were at risk of haemophilia A, 19 haemophilia B, and four von Willebrand's disease. There was only one reported error: a fetus with haemophilia was not detected *in utero*. There were seven fetal losses (3%), which suggests that the risk of haemophilia does not increase the likelihood of fetal loss following fetal blood sampling.

Recently the overall experience of prenatal diagnosis of thalassaemia and the haemoglobinopathies in Greece between 1977 and 1988 has been summarized (Old *et al.*, 1989). Altogether 3712 cases were diagnosed using fetal blood analysis. There were only 17 definite and three probable errors, and 33 instances in which it was impossible to obtain a sample. The overall fetal loss rate was approximately 2.5%.

Thus it appears that fetal blood sampling is still associated with appreciable fetal loss but that, provided the laboratory techniques are well developed, it is a remarkably successful approach to the prenatal diagnosis of common haemoglobin disorders. However, it has the major disadvantage of a long period of uncertainty for the mother and a difficult middle trimester termination of pregnancy, if indicated.

Fetal DNA analysis

Prenatal diagnosis using fetal DNA was first described by Kan and Dozy (1978) and early experiences were summarized by Boehm *et al.* (1983) and Old *et al.* (1984). The first successful prenatal diagnoses of sickle cell anaemia and β thalassaemia using DNA derived by CVS, and thus late in the first trimester, were reported by Old *et al.* (1982) and Goossens *et al.* (1983).

Recent results for first trimester prenatal diagnosis of the haemoglobin disorders have been summarised by Old *et al.* (1989). In Sardinia, where the majority of cases of β thalassaemia result from one mutation, over 1000 prenatal diagnoses have been carried out using either direct detection of the mutation by oligonucleotide probes or, more recently, by dot-blot analysis.

There have been no mis-diagnoses and the fetal loss is in the region of 2%. In the UK up to the end of 1988, over 600 prenatal diagnoses had been carried out by DNA analysis. In this population, the patients come from many different racial backgrounds and therefore many different β thalassaemia mutations have to be identified. The majority of cases of β thalassaemia were analysed by RFLP linkage studies, with a smaller proportion being diagnosed using oligonucleotide probes. In this series there were 14 fetal losses and five mis-diagnoses with six failures. In both these series the failure rates were greater if DNA had been obtained from amniotic fluid.

It appears, therefore, that first-trimester prenatal diagnosis is feasible and that it should be possible to achieve an error rate of under 1%. Possible sources of error include contamination of chorionic tissue with maternal tissue, plasmid contamination, failure of DNA digestion, recombination if RFLP probes that are not within a particular gene are used, and incorrect assignment of parental genotype. Recent studies in the author's laboratory suggest that maternal contamination is present in less than 2% of all samples received. Another important source of error is non-paternity, and it is becoming apparent that it will be necessary to run a paternity test using DNA fingerprinting technology if the overall error rates for DNA diagnosis are to be reduced to a minimum.

There has been less experience in first-trimester prenatal diagnosis of other haematological disorders using DNA analysis. Recent data are summarized by Galjaard (1987). It has been possible to diagnose haemophilia and Christmas disease using either RFLP linkage analysis (Harper *et al.*, 1984) or PCR amplification (Kogan *et al.*, 1987). It should be remembered that a proportion of cases of haemophilia are due to new mutations, but quite recently an ingenious approach to screening for mutations of large

Table 10.5 Some of the haematological disorders for which gene probes are available.

Haemoglobin disorders	*Coagulation and thrombosis*
α-globin	Factor VIII
β-globin	Factor IX
γ-globin	All other factors
Many others spanning globin gene clusters	Antithrombin III
	α_1-Antitrypsin (and variants)
	Protein C
Red-cell enzyme deficiencies	von Willebrand factor
Glucose-6-phosphate dehydrogenase	
Phosphoglycerate kinase	*Miscellaneous*
Pyruvate kinase	Erythropoietin
Many others	Transferrin and receptor
	Various cellular oncogenes
Red-cell membrane proteins	Complement (various components)
Spectrins, actin, band 4.1.	Haptoglobin
Others	Immunoglobins and T cell receptors
	Human T lymphocyto viruses (HTLVs)
Immunodeficiency	Platelet derived growth factor; G-CSF; GM-CSF; various interleukins
Adenosine deaminase	

genes like those for factor VIII or dystrophin has been described (Chamberlain *et al.*, 1988). Thus it seems likely that DNA analysis will be applied increasingly widely for both carrier detection and prenatal diagnosis of haemophilia and Christmas disease (Tuddenham, 1989). The same approaches can be used for any haematological disorder for which a gene probe is available. The principles will be exactly the same as those outlined for the haemoglobin disorders and haemophilia. If the mutation is known, an oligonucleotide probe can be constructed and the appropriate part of the gene amplified by PCR. If the mutation is not known, the disorder can be identified by RFLP linkage analysis, providing appropriate polymorphisms can be defined, and the affected chromosomes determined by a previous family study. A partial list of haematological disorders for which gene probes are now available is shown in Table 10.5.

PRACTICAL CONSIDERATIONS

Screening programmes

For the majority of genetic disorders of the blood the first antenatal clinic visit will remain the major point of screening. Since most of these conditions are rare it is unlikely that routine screening procedures will be incorporated into antenatal care programmes. Thus screening will consist of an adequate family history for any inherited blood disorders, and a routine blood count. In the case of haemoglobin disorders, however, the gene frequency is so high in certain populations that screening should become part of routine antenatal care (World Health Organization, 1982; Weatherall, 1990).

Haemoglobin disorders

In most countries, antenatal screening for the haemoglobin disorders will be restricted to maternal screening at the first antenatal visit. If first-trimester prenatal diagnosis becomes established, and women cannot be persuaded to present early in pregnancy, it may be necessary to set up population screening programmes, for school leavers for example. In high-incidence countries it is becoming routine to screen all pregnant women for thalassaemia or the sickle cell trait, depending on the particular population at risk. In countries with large immigrant populations it is equally important to screen women of appropriate racial backgrounds. The patient's name may not always give an indication of their race and in a busy antenatal clinic it is easy to miss patients who should be screened. This is not such a serious problem in the case of thalassaemia, since all pregnant women have an initial haematological screen, which, in most countries, includes an assessment of the red cell size on a Coulter counter. However, it is important that women of African origin are screened for the sickle cell trait. Furthermore, it should be remembered that this gene is not confined to black populations but occurs quite frequently in the Mediterranean region and Middle East.

Table 10.6 Haematological findings in α^0 or β thalassaemia heterozygotes, α^+ thalassaemia homozygotes, and $\alpha\beta$ thalassaemia heterozygotes.*

	Mean cell haemoglobin pg (± 1 S.D.)	Mean cell volume fl (± 1 S.D.)	Hb A_2
β thal trait	21 ± 1	70 ± 4	Raised
Normal Hb A_2 β thal trait†	22 ± 2	73 ± 6	Normal
α^0 thal‡ trait (--/$\alpha\alpha$)	22 ± 4	70 ± 8	Normal
Homozygous α^+ thal§ (-α/-α)	23 ± 1	72 ± 5	Normal
β thal trait/homozygous α^+ thal	25 ± 1	76 ± 3	Raised
β thal trait/α^0 thal trait	—‖	—‖	?Raised

* Data from Kattamis *et al.* (1979), Weatherall and Clegg (1981), Kanavakis *et al.* (1982), Higgs and Weatherall (1983), Rosatelli *et al.* (1984). Only cases of α thalassaemia analysed by gene mapping are included.
† Heterogeneous condition; a disorder with these findings interacts with β thalassaemia to produce thalassaemia major.
‡ Also known as α thalassaemia 1.
§ Also known as α thalassaemia 2.
‖ Data not available on cases confirmed by mapping. Likely to be similar to β thal trait with homozygous α^+ thal.

The haematological findings in the carrier states for the common forms of thalassaemia are summarized in Table 10.6. The key indices are the mean corpuscular haemoglobin (MCH) and mean corpuscular volume (MCV). If these are reduced, particularly if the haemoglobin level is normal or only slightly low, thalassaemia should be suspected. Although various mathematical treatments have been used to distinguish thalassaemia from iron deficiency, they are not very reliable in practice and an independent method should be used for assessing a women's iron status. The key question is below which values for the MCV and MCH should further studies to confirm the diagnosis of thalassaemia be instigated. Although it used to be recommended that an MCV of less than 70 fl, or an MCH of less than 25 pg, were indications for further study, subsequent experience suggests that these values are too low (Table 10.6). Ideally, the cut-off values should be 80 fl and 27 pg, respectively. Although this may entail a number of unnecessary investigations, it is particularly important to look for thalassaemia in women with slightly reduced red-cell indices in populations in which both α and β thalassaemia are common (this question is discussed later).

If the MCV and MCH are low, a haemoglobin A_2 estimation should be carried out. If the haemoglobin A_2 value is elevated, the diagnosis is β thalassaemia trait and the woman's husband should be studied. If both are β thalassaemia carriers, appropriate genetic counselling could be instituted.

The two main practical problems arising in antenatal screening of thalassaemia are the finding of a thalassaemic blood picture with a normal haemoglobin A_2 level, and the problem of identifying β thalassaemia in women who are heterozygous for both α and β thalassaemia. If a woman is found to have a typical thalassaemic blood picture with a normal haemoglobin A_2 level, the best approach in practice is to analyse the husband's blood. If it is normal the fetus is not at risk and the mother's thalassaemia genotype can be worked out at leisure. On the other hand, if the husband has a similar blood picture to his wife, or if he has β thalassaemia trait, the couple should be referred immediately to a laboratory that is able to sort out the different forms of α thalassaemia and the rare β thalassaemia variants.

A woman who has thalassaemic red-cell indices with a normal haemoglobin A_2 level is likely to have α thalassaemia. Furthermore, if her red-cell indices are similar to those of a β thalassaemia heterozygote, she is probably missing two out of the normal four α globin genes. However, identification of the chromosomes from which the α genes are deleted has important implications for the prognosis of her children. The normal α-globin genotype can be written *αα/αα*. In the more severe form of α thalassaemia, α^0 thalassaemia, both α globin genes on the same chromosome 16 are deleted; the heterozygous genotype is written --/αα, where -- indicates the chromosome from which both α genes have been lost (Figure 10.7). There is a milder and much commoner α thalassaemia determinant called α^+ thalassaemia. In this case only one of the α genes is lost; the heterozygous genotype is written *-α/αα*. Carriers for this condition are haematologically normal or have a very slight reduction in MCH and MCV values. However, α thalassaemia is so common that it is not unusual to encounter homozygotes with the genotype *-α/-α* (Figure 10.8). As shown in Table 10.6, the red-cell indices in such cases are indistinguishable from those of α^0

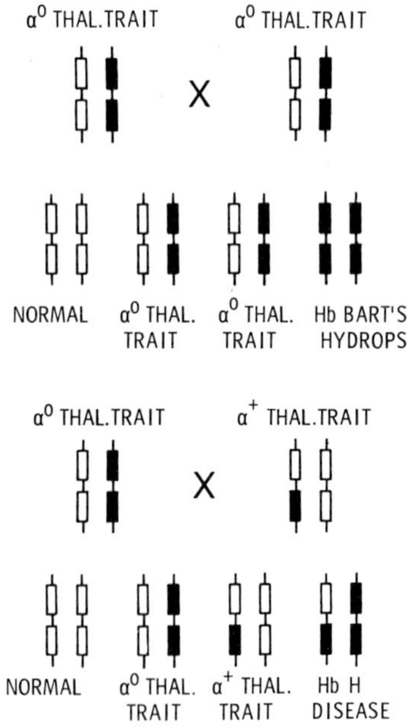

Figure 10.7 The genetics of α thalassaemia.

Figure 10.8 A comparison of the genotypes in heterozygous α^0 thalassaemia and homozygous α^+ thalassaemia.

thalassaemia heterozygotes. The deletion of two α genes produces the same phenotype, regardless of whether they are lost from the *same* or *opposite* pairs of homologous chromosome 16.

The genetic counselling implications of the interactions of the different α thalassaemia determinants are shown in Figure 10.7 and 10.8. A mating between two α^0 thalassaemia heterozygotes has a one in four chance of producing an infant with the haemoglobin Bart's hydrops syndrome. Apart from death in the third trimester or at term, this condition is also associated with a high incidence of toxaemia and post-partum haemorrhage. It is, therefore, a disorder for which prenatal diagnosis should be offered. On the other hand, an α^+ thalassaemia homozygote cannot have a child with haemoglobin Bart's hydrops: at worst they can have a child with haemoglobin H disease, which is relatively innocuous. The practical implication is that, if a couple are both found to have thalassaemic red cell indices with a normal haemoglobin A_2 level, it is important to sort out the arrangement of their missing α globin genes. Knowledge of their racial background is helpful; α^0 thalassaemia is found in Orientals and some Mediterranean populations, but it is quite uncommon in other racial groups. If a woman who is an α^0 thalassaemia carrier or an α^+ thalassaemia homozygote is married to a man who is a β thalassaemia heterozygote there are no risks for the children; αβ thalassaemia is always an innocuous interaction.

In some Mediterranean populations there is a form of β thalassaemia in which the haemoglobin A_2 level is normal (Kattamis *et al.*, 1979). This is a heterogeneous and still little-understood disorder, but there is no doubt that it can interact with the high haemoglobin A_2 form of β thalassaemia to produce a child with thalassaemia major. This is why it is important to be sure that, if they are married to a man with β thalassaemia, women who have a clinical picture of heterozygous thalassaemia and a normal haemoglobin A_2 are referred to a centre for globin chain synthesis studies. The α/β globin chain synthesis ratio in the severe types of normal haemoglobin A_2 β thalassaemia is identical to that in high haemoglobin A_2 β thalassaemia (Kattamis *et al.*, 1979).

Finally, it has become apparent in recent years that β thalassaemia heterozygotes who are also heterozygous for α^0 thalassaemia, or homozygous for α^+ thalassaemia, have MCH and MCV values which are very much higher than those of simple β thalassaemia heterozygotes. They also have elevated haemoglobin A_2 levels. The practical implication of this observation is that in populations in which α thalassaemia and β thalassaemia occur together, such as those of South-east Asia, the Middle East and the

Mediterranean region, a proportion of β thalassaemia heterozygotes may have much higher MCH and MCV values than is usually the case in other races. This is probably the basis for the condition that used to be called 'isolated high haemoglobin A_2'. If screening relies on red-cell indices, such patients may be missed and yet they are at risk of having children with thalassaemia major. Thus, in any population in which α and β thalassaemia occur together, the best method of screening for thalassaemia in pregnancy is to measure the haemoglobin A_2 level. If this is impractical, at least every woman with haemoglobin below 27 pg and MCV below 80 fl should have a haemoglobin A_2 estimation.

In summary, the majority of β thalassaemia heterozygotes, α^0 thalassaemia heterozygotes, and α^+ thalassaemia homozygotes can easily be identified from studies of red-cell indices and a haemoglobin A_2 estimation. Because of the common occurrence of α thalassaemia in populations where β thalassaemia is also common, a number of women will be encountered whose red-cell indices are only just below normal because of the interaction of the two genes. Thus a strong case can be made for screening all women from these racial groups with a haemoglobin A_2 estimation. If it is impractical, their haemoglobin A_2 level should be determined if their red-cell indices are slightly reduced.

Antenatal screening for other genetic haematological disorders

Since other genetic blood disorders are so rare as to make routine antenatal screening impracticable, further haematological studies are only indicated in families in which there is a history of inherited blood disease. In women with a haemolytic anaemia an accurate diagnosis should be made in a laboratory capable of assaying the appropriate red-cell enzymes; in cases with a dominant inheritance the risk to the fetus is 50%. In recessive disorders in which heterozygotes can be identified, the husband should be studied at the same time. Most red-cell enzymes can be assayed by fetal blood sampling, but gene probes for first-trimester diagnosis of these conditions are becoming increasingly available. In fact, except for those that are associated with multisystem disease, many genetic red-cell enzyme deficiencies are so mild that most parents would not opt for prenatal diagnosis.

The technical difficulties in identifying the carrier state for haemophilia in pregnancy are reviewed by Weatherall and Letsky (1984). RFLPs close to the factor VIII locus have been defined and, in suitable families, establishing whether a woman has inherited a haemophilia gene may be possible by linkage analysis using Southern blotting (Harper *et al.*, 1984) or by direct detection of an RFLP or mutation by PCR (Kogan *et al.*, 1987). Similarly, gene probes are now available for identifying carriers of the factor IX gene (Gianelli *et al.*, 1984; Giannelli, 1989). A partial list of other conditions that can be identified in the fetus, and that should be looked for in pregnant women, is shown in Tables 10.1 and 10.5.

Strategy for prenatal diagnosis programmes

The pace of development of prenatal diagnosis technology has been so fast over the last few years that its role in clinical practice is still not fully defined. The field is still in a state of flux, and both sampling and analytical techniques require further evaluation. What should be done in practice during this uncertain period? Again, it is easier to consider this problem by using the haemoglobin disorders as a model (Weatherall and Old, 1983; Old *et al*, 1989).

Haemoglobin disorders

As mentioned earlier, in most of the developed countries appropriate screening facilities for the common haemoglobin disorders are already established in haematology laboratories. It is essential that there is an adequate flow of information from laboratories to obstetricians, and that centres with expertise in counselling patients about the potential outcome of at risk pregnancies are developed.

The importance of developing adequate counselling facilities cannot be over-emphasized. In many ways, the field of prenatal detection of genetic disease has been running before it could walk. Thus, while we have sophisticated methods for screening and prenatal detection of the major haemoglobin disorders, the development of population programmes, both in the United States and in Great Britain, have been hampered by lack of adequate screening facilities. It is no use developing all this powerful technology if patients are to be left confused and improperly educated about the diseases for which these methods are being applied.

Currently, it is fairly clear that at least for the forseeable future fetal DNA analysis following CVS will become the mainstay of prenatal diagnosis programmes. In determining the most cost-effective and simple laboratory technology a number of problems will have to be addressed. In particular, it is becoming apparent that many genetic diseases such as thalassaemia and haemophilia are extremely heterogeneous at the molecular level. Thus, while one gene probe or restriction enzyme is adequate for the diagnosis of sickle cell anaemia, other technologies will have to be developed to cover the 60 or more β thalassaemia mutations that underlie this important disease. Such heterogeneity raises a number of practical issues. In the United Kingdom, for example, the thalassaemias are seen in individuals from Cyprus, other Mediterranean regions, the Middle East, the Indian subcontinent, South-east Asia and from many other parts of the world. Many different mutations are thus encounterd and many potentially affected children will be compound heterozygotes for different mutations (Weatherall and Clegg, 1981). This problem is made worse by the fact that many women present late in the first trimester and very little time is available for determining parental genotypes and carrying out fetal DNA analysis. Thus while it may be possible, in the long-term, to identify the different mutations as part of a national screening programme, the provision of a comprehensive prenatal diagnosis service will, for the immediate future,

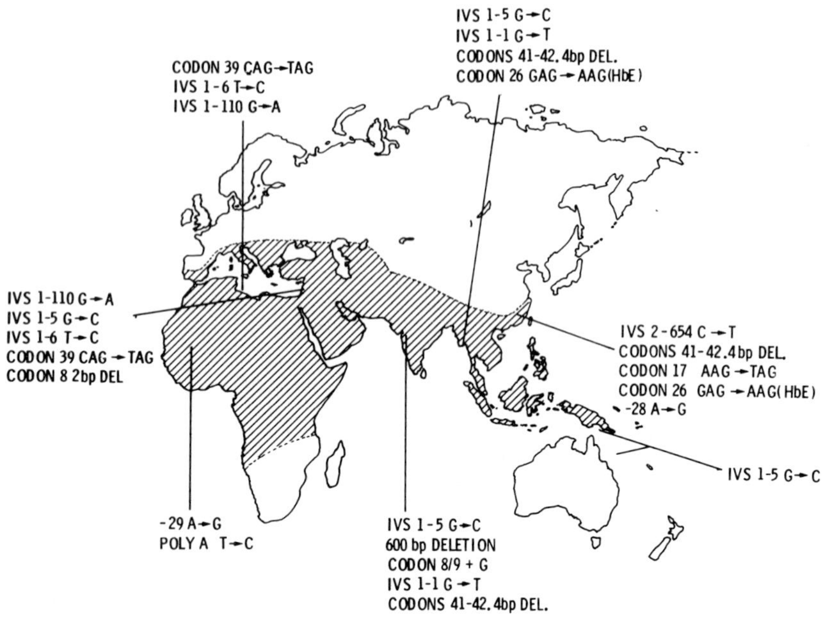

Figure 10.9 The common β thalassaemia mutations in different racial groups.

require considerable flexibility of technical approach. And there is a further problem. To provide a fully comprehensive prenatal diagnosis programme it must be possible to give accurate genetic counselling to prospective parents. Children who receive two β thalassaemia genes may have a clinical disorder ranging from a life-threatening anaemia during the first year to an extremely mild condition compatible with normal development and survival. Recent studies (Thein *et al.*, 1988) have suggested that, by and large, it will be possible to determine most of the interactions that cause either severe or mild β thalassaemia. This kind of analysis will have to be incorporated into prenatal diagnosis programmes in the future.

Given these problems, how should a programme be set up? First, it is important to attempt to determine the main thalassaemia mutations in any particular population. Most races have a handful of common mutations together with varying numbers of rare ones, so the ideal basis for a prenatal diagnosis programme will be to develop gene probes for the common mutations and to carry out fetal DNA analysis following CVS using PCR with oligonucleotide probes or, where the mutation can be detected directly, using appropriate enzymes on amplified DNA. This technology can be converted to simple dot-blot analysis with increasing experience. Laboratories with a sufficient expertise may be able to develop rapid sequencing methods for identifying unusual β thalassaemia mutations. But there will still be a necessity to carry out RFLP linkage studies in families in which the mutations cannot be identified, and it will probably be necessary for laboratories with a large population of thalassaemics to retain the ability to carry out fetal blood sampling and globin-chain synthesis for those rare cases in which DNA analysis is not possible.

Ultimately this type of programme should be applicable to the large, rural populations of India and South-east Asia. The best approach will be to set up diagnostic centres in various parts of the community, as has already been done in Thailand for example. While expertise in CVS is being developed it should be possible to define the common mutations in the population (Figure 10.9). Once this has been done, it should be feasible to develop prenatal diagnosis programmes, particularly if simple dot-blot technology can be used, perhaps in the form of a kit.

Other disorders

Prenatal detection of other haematological disorders follow the same lines as the thalassaemias. While gene probes are being developed, fetal blood sampling will remain the mainstay for the prenatal detection of many red cell, white cell and coagulation disorders. The rapid diagnostic techniques for determining mutations, such as have been applied to the factor VIII and IX genes, should make it possible to apply DNA technology widely for the detection of heterozygotes and for the prenatal diagnosis of haemophilia and Christmas disease. This can be carried out either by RFLP linkage analysis or by direct detection of the mutation as outlined in previous sections.

How long will it take to obtain gene probes for most of the common inherited blood diseases? It is beyond the scope of this chapter to describe in detail the methods being employed. Where the gene product is known, it is possible to make appropriate oligonucleotide probes to use in screening libraries for the appropriate gene. If nothing is known about the gene product, the general approach is to carry out RFLP linkage studies to try to detect approximately where the gene is. It is then possible to move along the chromosome to the affected locus and to determine its product by reverse genetics, a method that has been used successfully to define the genes for Duchenne muscular dystrophy, chronic granulomatous disease and, most recently, for cystic fibrosis. These methods, and current moves to produce a complete map of the human genome, are described for the general reader in a recent review of the overall possibilities of the new genetics (Weatherall, 1990).

REFERENCES

Alter BP (1980) Prenatal diagnosis of hemoglobinopathies. In *Progress in Pediatric Hematology/Oncology*, Vol. III (Schwarz F, (ed.), pp 123–146. Littleton, PSG Publishing

Alter BP (1981) Prenatal diagnosis of haemoglobinopathies: a status report. *The Lancet* **ii**: 1152–1155.

Alter BP (1984) Advances in the prenatal diagnosis of hematologic disease. *Blood* **64**: 329–340.

Alter BP (1989) Examination of fetal blood for hemoglobinopathies. In Perinatal Hematology (Alter BP, ed.), *Methods in Hematology* **21**: 13–29. New York: Churchill Livingstone.

Alter BP, Metzger JB, Yock PG, Rothchild SD and Dover GJ (1979) Selective hemolysis of adult red blood cells: an aid to prenatal diagnosis of hemoglobinopathies. *Blood* **53**: 279–287.

Antonarakis SE (1989) Diagnosis of genetic disorders at the DNA level. *New England Journal of Medicine* **320**: 153–163.

Antonarakis, SE, Boehm CD, Giardina PJV and Kazazian HH (1982) Non random association of polymorphic restriction sites in the β-globin gene complex. *Proceedings of the National Academy of Sciences of the United States of America* **79**: 137–141.

Auerbach AD, Liu Q, Ghosh R, Pollack MS, Douglas GW and Broxmeyer HE (1990) Prenatal identification of potential donors for umbilical cord blood transplantation for Fanconi's anaemia. *Transfusion* **30**: (in press).

Boehm CD, Antonarakis SE, Phillips JA, Stetten G and Kazazian HH Jr (1983) Prenatal diagnosis using DNA polymorphisms. Report on 95 pregnancies at risk for sickle-cell disease or β-thalassaemia. *New England Journal of Medicine* **308**: 1054–1058.

Borregaard N, Bang J, Berthelsen JG *et al.* (1982) Prenatal diagnosis of chronic granulomatous disease. *The Lancet* **i**: 114.

Canadian Collaborative CVS–Amniocentesis Clinical Trial Group (1989) Multicentre randomised clinical trial of chorion villus sampling and amniocentesis. *Lancet* **i**: 1–6.

Caskey CT, Gibbs RA, Witowski JA and Hejtmanick JF (1988) Diagnosis of human inheritable defects by recombinant DNA methods. *Philosophical Transactions of the Royal Society of London, B* **319**: 353–360.

Chamberlain JS, Gibbs RA, Ranier JE *et al.* (1988) Deletion screening of the Duchenne muscular dystrophy locus via multiplex DNA amplification. *Nucleic Acids Research* **16**: 11141–11156.

Cividalli G, Nathan DG, Kan YW, Santamarina B and Frigoletto F (1974) Relation of beta to gamma synthesis during the first trimester: an approach to prenatal diagnosis of thalassemia. *Pediatric Research* **80**: 553–560.

Clegg JB, Naughton MA and Weatherall DJ (1965) An improved method for the characterization of human haemoglobin mutants; identification of $\alpha_2\beta_2$95Glu; haemoglobin N (Baltimore). *Nature* **207**: 945–947.

Conner BJ, Reyes AA, Morin C, Itakura K, Teplitz RL and Wallace RB (1983) Detection of sickle cell β^S-globin allele by hybridization with synthetic oligonucleotides. *Proceedings of the National Academy of Sciences of the United States of America* **80**: 278–282.

Daffos F, Capella-Pavlovsky M, Forestier F (1983) A new procedure for pure fetal blood sampling in utero. *Prenatal Diagnosis* **3**: 271–277.

Davies KE (1985) Molecular genetics of the human X chromosome. *Journal of Medical Genetics* **22**: 243–249.

Davies KE (ed.) (1988) *Genome Analysis, a Practical Approach*. Oxford: IRL Press.

Davies KE and Read AP (1988) *Molecular Basis of Inherited Disease*. Oxford: IRL Press.

Davies KE and Robson KJH (1987) Molecular analysis of human monogenic diseases. *BioEssays* **6**: 247–253.

Deybach JCh, Grandchamp B, Grelier M *et al.* (1980) Prenatal exclusion of congenital erythropoietic porphyria (Gunther's disease) in a fetus at risk. *Human Genetics* **53**: 217–221.

Durandy A, Oury C, Griscelli C *et al.* (1982) Prenatal testing for inherited immune deficiencies by fetal blood sampling. *Prenatal Diagnosis* **2**: 109–113.

Emery AEH (1984) *An Introduction to Recombinant DNA*. Chichester: John Wiley & Son.

Firshein SI, Hoyer LW, Lazarchick J *et al.* (1979) Prenatal diagnosis of classic hemophilia. *New England Journal of Medicine* **300**: 937–941.

Galjaard H (1987) Worldwide experience with first-trimester fetal diagnoses by molecular analysis. In *Human Genetics* (Vogel F and Springer K, eds), pp 611–621. Berlin: Springer-Verlag.

Giannelli F (1989) Factor IX. *Clinical Haematology* **2**: 821–848.

Giannelli F, Choo KH, Winship PR *et al.* (1984) Characterisation and use of an intragenic polymorphic marker for detection of carriers of haemophilia B (factor IX deficiency). *Lancet* **i**: 239–241.

Gluckman E, Broxmeyer HE, Auerbach AD *et al.* (1989) Hematopoietic reconstitution in a patient with Fanconi's anemia by means of umbilical-cord blood from an HLA-identical sibling. *New England Journal of Medicine* **321**: 1174–1178.

Goossens M, Dumez Y, Kaplan *et al.* (1983) Prenatal diagnosis of sickle-cell anaemia in the first trimester of pregnancy. *New England Journal of Medicine* **309**: 831–833.

Halley DJ, Keijzer W, Jasers NG *et al.* (1979) Prenatal diagnosis of xeroderma pigmentosum (group C) using assays of unscheduled DNA synthesis and postreplication repair. *Clinical Genetics* **16**: 137–142.

Handyside AH, Pattinson JK, Penketh RJA *et al.* (1989) Biopsy of human preimplantation embryos and sexing by DNA amplification. *The Lancet* **i**: 347–349.

Harper K, Winter R, Pembrey M, Hartley D, Davies KE and Tuddenham E (1984) A clinically useful DNA probe closely linked to haemophilia A. *The Lancet* **ii**: 6–8.

Hecht F and Cadien JD (1984) Tay–Sachs disease and other fatal metabolic disorders. In *Antenatal and Neonatal Screening* (Wald N, ed.), pp 129–154. Oxford: Oxford University Press.

Higgs DR and Weatherall DJ (1983) Alpha thalassemia. *Current Topics in Hematology* **4**: 37–97.

Higgs DR, Vickers MA, Wilkie AOM *et al.* (1989) A review of the molecular genetics of the human α-globin gene cluster. *Blood* **73**: 1081–1104.

Hobbins JC and Mahoney MJ (1974) In utero diagnosis of hemoglobinopathies. *New England Journal of Medicine* **290**: 1065–1067.

Holmberg L, Gustavii B and Jonsson A (1983) A prenatal study of fetal platelet count and size with application to fetus at risk for Wiskott–Aldrich syndrome. *Journal of Pediatrics* **102**: 773–776.

Hoyer LW, Lindsten J, Blomback M *et al.* (1979) Prenatal evaluation of fetus at risk for severe von Willebrand's disease. *Lancet* **ii**: 191–192.

Jeffreys AJ (1979) DNA sequence variants in the $^{G}\gamma$-, $^{A}\gamma$-, δ- and β-globin genes of man. *Cell* **18**: 1–10.

Junien C, Lerous A, Lostanlen D *et al.* (1981) Prenatal diagnosis of congenital enzymopenic methaemoglobinaemia with mental retardation due to generalized cytochrome b_5 reductase deficiency: first report of two cases. *Prenatal Diagnosis* **1**: 17–22.

Kan YW and Dozy AM (1978) Antenatal diagnosis of sickle-cell anaemia by DNA analysis of amniotic-fluid cells. *Lancet* **ii**: 910–912.

Kan YW, Valenti C, Carnazza V, Guidotti R and Reider RF (1974) Fetal blood-sampling in utero. *Lancet* **i**: 7–80.

Kan YW, Lee KY, Furbetta M, Angius A and Cao A (1980) Polymorphism of DNA sequences in the beta globin gene region. Application to prenatal diagnosis of β^0 thalassemia in Sardinia. *New England Journal of Medicine* **302**: 185–188.

Kanavakis E, Wainscoat JS, Wood WG *et al.* (1982) The interaction of α thalassaemia with heterozygous β thalassaemia. *British Journal of Haematology* **52**: 465–473.

Kattamis C, Metaxatou-Mavromati A, Wood WG, Nash JR and Weatherall DJ (1979) The heterogeneity of normal Hb A_2-β thalassaemia in Greece. *British Journal of Haematology* **42**: 109–123.

Kogan SC, Doherty M and Gitschier J (1987) An improved method for prenatal diagnosis of genetic diseases by analysis of amplified DNA sequences. *New England Journal of Medicine* **317**: 985–990.

Lestas AN, Rodeck CH and White JM (1982) Normal activities of glycolytic enzymes in the fetal erythrocytes. *British Journal of Haematology* **50**: 439–444.

Levinsky RJ, Linch DC and Rodeck CH (1982) Prenatal exclusion of severe combined immunodeficiency. *Archives of Diseases in Childhood* **57**: 958–960.

Linch DC, Beverley PC, Levinsky RJ and Rodeck CH (1982a) Phenotypic analysis of fetal blood leukocytes: potential for prenatal diagnosis of immunodeficiency. *Prenatal Diagnosis* **3**: 211–218.

Linch DC, Knott LJ, Rodeck CH and Huehns ER (1982b) Studies of circulating hemopoietic progenitor cells in human fetal blood. *Blood* **59**: 976–979.

Ljung R, Holmberg L, Gustavii B, Philip B and Bang J (1982) Haemophilia A and B — two years experience of genetic counselling and prenatal diagnosis. *Clinical Genetics* **22**: 70–82.

Luthy DA, Hall JG and Graham CB (1979) Prenatal diagnosis of thrombocytopenia with absent radii. *Clinical Genetics* **15**: 495–499.

Mibashan RS, Peake IR, Rodeck CH *et al.* (1980) Dual diagnosis of prenatal haemophilia A by measurement of fetal factor VIIIC and VIIIC antigen (VIIIC Ag). *Lancet* **ii**: 944–997.

Mibashan RS, Rodeck CH and Thumpston JK (1982) Prenatal diagnosis of the hemophilias. In *Methods in Hematology: The Hemophilias* (Bloom AL ed.), p 176. Edinburgh: Churchill Livingstone.

Mibashan RS, Peake IR and Nicolaides KA (1989) Prenatal diagnosis of hemostatic disorders. In *Perinatal Hematology* (Alter BP ed.), *Methods in Hematology* **21**: 64–107, New York: Churchill Livingstone.

Newburger PE, Cohen HJ, Rothchild SB *et al.* (1979) Prenatal diagnosis of chronic granulomatous disease. *New England Journal of Medicine* **300**: 178–181.

Newton CR, Graham A, Heptinstall LE *et al.* (1989) Analysis of any point mutation in DNA. The amplification refractory mutation system (ARMS). *Nucleic Acids Research* **17**: 2503–2516.

Old JM and Higgs DR (1983) Gene analysis. *Methods in Hematology*, vol. 6. *The Thalassemias* (Weatherall DJ, ed.), pp 74–102. Edinburgh: Churchill Livingstone.

Old JM, Ward RHT, Petrou M, Karagozlu F, Modell B and Weatherall DJ (1982) First trimester diagnosis for haemoglobinopathies: a report of 3 cases. *The Lancet* **ii**: 1413– 1416.

Old JM, Petrou M, Modell B and Weatherall DJ (1984) Feasibility of antenatal diagnosis of β thalassaemia by DNA polymorphisms in Asian Indian and Cypriot populations. *British Journal of Haematology* **57**: 255–264.

Old JM, Thein SL, Weatherall DJ, Cao A and Loukopoulos D (1989) Prenatal diagnosis of the major haemoglobin disorders. *Molecular Biology and Medicine* **6**: 55–63.

Orkin SH (1984) Prenatal diagnosis of hemoglobin disorders by DNA analysis. *Blood* **63**: 249–253.

Orkin SH and Kazazian HH (1984) The mutation and polymorphism of the human β-globin gene and its surrounding DNA. *Annual Review of Genetics* **18**: 131–171.

Orkin SH, Kazazian HH, Antonarakis SE *et al.* (1982) Linkage of β-thalassaemia mutations and β-globin gene polymorphisms with DNA polymorphisms in human β-globin gene cluster. *Nature* **296**: 627–631.

Orkin SH, Antonarakis SE and Kazazian HH (1983) Polymorphism and molecular pathology of the human β-globin gene. *Progress in Hematology* **13**: 49–73.

Palmiter RD and Brinster RL (1985) Transgenic mice. *Cell* **41**: 343–345.

Piratsu M, Kan YW, Cao A, Conner BJ, Teplitz RL and Wallace RB (1983) Prenatal diagnosis of β-thalassemia. Detection of a single nucleotide mutation in man. *New England Journal of Medicine* **309**: 284–287.

Rodeck CH (1980) Fetoscopy guided by real-time ultrasound for pure fetal blood samples, fetal skin samples, and examination of the fetus in utero. *British Journal of Obstetrics and Gynaecology* **87**: 449–456.

Rodeck CH and Morsman JM (1983) First-trimester chorion biopsy. *British Medical*

Bulletin **39**: 338–342.

Rodeck CH and Nicolini U (1989) Obstetric approaches to fetal hematology. In *Perinatal Hematology* (Alter BP ed.), *Methods in Hematology* **21**: 1–12. New York: Churchill Livingstone.

Rosa R, Prehu MO, Calvin MC *et al.* (1984) New cases of hereditary triose-phosphate isomerase deficiency (TPI): possibility of prenatal diagnosis. *Blood* **64**: 35a.

Rosatelli C, Falchi AM, Scalas MT, Tuveri T, Furbetta M and Cao A (1984) Hematological phenotype of the double heterozygous state for alpha and beta thalassemia. *Hemoglobin* **8**: 25–35.

Saiki RK, Scharf S, Faloona F *et al.* (1985) Enzymatic amplification of β-globin genomic sequences and restriction site analysis for diagnosis of sickle cell anemia. *Science* **230**: 1350–1354.

Saiki RK, Gelfand DH, Stoffel S *et al.* (1988) Primer-directed enzymatic amplification of DNA with a thermostable DNA polymerase. *Science* **239**: 487–491.

Shaham M, Voss R, Becker Y, Yarconi S, Ornoy AS and Kohn G (1982) Prenatal diagnosis of ataxia telangiectasia. *Journal of Pediatrics* **100**: 134–137.

Simmonds HA, Fairbanks LD, Webster DR *et al.* (1983) Rapid prenatal diagnosis of adenosine deaminase deficiency and other purine disorders using foetal blood. *Bioscience Reports* **3**: 31–33.

Thein SL and Weatherall DJ (1988) The Thalassaemias. In *Recent Advances in Haematology*, vol. 5 (Hoffbrand AV, ed.), pp 43–74. Edinburgh: Churchill Livingstone.

Thein SL, Hesketh C, Wallace RB and Weatherall DJ (1988) The molecular basis of thalassaemia major and intermedia in Indians; application to prenatal diagnosis. *British Journal of Haematology* **70**: 225–231.

Trent RJ, Davis B, Wilkinson T and Kronenberg H (1985) Identification of β variant hemoglobin by DNA restriction endonuclease mapping. *Hemoglobin* **8**: 443–462.

Tuddenham EGD (1989) Factor VIII and haemophilia A. *Clinical Haematology* **2**: 849–878.

Valentine WN and Paglia DE (1984) Erythrocyte enzymopathies, hemolytic anemia, and multisystem disease: an annotated review. *Blood* **64**: 583–591.

Wainscoat JS, Old JM, Thein SL and Weatherall DJ (1984) A new DNA polymorphism for prenatal diagnosis of β thalassaemia in Mediterranean populations. *The Lancet* **i**: 1299–1301.

Wallace RB, Schold M, Johnson MJ, Dembeck P and Itakura K (1981) Oligonucleotide directed mutagenesis of the human β-globin gene: a general method for producing specific point mutations in cloned DNA. *Nucleic Acids Research* **9**: 3647–3656.

Weatherall DJ (1985) Prenatal diagnosis of inherited blood diseases. *Clinics in Haematology* **14**: 747–774.

Weatherall DJ (1990) *The New Genetics and Clinical Practice*, 3rd edn. Oxford: Oxford University Press (in press).

Weatherall DJ and Clegg JB (1981) *The Thalassaemia Syndromes*, 3rd edn. Oxford: Blackwell Scientific Publications.

Weatherall DJ and Letsky EA (1984) Genetic haematological disorders. In *Antenatal and Neonatal Screening for Disease* (Wald N, ed.), pp 155–191. Oxford: Oxford University Press.

Weatherall DJ and Old JM (1983) Antenatal diagnosis of the haemoglobin disorders by analysis of foetal DNA. *Molecular Biology and Medicine* **1**: 151–155.

Weatherall DJ, Clegg JB and Naughton MA (1965) Globin synthesis in thalassemia: an *in vitro* study. *Nature* **208**: 1061–1065.

White TJ, Arnheim N and Erlich HA (1989) The polymerase chain reaction. *Trends in Genetics* **5**: 185–189.

Whitelaw AGL, Rogers PA, Hopkinson FDA *et al.* (1979) Congenital haemolytic anaemia resulting from glucose phosphate isomerase deficiency: genetics,

clinical picture and prenatal diagnosis. *Journal of Medical Genetics* **16**: 189–196.
World Health Organization (1982) Report on the community control of hereditary anaemias. Memorandum from a WHO meeting. *Bulletin of the World Health Organization* **61**: 63–80.

Index